ATLS®

Advanced
Trauma
Life
Support®
Course for Physicians

This Fifth Edition of the *ATLS® Student Manual* is dedicated to the
memory of our colleagues and friends,

RAYMOND H. ALEXANDER, MD, FACS
and
HERBERT J. PROCTOR, MD, FACS

This program is dedicated to the care of all victims of trauma.

Published 1993. Third Impression, 1995.
Printed in the United States of America.

Advanced Trauma Life Support® Student Manual   ISBN 1-880696-01-0

The Role of the Committee on Trauma of the American College of Surgeons

The American College of Surgeons (ACS), founded to improve the care of the surgical patient, has long been a leader in establishing and maintaining the high quality of surgical practice in North America. In accordance with that role, and recognizing that **trauma is a surgical disease**, the ACS Committee on Trauma has worked to establish standards for the care of the trauma patient.

Accordingly, the Committee sponsors and contributes to the continued development of the Advanced Trauma Life Support (ATLS) Course for Physicians. The ATLS Course does not present new concepts in the field of trauma care. However, it does teach well-established treatment methods and approaches trauma care in a systematized manner, presenting to the physician a concise method of establishing assessment and management priorities in the care of the trauma patient.

This edition has been prepared for the ACS by members of the Subcommittee on ATLS and the ACS Committee on Trauma, other individual Fellows of the College, and nonsurgical consultants to the Subcommittee who were selected for their special competence in the first hour of trauma care and for their expertise in medical education. The Committee believes that those having the responsibility for such patients will find the information valuable. It must be recognized that injured patients present a wide range of complex problems. Accordingly, the authors have presented a concise approach to assessing and managing the multiply injured patient in the **first hour**. The course presents physicians with knowledge and techniques that are comprehensive and easily adapted to fit their needs. The skills presented in this manual recommend **one, safe way** to perform each technique. The ACS recognizes that there are other acceptable approaches.

Revision of the ATLS core content material is conducted every four years by the Subcommittee on ATLS of the ACS Committee on Trauma. Thus, the material represents an educational guideline and a timely approach to the early care of the trauma patient. By introducing this course and maintaining its high quality, the Committee hopes to provide another instrument by which to reduce the mortality and morbidity related to trauma. The Committee on Trauma recommends that physicians participating in the ATLS Student Course reverify their status every four years to maintain both their current status in the program and their knowledge of state-of-the-art trauma care.

Subcommittee on Advanced Trauma Life Support of the American College of Surgeons Committee on Trauma 1988-1992

Max L. Ramenofsky, MD, FACS
Chairman

Raymond H. Alexander, MD, FACS (D)
Jameel Ali, MD, FACS
Charles Aprahamian, MD, FACS
Richard M. Bell, MD, FACS
Rea Brown, MD, FACS
Paul E. Collicott, MD, FACS
Brent E. Krantz, MD, FACS

Gregory J. Jurkovich, MD, FACS
Kimball I. Maull, MD, FACS
William F. McManus, MD, FACS
Herbert J. Proctor, MD, FACS (D)
Stuart A. Reynolds, MD, FACS
James M. Salander, MD, FACS

American College of Surgeons Committee on Trauma

A. Brent Eastman, MD, FACS
Chairman

Editorial Notes

The ACS Committee on Trauma hereafter is referred to as the Committee, and State/Provincial Chairman(men) referred to as S/P Chairman(men).

Throughout this manual, masculine pronouns are used for simplification. These pronouns are used to embrace both genders.

Advanced Trauma Life Support® and ATLS® are proprietary trademarks and service marks owned by the American College of Surgeons and cannot be used by individuals or entities outside the ACS Committee on Trauma organization for their goods and services without ACS approval. Accordingly, any reproduction of either or both marks in direct conjunction with the ACS ATLS Program within the ACS Committee on Trauma organization must be accompanied by the common law symbol of trademark ownership.

Contributing Authors

The Committee gratefully acknowledges these individuals for their medical expertise and support in the development of the ATLS Course materials.

Raymond H. Alexander, MD, FACS (D)
Professor of Surgery, Associate Chairman of Department of Surgery, University of Florida Health Science Center, Jacksonville, Florida.

Jameel Ali, MD, FACS
Professor of Surgery, Director of Postgraduate Education, Department of Surgery, University of Toronto, Toronto, Ontario, Canada.

Charles Aprahamian, MD, FACS
Professor of Surgery, Chief of Trauma Service and Emergency Surgery, Medical College of Wisconsin, Milwaukee, Wisconsin.

Richard M. Bell, MD, FACS
Professor of Surgery, University of South Carolina School of Medicine, Columbia, South Carolina.

Emidio Bianco, MD, JD
Assistant Chairman, Professional Affairs, Department of Legal Medicine, Armed Forces Institute of Pathology, Washington, DC.

Rea Brown, MD, FACS
Director of General Surgery, Director of Critical Care Trauma Unit, Montreal General Hospital; Professor of Surgery, McGill University, Montreal, Ontario, Canada.

Paul E. Collicott, MD, FACS
Clinical Assistant Professor of Surgery, University of Nebraska College of Medicine, Omaha, Nebraska; Chairman, Department of Trauma, Lincoln General Hospital, Lincoln, Nebraska.

Frank X. Doto, MS
Professor of Health Education, County College of Morris, Randolph, New Jersey.

John H. George, PhD
Physician Liaison, Lincoln General Hospital, Lincoln, Nebraska.

Irvene K. Hughes, RN
Manager, ATLS Division, ACS Trauma Department, American College of Surgeons, Chicago, Illinois.

Richard L. Judd, PhD
Executive Dean and Professor of Emergency Medical Sciences, Central Connecticut State University, New Britain, Connecticut.

Gregory J. Jurkovich, MD, FACS
Associate Professor of Surgery, University of Washington; Director, Emergency Room Surgical Services, Harborview Medical Center, Seattle, Washington.

Brent E. Krantz, MD, FACS
Director of Trauma, St Luke's Hospital, Fargo, North Dakota.

Francis G. Lapiana, MD, FACS
Professor of Surgery, Uniformed Services University of the Health Sciences; Director, Ophthalmic, Plastic, Reconstruction, and Orbital Surgery, Walter Reed Army Medical Center, Washington, DC.

Kimball I. Maull, MD, FACS
Director, R Adams Cowley Shock Trauma Center, Maryland Institute for Emergency Medical Services Systems, Baltimore, Maryland.

James A. McGehee, DVM, MS
Deputy Director, Clinical Investigation, David Grant Medical Center, Travis Air Force Base, California.

William F. McManus, MD, FACS
Clinical Professor of Surgery, University of Texas Health Science Center at San Antonio, Texas, and Uniformed University of the Health Sciences, Bethesda, Maryland; Chief, Clinical Division, United States Army Institute of Surgical Research, Fort Sam Houston, Texas.

Norman E. McSwain, Jr., MD, FACS
Professor of Surgery, Director of Trauma Services, Tulane University School of Medicine, New Orleans, Louisiana.

Cynthia L. Meyer, MD
Chief of Otolaryngology, Head and Neck Surgery, 2nd General Hospital, Landstuhl, Germany; Associate Clinical Instructor, Department of Surgery (ENT), Head and Neck Surgery, Uniformed Services University of the Health Sciences, Bethesda, Maryland.

James B. Nichols, DVM, MS
Director, Animal Care, University of Vermont, Burlington, Vermont.

Frank Olson, EdD
Professor of Education and Chairman of Secondary Education, Pacific Lutheran University, Tacoma, Washington.

Andrew B. Peitzman, MD, FACS
Associate Professor of Surgery, Director of Trauma and Emergency Services, Presbyterian University Hospital, Pittsburgh, Pennsylvania.

Herbert Proctor, MD, FACS (D)
Professor of Surgery; Head, Trauma Section, University of North Carolina, Chapel Hill, North Carolina.

Max L. Ramenofsky, MD, FACS
Professor and Chief, Division of Pediatric Surgery, State University of New York, Health Sciences Center at Brooklyn, Brooklyn, New York.

Stuart A. Reynolds, MD, FACS
Chief of Surgery, Northern Montana Hospital, Havre, Montana.

James M. Salander, MD, FACS
Associate Professor of Surgery, Uniformed Services University of the Health Sciences, Bethesda, Maryland.

Richard C. Simmonds, DVM, MS
Director of Laboratory Animal Medicine, University of Nevada System; Professor of Physiology, University of Nevada School of Medicine, Reno, Nevada.

Joseph J. Tepas, III, MD, FACS
Professor of Surgery, Department of Surgery and Chief of Division of Pediatric Surgery, University of Florida Health Science Center, Jacksonville, Florida.

Peter G. Trafton, MD, FACS
Associate Professor, Department of Orthopedics, Brown University; Surgeon in Charge, Division of Trauma, Department of Orthopedics, Rhode Island Hospital; Providence Veterans Administration Medical Center, Providence, Rhode Island.

Clark Watts, MD, FACS
Professor of Surgery (Neurosurgery), Department of Surgery, University of Maryland School of Medicine; Director of Neurosurgery, Maryland Institute for Emergency Medical Services Systems, Baltimore, Maryland.

John West, MD, FACS
Orange, California.

Acknowledgments

The Committee also gratefully acknowledges these individuals who reviewed the core medical content for its validity and relevance to private and academic practice and/or contributed to media resources for the course materials.

ATLS Working Party for the
Royal College of Surgeons of England
David V. Skinner, FRCS(Ed), FRCS(Eng)
Chairman

Ian Haywood, FRCS(Eng), MRCS, LRCP
Miles H. Irving, FRCS(ED), FRCS(Eng)
J.W. Rodney Peyton, FRCS(Ed), MRCP
Bernard Riley, FFARCS
James M. Ryan, MCh, FRCS(Eng),
  RAMC
Peter H. Worlock, DM, FRCS(Ed),
  FRCS(Eng)

James Barone, MD, FACS
Stamford, Connecticut

John Barrett, MD, FACS
Chicago, Illinois

Richard E. Burney, MD, FACS
Ann Arbor, Michigan

David E. Clark, MD, FACS
Portland, Maine

Cook County Hospital
Chicago, Illinois

Martin R. Eichelberger, MD, FACS
Washington, DC

John Fildes, MD, FACS
Chicago, Illinois

Ronald P. Fischer, MD, FACS
Houston, Texas

Stevenson Flanigan, MD, FACS
Little Rock, Arkansas

Richard Gamelli, MD, FACS
Maywood, Illinois

Roger Gilbertson, MD
Fargo, North Dakota

Burton H. Harris, MD, FACS
Boston, Massachusetts

June E. Heilman, MD, FACS
Pocatello, Idaho

David B. Hoyt, MD, FACS
San Diego, California

Mary C. McCarthy, MD, FACS
Dayton, Ohio

Avraham Rivkind, MD
Jerusalem, Israel

William P. Schecter, MD, FACS
San Francisco, California

Marc J. Shapiro, MD, FACS
St. Louis, Missouri

Thomas E. Shaver, MD, FACS
Mission Viejo, California

St. Luke's Hospitals MeritCare
Fargo, North Dakota

Gregory A. Timberlake, MD, FACS
Morgantown, West Virginia

Stanley Trooskin, MD, FACS
Brooklyn, New York

John A. Weigelt, MD, FACS
Dallas, Texas

Bradley D. Wong, MD, FACS
Honolulu, Hawaii

Table of Contents

The Role of the ACS Committee on Trauma iii
Editorial Notes...iv
Contributing Authors..v
Acknowledgments...viii

COURSE OVERVIEW: THE PURPOSE, HISTORY, AND CONCEPTS 9–16
   Program Goals...9
   Course Objectives 10
     I. The Need 11
     II. Nebraska Conception and Inception 11
     III. The Concept 13
     IV. The Course Overview...13
     V. Course Development and Dissemination....................................14
     VI. Acknowledgments...15
     VII. Summary 16
   Bibliography..16

CHAPTER 1 INITIAL ASSESSMENT AND MANAGEMENT 17–37
   Objectives 17
     I. Introduction..19
     II. Preparation—Prehospital/Inhospital...19
     III. Triage 20
     IV. Primary Survey—ABCs 21
     V. Resuscitation—ABCs 24
     VI. Roentgenograms...27
     VII. Secondary Survey—History/Physical Examination 27
   Table 1, Mechanisms of Injury...29
     VIII. Re-evaluation..34
     IX. Definitive Care 35
     X. Disaster...35
     XI. Records and Legal Considerations...35
     XII. Summary 36
   Bibliography..37
Skill I   **Initial Assessment and Management** 39–46

CHAPTER 2 AIRWAY AND VENTILATORY MANAGEMENT 47–59
   Objectives 47
     I. Introduction..49
     II. Airway—Problem Recognition/Objective Signs 49
     III. Ventilation—Problem Recognition/Objective Signs 50
     IV. Management—Airway Maintenance Techniques/Definitive
        Airway/Ventilation and Oxygenation....................................51
   Table 1, PaO_2 versus O_2 Saturation Levels....................................56
   Figure 1, Airway Algorithm..57
     V. Summary 58
   Bibliography..58
Skill II   **Airway and Ventilatory Management**...61–68
     Oropharyngeal Airway Insertion..63

Table of Contents continued

	Nasopharyngeal Airway Insertion	63
	Ventilation Without Intubation	63
	Adult Orotracheal Intubation	64
	Adult Nasotracheal Intubation	65
	Infant Endotracheal Intubation	67
Skill III	**Cricothyroidotomy**	**69–73**
	Needle Cricothyroidotomy	71
	Surgical Cricothyroidotomy	72
	Figure 1, Surgical Cricothyroidotomy	73

CHAPTER 3	**SHOCK**	**75–94**
	Objectives	75
I.	Introduction	77
II.	Initial Patient Assessment—Recognition/ Clinical Differentiation of Etiology	77
III.	Hemorrhagic Shock—Pathophysiology/Definition/Direct Effects/ Fluid Changes Secondary to Soft-Tissue Injury	80
IV.	Initial Management—Physical Examination/Vascular Access Lines/ Initial Fluid Therapy	83
V.	Evaluation of Fluid Resuscitation and Organ Perfusion— General/Urinary Output/Acid/Base Balance	85
	Table 1, Estimated Fluid and Blood Losses	86
VI.	Therapeutic Decisions Based on Fluid Resuscitation Response—Rapid/Transient/Minimal	86
VII.	Blood Replacement—PRBCs versus Whole Blood/ Crossmatched, Type-specific and Type O Blood/ Blood Filters/Warming Fluids/Autotransfusion/ Coagulopathy/Calcium Administration	87
	Table 2, Responses to Initial Fluid Resuscitation	88
VIII.	Pneumatic Antishock Garment—Indications/Contraindications/ Dangers/Deflation and Removal	89
IX.	Pitfalls in Diagnosis and Treatment—Equating Blood Pressure with Cardiac Output/Age/Athletes/ Medications/Hypothermia/Pacemaker	90
X.	Reassessing Patient Response and Avoiding Complications—Continued Hemorrhage/ Fluid Overload and CVP Monitoring/Recognition of Other Problems	91
XI.	Summary	93
	Bibliography	93
Skill IV	**Vascular Access and Monitoring**	**95–106**
	Subclavian Venipuncture: Infraclavicular Approach	97
	Figure 1, Subclavian Venipuncture: Infraclavicular Approach	98
	Internal Jugular Venipuncture	98
	Figure 2, Internal Jugular Venipuncture	99
	Femoral Venipuncture, Seldinger Technique	100
	Figure 3, Femoral Venipuncture, Seldinger Technique	101
	Intraosseous Puncture/Infusion	102

Table of Contents continued

Figure 4, Intraosseous Puncture...103
    Pulse Oximetry Monitoring 104
Figure 5, PaO$_2$ and %SaO$_2$ Relationship 106
Skill V   **Venous Cutdown** 107–110
    Figure 1, Saphenous Venous Cutdown 110

CHAPTER 4 THORACIC TRAUMA...**111–125**
    Objectives 111
    I. Introduction—Incidence/Pathophysiology/
       Initial Assessment and Management 113
    II. Primary Survey of Life-threatening Injuries—ABCs/Thoracotomy 114
    III. Life-threatening—Airway Obstruction/Tension Pneumothorax/
       Open Pneumothorax/Massive Hemothorax/Flail Chest/Cardiac
       Tamponade 115
    IV. Potentially Lethal—Pulmonary Contusion with or without
       Flail/Myocardial Contusion/Traumatic Aortic
       Rupture/Traumatic Diaphragmatic Hernia/
       Tracheobronchial Tree Injuries/Esophageal Trauma 118
    V. Other Manifestations—Subcutaneous Emphysema/
       Crushing Injury/Simple Pneumothorax/
       Hemothorax/Scapular and Rib Fractures/
       Other Indications for Chest Tube Insertion 123
    VI. Summary..125
    Bibliography...125
Skill VI   **Roentgenographic Identification of Thoracic Injuries**...............127–133
Skill VII   **Chest Trauma Management**...135–140
    Needle Thoracentesis 137
    Chest Tube Insertion 138
    Pericardiocentesis 139

CHAPTER 5 ABDOMINAL TRAUMA...**141–154**
    Objectives 141
    I. Introduction—High Index of Suspicion/
       Regions of Abdomen 143
    II. Assessment—History/Physical Examination/Intubation/
       Blood Sampling/Roentgenographic Studies/
       Special Diagnostic Studies 143
    Table 1, Associated Injuries 146
    Table 2, DPL versus CT..148
    III. Indications for Celiotomy 148
    IV. Special Problems—Blunt Trauma/Penetrating Trauma/
       Pelvic Fractures and Associated Injuries....................................149
    V. Summary 152
    Bibliography...153
Skill VIII Diagnostic Peritoneal Lavage 155–158

CHAPTER 6 HEAD TRAUMA **159–183**
    Objectives 159

Table of Contents continued

    I. Introduction 161

    II. Anatomy and Physiology—Scalp/Skull/Meninges/
        Brain/Cerebrospinal Fluid/Tentorium/
        Consciousness/Intracranial Pressure 161

    III. Assessment—History/ABCs/Vital Signs/AVPU +
        Minineurologic Examination/GCS/
        Special Assessment 164

    IV. Specific Types—Fractures/Diffuse
        Brain Injuries/Focal Injuries 169

    V. Emergency Management—Establishing Specific
        Diagnosis/Emergency Management 174

    Table 1, Approximate % of Patients Requiring Surgery 174

    Figure 1, Head Injury Triage Scheme 176

    Table 2, Relative Risk of Intracranial Lesion 177

    VI. Other Manifestations—Seizures/Restlessness/Hyperthermia ...179

    VII. Scalp Wounds—Blood Loss/Inspection/Repair 180

    VIII. Definitive Surgical Management 181

    IX. Summary 182

    Bibliography 183

Skill IX   **Head and Neck Trauma Assessment and Management** 185–190

    Assessment and Management of Head Trauma 187

    Application of Cervical Traction Tongs (Optional) 189

CHAPTER 7 SPINE AND SPINAL CORD TRAUMA **191–203**

    Objectives 191

    I. Introduction 193

    II. History 193

    III. Assessment—General/Vertebral/Neurologic/
        Neurogenic and Spinal Shock/Effect on
        Other Organ Systems/Roentgenograms 193

    IV. Types of Injuries—Fracture and Fracture-
        Dislocation/Open Wounds 197

    V. Treatment—Immobilization/IV Fluids/Medications/
        Transfer 201

    VI. Summary 202

    Bibliography 202

Skill X   **Roentgenographic Identification of Spine Injuries** 205–209

Skill XI   **Immobilization Techniques for Neck and Spinal Trauma** 211–218

    Assessment of Neck and Spine Injuries 213

    Immobilization/Modified Log-roll Technique 214

    Application and Use of Scoop Stretcher (Optional) 217

CHAPTER 8 EXTREMITY TRAUMA **219–239**

    Objectives 219

    I. Introduction—Primary Survey and Resuscitation/
        Secondary Survey/Early Management 221

Table of Contents continued

II. Assessment—History/Physical Examination/
     Vascular Injuries/Traumatic Amputation/Open
     Wound/Compartment Syndrome/Nerve Injury/
     Joint Injury/Fractures 222
  Table 1, Peripheral Nerve Assessment, Lower Extremities..................229
  Table 2, Peripheral Nerve Assessment, Upper Extremities 229
  Table 3, Open Fracture Grading 231
III. Management—Vascular Injuries/Traumatic Amputation/
     Open Wounds/Compartment Syndrome/
     Nerve Injury/Joint Injury/Fractures/
     Pain Control 233
IV. Principles of Immobilization—Femoral Fractures/
     Knee Injuries/Tibia Fractures/Ankle Fractures/
     Upper Extremity and Hand Injuries.................................236
  V. Summary 238
  Bibliography...238

**Skill XII   Principles and Techniques of Immobilization for Extremity
              Trauma** 241–244
     Principles of Extremity Immobilization 243
     Application of Leg Traction Splint 243

CHAPTER 9   INJURIES DUE TO BURNS AND COLD............245–259
  Objectives 245
  I. Introduction...247
  II. Immediate Life-saving Measures—Airway/Stop
      Burning Process/IV Lines...247
  III. Assessment—History/BSA/Depth 248
  IV. Stabilizing—ABCs/Physical Examination/Flow Sheet/
      Baseline Determinations/Circumferential
      Burns/NG Tube Insertion/Narcotics,
      Analgesics, Sedatives/Wound Care 249
  Figure 1, "Rule of Nines" 250
  Figure 2, Depth of Burn 251
  V. Special Burn Requirements—Chemical/Electrical..............254
  VI. Criteria for Transfer—Types/Transfer Procedure 255
  VII. Cold Injury—Types of Frostbite and Nonfreezing Injury/
       Management..256
  VIII. Hypothermia—Signs/Management..................................257
  IX. Summary 258
  Bibliography...259

CHAPTER 10   PEDIATRIC TRAUMA...............................261–281
  Objectives 261
  I. Introduction—Size and Shape/Skeleton/Surface Area/
     Psychologic Status/Long-term Effects/
     Equipment 263
  II. Airway—Anatomy/Management 264

Table of Contents continued

   III. Shock—Recognition/Fluid Resuscitation/Blood
       Replacement/Venous Access/
       Thermoregulation 266
Table 1, Systemic Responses to Blood Loss 267
Table 2, Vital Signs 267
Table 3, Resuscitation Flow Diagram..269
Figure 1, Site for Intraosseous Infusion 270
   IV. Chest Trauma 271
    V. Abdominal Trauma—Assessment/DPL/CT/
       Nonoperative Management 271
   VI. Head Trauma—Assessment/Management..273
Table 4, Pediatric Verbal Score 274
  VII. Spinal Cord Injury—Anatomic Differences/
       Roentgenographic Considerations 275
 VIII. Extremity Trauma—History/Blood Loss/Physeal
       Fractures/Unique Fractures/
       Immobilization Principles 276
   IX. The Battered, Abused Child 277
    X. Epidemiology of Pediatric Injury/Strategies for Injury Control 278
   XI. Summary 279
Bibliography...279
Table 5, Pediatric Equipment...281

CHAPTER 11 TRAUMA IN PREGNANCY **283–292**
Objectives 283
    I. Introduction..285
   II. Anatomic and Physiologic Alterations—Anatomic/
       Hemodynamic/Blood Volume and Composition/
       Respiratory/Gastrointestinal/Urinary/
       Endocrine/Musculoskeletal/Neurologic..285
   III. Mechanisms of Injury—Penetrating/Blunt..288
   IV. Severity of Injuries..288
    V. Diagnosis and Management—Primary and Secondary
       Assessment/Monitoring/Definitive Care..289
   VI. Summary 291
Bibliography...292

CHAPTER 12 STABILIZATION AND TRANSPORT..............................**293–303**
Objectives 293
    I. Introduction..295
   II. Determining the Need for Transfer 295
   III. Transfer Responsibilities—Referring Physician/
       Receiving Physician...296
   IV. Modes of Transportation 297
    V. Transfer Protocols—Referring Physician/Transfer
       Personnel/Documentation/Prior to Transfer/
       Management During Transfer 297
Table 1, Interhospital Triage Criteria...298

Table of Contents continued

VI. Transfer Data..301
VII. Summary..301
Bibliography..301
Chart 1, Sample Transfer Form 302
Chart 2, Revised Trauma Score 303

RESOURCE DOCUMENTS **305–396**
    Contents 305
     1. Trauma Prevention..307
     2. Prehospital Triage Criteria...317
     3. Kinematics of Trauma 319
     4. Protection of Personnel from Communicable Diseases 333
     5. Roentgenographic Studies 335
     6. Tetanus Immunization 353
     7. Pediatric Trauma Score 359
     8. Sample Trauma Flow Sheet..361
     9. Sample Transfer Agreement 365
    10. Sample Transfer Record Information 367
    11. Organ and Tissue Donation 369
    12. Preparations for Disaster..371
    13. Ocular Trauma (Optional Lecture) 373
    14. ATLS and the Law (Optional Lecture) 381

American College of Surgeons

Course Overview:
The Purpose, History, and
Concepts of the ATLS Program
for Physicians

Program Goals:

The Advanced Trauma Life Support Course provides the physician with a safe, reliable method for immediate management of the injured patient and the basic knowledge necessary to:

1. Assess the patient's condition rapidly and accurately.

2. Resuscitate and stabilize the patient on a priority basis.

3. Determine if the patient's needs will likely exceed a facility's capabilities.

4. Arrange for the patient's interhospital transfer.

5. Assure that optimum care is provided each step of the way.

Course Objectives:

The purpose of this course is to orient physicians to the initial assessment and management of the trauma patient. In general, the content and skills presented in the materials are designed to assist physicians in providing the **first hour** of emergency care for the trauma patient. Therefore, this course represents the minimum information necessary to manage the trauma patient in the first hour.

Upon completion of the Advanced Trauma Life Support Course, the physician participant will be able to:

A. Demonstrate concepts and principles of primary and secondary patient assessment.

B. Establish management priorities in a trauma situation.

C. Initiate primary and secondary management necessary within the first hour of emergency care for acute life-threatening emergencies.

D. Demonstrate, in a given simulated clinical and surgical skill practicum, the following skills used in the initial assessment and management of patients with multiple injuries:

   1. Primary and secondary assessment of a patient with simulated, multiple injuries

   2. Establishing a patent airway and initiating one- and two-man ventilation

   3. Orotracheal and nasotracheal intubation on adult and infant manikins

   4. Cricothyroidotomy

   5. Initiation of percutaneous venous access, central intravenous lifelines with central venous pressure monitoring, intraosseous infusion, and pulse oximetry monitoring

   6. Venous cutdown

   7. Pleural decompression via needle thoracentesis and chest tube insertion

   8. Pericardiocentesis

   9. Roentgenographic identification of thoracic injuries

   10. Peritoneal lavage

   11. Application of cervical traction tongs (optional)

   12. Roentgenographic identification of spine injuries

   13. Immobilization and stabilization of spinal injuries

   14. Immobilization and stabilization of extremity injuries

I. The Need

The first edition of this manual appeared in 1980. Since that time many dramatic and significant changes have taken place in the care of the injured patient, none more so than the Advanced Trauma Life Support (ATLS) Program for Physicians. Nevertheless, trauma remains the leading cause of death in the first four decades of life (ages 1 through 44 years), surpassed only by cancer and atherosclerosis as the major cause of death in all age groups. As great as the death rate from injury is, about 145,000 deaths annually in the United States, disability from injury dwarfs the mortality by three to one. The societal cost is staggering, as is the amount of human suffering. The need for improved methods of caring for injured patients is as great now as it ever has been.

Approximately 60 million injuries occur annually in the United States. Approximately 30 million (50%) of these injuries require medical care, and 3.6 million (12% of 30 million) require hospitalization. Nearly nine million of these injuries are disabling— 300,000 permanent disabilities and 8,700,000 temporary disabilities.

Trauma-related costs are in excess of $100 billion annually—approximately 40% of the health care dollar. This cost is accounted for by lost wages, medical expenses, insurance administration costs, property damage, fire loss, and indirect loss from work accidents. Yet with these staggering costs, less than four cents of each federal research dollar is expended on trauma research. As monumental as these data are, the true cost to society can be measured only when it is realized that trauma strikes down its youngest and potentially most productive members. As tragic as is any "accidental" death, the loss of life in the early years is the most tragic of all. If there was a disease that primarily struck down the young, society would not tolerate such an occurrence for long. Yet, trauma is such a disease.

There are methods and modalities available to prevent most injuries. To this point in time, these methods have been marginally effective. Barring effective prevention modalities, the ATLS treatment method is all the more necessary.

II. Nebraska Conception and Inception

The year 1978 was a banner year, which in retrospect foreshadowed a new approach to provision of care to individuals suffering major, life-threatening injury. This was the year in which the first Advanced Trauma Life Support Course was conducted. This prototype ATLS Course was field-tested in conjunction with the Southeast Nebraska Emergency Medical Services. One year later in 1979, the American College of Surgeons (ACS) Committee on Trauma (COT), recognizing trauma as a surgical disease, enthusiastically adopted the course under the imprimatur of the College and incorporated it as an educational program of the College.

Before 1980 the delivery of trauma care by physicians in the United States was at best inconsistent. There was not a standardized program to train physicians in trauma care anywhere in the world. As often happens, a tragedy occurred in February 1976 that changed the face of trauma care in the first hour for the injured patient in the United States and potentially in much of the rest of the world. An orthopedic surgeon, piloting his own private plane, crashed in a rural Nebraska cornfield. The surgeon sustained serious injuries, three of his children sustained critical injuries, and one child sustained minor injuries. His wife was killed instantly. The care he and his family received was woefully inadequate by today's standards.

The surgeon, recognizing how inadequate his treatment was, stated: "When I can provide better care in the field with limited resources than what my children and I received at the primary care facility—there is something wrong with the system and the system has to be changed." Indeed the system has been changed!

A group of private-practice surgeons and physicians in Nebraska, the Lincoln Medical Education Foundation (LMEF), and the Lincoln-area Mobile Heart Team Nurses with the help of the University of Nebraska Medical Center, the Nebraska State Committee on Trauma of the ACS and Southeast Nebraska Emergency Medical Services identified the need for training in advanced trauma life support. A combined educational format of lectures, associated with life-saving skill demonstrations and practical laboratory experiences formed the first prototype ATLS Course for physicians.

This prototype course was based on a rather major assumption—that appropriate and timely care given early could improve the outcome of the injured significantly. It was not until five years later that this assumption was proven to be correct by the identification of the trimodal distribution of death due to trauma.

The trimodal distribution of death due to injury was described in 1982. Death due to injury occurs in one of three time periods. The **first peak** of death is within seconds to minutes from injury. During this early period deaths are generally due to lacerations of the brain, brain stem, high spinal cord, heart, aorta, and other large blood vessels. Very few of these patients can be salvaged due to the severity of their injuries. Salvage after injury during this peak can be achieved only in certain large urban areas where rapid prehospital care and transport are available. The optimum salvage during this peak of traumatic deaths can best be accomplished by effective prevention methodologies.

The **second peak** occurs within minutes to several hours following injury. The ATLS Course focuses primarily on this peak. Deaths occurring during this period are usually due to subdural and epidural hematomas, hemopneumothorax, ruptured spleen, lacerations of the liver, pelvic fractures, and/or other multiple injuries associated with significant blood loss. The first hour of care following injury is characterized by rapid assessment and resuscitation which are the fundamental principles of the ATLS Program.

The **third death peak**, occurring several days to weeks after the initial injury, is most often due to sepsis and multiple organ system failure. Care provided during each of the preceding time periods impact on outcome during this stage. Thus, the first and every subsequent individual to see the injured patient have a direct effect on long-term outcome.

The original intent of the ATLS Program was that it be targeted for physicians who do not manage major trauma on a daily basis. The original audience for the course has not changed. However, today the ATLS method is accepted as a gold standard for the first hour of trauma care by all who provide care for the injured, whether the patient is treated in an isolated rural area or a state-of-the-art Level 1 Trauma Center.

III. The Concept

The concept behind the course was, as with all lasting concepts, simple yet profound. The approach to the injured patient, which was being taught in medical schools, was the same approach one would utilize for a patient with a previously undiagnosed medical condition, ie, extensive history including past medical history, physical examination starting at the top of the head and progressing down the body, and development of a differential diagnosis and a list of ancillary diagnostic modalities to identify or exclude the differential diagnosis. Although this approach was quite adequate for a patient with diabetes mellitus or even many acute surgical illnesses, it did not satisfy the needs of the trauma patient suffering severe injury. The approach itself required change.

There were several underlying concepts to the development of the ATLS Program that were initially anathematic to physicians not accustomed to seeing and treating trauma victims. The most important was to treat the greatest threat to life first. The next was that the lack of a definitive diagnosis should never impede the application of an indicated treatment. The final concept was that a detailed history was not the essential prerequisite to begin the evaluation of an acutely injured patient. The result was the development of the "ABCs" approach to the evaluation and treatment of the injured.

The ATLS Course teaches that life-threatening injury kills and maims in certain reproducible time frames. For example, the loss of an airway kills more quickly than does the loss of the ability to breathe. The latter kills more quickly than loss of circulating blood volume. The presence of an expanding intracranial mass lesion is the next most lethal problem. Thus, the mnemonic "ABCDE" defines the specific, ordered, prioritized evaluations and interventions that should be followed in all injured patients:

A   Airway with cervical-spine control
B   Breathing
C   Circulation
D   Disability or neurologic status
E   Exposure (undress) with temperature control

IV. The Course Overview

The ATLS Course emphasizes the first hour of initial assessment and primary management of the injured patient, starting at the point in time of injury and continuing through initial assessment, life-saving intervention, re-evaluation, stabilization, and when needed, transfer to a trauma center. The course consists of pre- and post-course tests, core content lectures, case presentations, discussions, development of life-saving manipulative skills, practical laboratory experience, and a final performance proficiency evaluation. Upon completion of the course, the physicians should feel confident in implementing the trauma skills taught in the ATLS Course.

Based on well-established principles and objectives of trauma management, the course is intended to provide the physicians with **one** acceptable method for **safe**, immediate management and the basic knowledge necessary to:

1. Assess the patient's condition rapidly and accurately.
2. Resuscitate and stabilize the patient on a priority basis.

3. Determine if the patient's needs will likely exceed a facility's capabilities.
4. Arrange for the patient's interhospital transfer.
5. Assure that optimum care is provided each step of the way.

Included in this manual, at the conclusion of the scientific core content, are a series of relevant resource documents designed to enhance the core content.

1. Trauma Prevention
2. Prehospital Triage Criteria
3. Kinematics of Trauma
4. Protection of Personnel from Communicable Diseases
5. Roentgenographic Studies
6. Tetanus Immunization
7. Pediatric Trauma Score
8. Trauma Flow Sheet
9. Transfer Agreement
10. Transfer Record
11. Organ and Tissue Donation
12. Preparations for Disaster
13. Ocular Trauma (Optional Lecture)
14. ATLS and the Law (Optional Lecture)

V. Course Development and Dissemination

A. The 1980s

The course was given nationally for the first time in January 1980. Canada became an active participant in the ATLS Program in 1981. Countries in Latin and South America joined the ACS Committee on Trauma in 1986 and implemented the ATLS Program. Under the auspices of the ACS Military Committee on Trauma, the program has been conducted for US military physicians in Germany, Guam, Panama, and Japan.

Since its inception, the program has grown both in number of courses and participants each year. By the end of the 1980s, the course had trained approximately 120,000 physicians in more than 5000 courses across North and South America. Currently, an average of 13,000 physicians are trained in the ATLS Course each year in 750 courses.

The text for the course is revised every four years incorporating new modalities of evaluation and treatment which have become accepted parts of the armamentarium of physicians treating trauma patients. To retain a current status in the ATLS Program, an individual must reverify with the latest edition of the materials every four years.

A parallel-type course to the ATLS Course is the Prehospital Trauma Life Support (PHTLS) Course sponsored by the National Association of Emergency Medical Technicians (NAEMT). The PHTLS Course, developed in cooperation with the ACS Committee on Trauma, is based on the concepts of the ACS ATLS Program for Physicians, and is conducted for emergency medical technicians, paramedics, and nurses who are providers of prehospital trauma care. In addition, trauma courses for nurses have been developed with similar concepts and philosophies. At present, the benefits of having both prehospital and inhospital trauma personnel speaking the same language are apparent.

B. The Future—International Dissemination

The ATLS Program was exported outside of North America, as a first-ever pilot project, in 1986 to the Republic of Trinidad and Tobago. The ACS Board of Regents gave permission in 1987 for promulgation of the ATLS program in other countries within strict guidelines. The program may be requested by a recognized surgical organization or ACS Chapter in another country by corresponding with the ATLS Subcommittee Chairman, care of the ACS ATLS Division. Since 1987, the program has been requested and approved for implementation by these organizations:

1. Royal College of Surgeons of England; implemented in November 1988

2. Royal Australasian College of Surgeons; implemented in December 1988 The ATLS Course has been termed "Early Management of Severe Trauma (EMST)"

3. Israeli Surgical Society; implemented in January 1990

4. Society of Surgeons of Trinidad and Tobago; piloted in 1986 and implemented in June 1990

5. Royal College of Surgeons in Ireland; implemented in May 1991

6. ACS Chapter of Saudi Arabia; implemented in October 1991

7. South African Trauma Society; implemented in 1992

8. Chapter of Surgeons of the Academy of Medicine, Singapore; implemented in 1992

Currently, 15 countries are actively providing the ATLS Course to their physicians. They include the United States and U.S. territories, Canada, Republic of Trinidad/Tobago, Mexico, Chile, Brazil, Bolivia, Argentina, United Kingdom, Australia, New Zealand, Israel, Ireland, Republic of South Africa, Saudi Arabia, and Republic of Singapore.

VI. Acknowledgments

The Committee on Trauma of the ACS and the ATLS Subcommittee gratefully acknowledge these organizations for their time and efforts in developing and field testing the Advanced Trauma Life Support concept: The Lincoln Medical Education Foundation, Southeast Nebraska Emergency Medical Services, the University of Nebraska College of Medicine, and the Nebraska State Committee on Trauma of the ACS. We also are indebted to those Nebraska physicians who supported the development of this course and to the Lincoln Area Mobile Heart Team Nurses who shared their time and ideas to help build it. Appreciation for their support of the world-wide promulgation of the course is extended to those organizations identified previously in this chapter.

VII. Summary

For those physicians who infrequently treat trauma, the ATLS Course provides an easily remembered method for evaluating and treating the victim of a traumatic event. For those physicians who treat traumatic disease on a frequent basis, the ATLS Course provides a scaffold for evaluation, treatment, education, and quality assurance—in short, a system of trauma care that is measurable, reproducible, and comprehensive.

The Committee on Trauma of the ACS anticipates that through the application of the skills taught in the ATLS Course, a significant reduction in trauma morbidity and mortality will be accomplished. The establishment of minimum standards of care in the early assessment and management of the trauma patient will bring about this expected outcome. Through the dedicated and committed efforts of health care professionals, this worthy goal can be achieved.

Bibliography

1. Committee on Trauma Research, Commission on Life Sciences, National Research Council, and the Institute of Medicine: **Injury in America**. Washington, DC, National Academy Press, 1985.

2. Committee to Review the Status and Progress of the Injury Control Program at Centers for Disease Control: **Injury Control**. Washington, DC, National Academy Press, 1988.

3. Trunkey DD: Trauma. **Scientific American** 1983;249:28-35.

Chapter 1:
Initial Assessment and Management

Objectives:

Upon completion of this topic, the physician will be able to demonstrate an ability to apply the principles of emergency medical care to the multiply injured patient. Specifically, the physician will be able to:

A. Identify the correct sequence of priorities to be followed in assessing the multiply injured patient.

B. Outline the primary and secondary evaluation surveys to be used in assessing the multiply injured patient.

C. Identify and discuss the key components of and rationale for obtaining the patient's history and the history of the trauma incident.

D. Explain guidelines and techniques to be used in the initial resuscitative and definitive-care phases of treatment of the multiply injured patient.

E. Conduct an initial assessment and management survey on a simulated multiply injured patient, using the correct sequence of priorities and explaining management techniques for primary treatment and stabilization.

**Chapter 1:
Initial
Assessment
and
Management**

I. Introduction

The treatment of the seriously injured patient requires rapid assessment of the injuries and institution of life-preserving therapy. Since time is of the essence, a systematic approach that can be reviewed and practiced is desirable. This process is termed "Initial Assessment" and includes:

1. Preparation

2. Triage

3. **Primary survey (ABCs)**

4. **Resuscitation**

5. **Secondary survey (head-to-toe)**

6. Continued postresuscitation monitoring and re-evaluation

7. **Definitive care**

The primary and secondary surveys should be repeated frequently to ascertain any deterioration in the patient's status, and necessary treatment instituted at the time an adverse change is identified.

This sequence is presented in this chapter as a longitudinal progression of events. **In the actual clinical situation, many of these activities occur in parallel or simultaneously.** The linear or longitudinal progression allows the physician an opportunity to mentally review the progress of an actual trauma resuscitation for completeness.

II. Preparation

Preparation for the trauma patient occurs in two different clinical settings. First, the **prehospital phase**, from which all events must be coordinated with the physicians at the receiving hospital. Second, the **inhospital phase**, during which preparations must be made to facilitate the rapid progression of resuscitating the trauma patient.

A. Prehospital Phase

Coordination with the prehospital agency can greatly expedite the treatment of the patient in the field. The prehospital system should be set up such that the receiving hospital is notified **before** the prehospital personnel transport the patient from the scene. Emphasis should be placed on airway maintenance, control of external bleeding and shock, immobilization of the patient, and immediate transport to the **closest, appropriate facility**, preferably a verified trauma center. Every effort should be made to minimize scene time. (See Resource Document 2, Prehospital Triage Criteria and Flow Chart 1, Triage Decision Scheme.) Emphasis also should be placed on obtaining and reporting pertinent information needed for triage at the hospital, time of injury, events related to the injury, and patient history. The mechanisms of injury can suggest the degree of injury as well as specific injuries for which the patient must be evaluated.

B. Inhospital Phase

Advanced planning for the trauma patient's arrival is essential. In the emergency department, preparation must be made for the patient's arrival. Ideally, a suitable area should be kept available for trauma patients. Proper airway equipment (laryngoscopes, tubes, etc) should be organized, tested, and set up in a place where they are immediately available. Warmed intravenous crystalloid solutions, eg, Ringer's lactate, should be available and hung in readiness. Appropriate monitoring capabilities should be immediately available. A method to summon extra medical assistance should be in place. A means to assure prompt response by laboratory and radiology personnel is necessary. Ideally, transfer agreements with a verified trauma center should be established and in place. (Reference: ACS Committee on Trauma, *Resources for Optimal Care of the Injured Patient.*) (See Resource Document 9, Transfer Agreement.)

All personnel who have contact with the patient must be protected from communicable diseases. Most prominent among these diseases are hepatitis and the Acquired Immune Deficiency Syndrome (AIDS). The Centers for Disease Control (CDC) and other health agencies strongly recommend the use of universal precautions (eg, face mask, eye protection, water-impervious apron, leggings, and gloves) when coming in contact with body fluids. The ACS Committee on Trauma considers these to be **minimum** precautions. (See Resource Document 4, Protection of Personnel from Communicable Diseases.)

III. Triage

Triage is the sorting of patients based on the need for treatment and the available resources to provide that treatment. Treatment is rendered based on the ABC priorities (**A**irway with cervical spine control, **B**reathing, and **C**irculation with hemorrhage control) as outlined later in this chapter.

Triage also pertains to the sorting of patients in the field and the medical facility to which they are to be transported. It is the responsibility of the prehospital personnel and their medical director to see that the appropriate patients arrive at the appropriate hospital. It is inappropriate for prehospital personnel to deliver a severely traumatized patient to a nontrauma center hospital if a trauma center is available. (See Resource Document 2, Prehospital Triage Criteria and Flow Chart 1, Triage Decision Scheme.) The Pediatric Trauma Score is helpful in identifying those severely injured patients who should be transported to a trauma center. (See Resource Document 7, Pediatric Trauma Score.)

To prevent inappropriate patient transfer, an attempt to triage or sort trauma patients in the field is desirable. The American College of Surgeons Committee on Trauma has published criteria based on physiologic indices and mechanism of injury. Many trauma systems have used these criteria or a modification thereof to triage patients to trauma and nontrauma hospitals.

Two types of triage situations usually exist:

1. The number of patients and the severity of their injuries do **not** exceed the ability of the facility to render care. In this situation, patients with life-threatening problems and those sustaining multiple-system injuries are treated first.

2. The number of patients and the severity of their injuries **exceed** the capability of the facility and staff. In this situation, those patients with the greatest chance of survival, with the least expenditure of time, equipment, supplies, and personnel, are managed first.

IV. Primary Survey

Patients are assessed and treatment priorities are established based on their injuries, the stability of their vital signs, and the injury mechanism. In the severely injured patient, logical sequential treatment priorities must be established based on overall patient assessment. The patient's vital functions must be assessed quickly and efficiently. Patient management must consist of a rapid primary evaluation, resuscitation of vital functions, a more detailed secondary assessment, and finally, the initiation of definitive care. This process constitutes the ABCs of trauma care and identifies life-threatening conditions.

A **A**irway maintenance with cervical spine control
B **B**reathing and ventilation
C **C**irculation with hemorrhage control
D **D**isability: Neurologic status
E **E**xposure/Environmental Control: Completely undress the patient, but prevent hypothermia

During the primary survey, life-threatening conditions are identified and management is begun **simultaneously**. The prioritized assessment and management procedures reviewed in this chapter are identified as sequential steps in order of importance and for the purpose of clarity. However, these steps are frequently accomplished simultaneously.

Priorities for the care of the pediatric patient are basically the same as for adults. Although the quantities of blood, fluids, and medications, the size of the child, degree of heat loss, and injury patterns may differ, assessment and priorities are the same. Specific problems of the pediatric trauma patient are addressed in Chapter 10.

A. Airway with Cervical Spine Control

Upon initial evaluation of the trauma patient, the airway should be assessed first to ascertain patency. This rapid assessment for signs of airway obstruction should include inspection for foreign bodies and facial, mandibular, or tracheal/laryngeal fractures that may result in airway obstruction. Measures to establish a patent airway should protect the cervical spine. The chin lift or jaw thrust maneuvers are recommended to achieve this task.

While assessing and managing the patient's airway, great care should be taken to prevent excessive movement of the cervical spine. The patient's head and neck should not be hyperextended, hyperflexed, or rotated to establish and maintain the airway. Based on the history of the trauma incident, the loss of integrity of the cervical spine should be suspected. Neurologic examination alone does not rule out a cervical spine injury. The integrity of the bony components of the cervical spine can be assessed initially by visualizing all seven cervical vertebrae, including the C-7 to T-1 interspace on a crosstable lateral cervical spine roentgenogram. The lateral cervical spine film does **not** exclude all cervical spine injuries. Immobilization of the patient's head and neck with appropriate cervical immobilization devices should be accomplished and maintained. If immobilizing devices must be removed temporarily, the head and neck should be stabilized with manual, in-line immobilization by one member of the trauma team. These devices should be left in place until cervical spine injury is excluded. **Remember: Assume a cervical spine injury in any patient with multisystem trauma, especially with an altered level of consciousness or a blunt injury above the clavicle.**

Pitfalls:
1. Foreign body in the airway
2. Mandibular or maxillofacial fracture
3. Tracheal or laryngeal disruption
4. Cervical spine injury

B. Breathing

Airway patency alone does not assure adequate ventilation. Adequate exchange of gases is mandatory to maximize oxygen transfer and carbon dioxide elimination. Ventilation involves adequate function of the lungs, chest wall, and diaphragm. Each component must be examined and evaluated rapidly.

The patient's chest should be exposed to assess ventilatory exchange adequately. Auscultation should be performed to assure air exchange in the lungs. Percussion may reveal the presence of air or blood in the chest. Visual inspection and palpation may reveal injuries to the chest wall that may compromise ventilation.

Injuries that may acutely impair ventilation are tension pneumothorax, flail chest with pulmonary contusion, and open pneumothorax. Hemothorax, simple pneumothorax, fractured ribs, and pulmonary contusion may compromise ventilation to a lesser degree.

Pitfalls:
1. Tension pneumothorax
2. Flail chest with pulmonary contusion
3. Open pneumothorax
4. Massive hemothorax

C. Circulation with Hemorrhage Control

1. Blood volume and cardiac output

Hemorrhage is the predominant cause of postinjury deaths that are amenable to effective and rapid treatment in the hospital setting. Hypotension following injury must be considered to be hypovolemic in origin until proved otherwise. Rapid and accurate assessment of the injured patient's hemodynamic status is therefore essential. Two elements of observation yield key information within seconds—level of consciousness and pulse.

a. Level of consciousness

When circulating blood volume is reduced, cerebral perfusion may be critically impaired, resulting in altered levels of consciousness. However, a conscious patient also may have lost a significant amount of blood.

b. Skin color

Skin color can be helpful in evaluating the hypovolemic injured patient. A patient with pink skin, especially in the face and extremities, is rarely critically hypovolemic after injury. Conversely, the ashen, gray skin of the face and the white skin of the exsanguinated extremities are ominous signs of hypovolemia. These latter signs usually indicate a blood volume loss of at least 30%, if hypovolemia is the cause.

c. Pulse

Pulses, usually an easily accessible central pulse (femoral or carotid), should be assessed bilaterally for quality, rate, and regularity. Full, slow, and regular peripheral pulses are **usually** signs of a relatively normovolemic patient. Rapid, thready pulses are early signs of hypovolemia, but may have other causes as well. An irregular pulse is usually a warning of cardiac impairment. Absent central pulses, not attributable to local factors, signify the need for immediate resuscitative action to restore depleted blood volume and effective cardiac output if death is to be avoided.

2. Bleeding

External, severe hemorrhage is identified and controlled in the primary survey.

Rapid, external blood loss is managed by direct manual pressure on the wound. Pneumatic splinting devices also may help control hemorrhage. These devices should be transparent to allow monitoring of underlying bleeding. Tourniquets should **not** be used because they crush tissues and cause distal ischemia. The use of hemostats is time-consuming, and surrounding structures, such as nerves and veins, can be injured. Hemorrhage into the thoracic or abdominal cavities, into muscles surrounding a fracture, or as a result of a penetrating injury can account for major, occult blood loss.

Pitfalls: Hypovolemia resulting from
1. Intra-abdominal or intrathoracic injury
2. Fractures of the femur and/or pelvis
3. Penetrating injuries with arterial or venous involvement
4. External hemorrhage from any source

D. Disability (Neurologic Evaluation)

A rapid neurologic evaluation is performed at the end of the primary survey. This neurologic evaluation establishes the patient's level of consciousness, and pupillary size and reaction. A simple mnemonic to describe the level of consciousness is the AVPU method.

A Alert
V Responds to Vocal stimuli
P Responds only to Painful stimuli
U Unresponsive

The Glasgow Coma Scale (GCS) is a more detailed neurologic evaluation that is quick, simple, and predictive of patient outcome. This evaluation can be done in lieu of the AVPU. If not done in the primary survey, the GCS should be performed as part of the more detailed, quantitative neurologic examination in the secondary survey. (See Chapter 6, Head Trauma and Chapter 12, Stabilization and Transport, Chart 2, Revised Trauma Score with Glasgow Coma Scale Score.)

A decrease in the level of consciousness may indicate decreased cerebral oxygenation and/or perfusion or may be due to direct cerebral injury. An altered level of consciousness indicates the need for immediate re-evaluation of the patient's oxygenation, ventilation, and perfusion status. Alcohol and/or other drugs also may alter the patient's level of consciousness. However, having excluded hypoxia and hypovolemia, changes in the level of consciousness should be considered to be of traumatic central nervous system origin until proven otherwise.

Pitfalls:
1. Head injury
2. Decreased oxygenation
3. Shock
4. Altered level of consciousness secondary to alcohol and/or other drugs **(This is a diagnosis of exclusion. Head injury, decreased oxygenation, and shock must be excluded first.)**

E. Exposure/Environmental Control

The patient should be completely undressed, usually by cutting off the garments to facilitate thorough examination and assessment of the patient. After the patient's clothing is removed, it is imperative to cover and protect the patient from becoming hypothermic in the emergency department. Warm blankets are useful, intravenous fluids should be warmed before administering to the patient, and a warm environment should be maintained.

V. Resuscitation

A. Airway

The airway should be protected in all patients and secured in those patients whose ventilation is not adequate. The jaw thrust or chin lift maneuver may suffice in some cases. The use of a nasopharyngeal airway may initially establish and maintain airway patency in the conscious patient. If the patient is unconscious and has no gag reflex, an oropharyngeal airway may be helpful.

B. Breathing/Ventilation/Oxygenation

Definitive control of the airway in patients who have compromised airways due to mechanical factors, who have ventilatory problems, or who are unconscious is achieved by endotracheal intubation, either nasally or orally. This procedure should be accomplished with control of the cervical spine. A surgical airway can be performed if oral or nasal intubation is contraindicated or cannot be accomplished due to technical reasons. (See Chapter 2, Airway and Ventilatory Management.)

A tension pneumothorax compromises ventilation, and if suspected, chest decompression should be accomplished immediately.

Every injured patient should receive supplemental oxygen therapy. If not intubated, the patient ideally should have oxygen delivered by a mask/reservoir device to achieve optimal oxygenation. (See Chapter 2, Airway and Ventilatory Management.)

C. Circulation

A minimum of two large-caliber intravenous catheters (IVs) should be established. The maximum rate of fluid administration is determined by the internal diameter of the catheter and inversely by its length, not by the size of the vein in which the catheter is placed. Initiation of upper extremity peripheral intravenous lines is preferred in most cases. Other peripheral lines, cutdowns, and central venous lines should be utilized and performed as necessary in accordance with the skill level of the physician caring for the patient. (See Skill Station IV, Vascular Access and Monitoring and Skill Station V, Venous Cutdown in Chapter 3, Shock.)

When initiating the intravenous lines, blood should be drawn for type and crossmatch and for baseline hematologic studies, including a pregnancy test for all females of childbearing age.

Vigorous intravenous fluid therapy with a balanced salt solution should be initiated. Ringer's lactate solution is preferred as the initial crystalloid solution and should be administered rapidly in the adult patient. Such bolus intravenous therapy may require the administration of two to three liters of solution to achieve an appropriate patient response.

The shock state associated with trauma is most often hypovolemic in origin. If the patient remains unresponsive to bolus intravenous therapy, type-specific blood may be administered as necessary. If type-specific blood is not available, low titer type O or O-negative blood must be considered as a substitute. For life-threatening blood loss, the use of unmatched, type-specific blood is preferred over type O blood unless multiple, unidentified casualties are being treated simultaneously. Hypovolemic shock should **not** be treated by vasopressors, steroids, or sodium bicarbonate.

Hypothermia can be produced quickly in the emergency department by leaving the patient uncovered and by rapid administration of room temperature fluids or four-degree centigrade blood. The use of a high-flow fluid warmer or microwave oven to heat crystalloid fluids to 39 degrees centigrade is recommended. Blood, plasma, and glucose-containing solutions should not be warmed in a microwave oven. (See Chapter 3, Shock.)

Careful **electrocardiographic** (ECG) monitoring of all trauma patients is required. Dysrhythmias, including unexplained tachycardia, atrial fibrillation, premature ventricular contractions, and ST segment changes, may indicate cardiac contusion. Electromechanical dissociation (EMD) may indicate cardiac tamponade, tension pneumothorax, and/or profound hypovolemia. When bradycardia, aberrant conduction, and premature beats are present, hypoxia and hypoperfusion should be suspected immediately. Hypothermia also produces these dysrhythmias.

D. Urinary and Gastric Catheters

The placement of urinary and gastric catheters should be considered as part of the resuscitation phase. Urine should be submitted for routine laboratory analysis.

1. Urinary catheters

Urinary output is a sensitive indicator of the volume status of the patient. Urinary catheterization is contraindicated in patients in whom urethral transection is suspected. Urethral injury should be suspected if there is (1) blood at the penile meatus, (2) blood in the scrotum, and (3) the prostate is high-riding or cannot be palpated. Accordingly, urinary catheter insertion should not be attempted before an examination of the rectum and genitalia has been performed, and associated injuries have been excluded.

2. Gastric catheters

A gastric tube is indicated to reduce stomach distention and decrease the risk of aspiration. However, thick or semisolid gastric contents will not return through the tube, and actual passage of the tube may induce vomiting. For the tube to be effective, it must be positioned properly, attached to appropriate suction, and be functioning. Blood in the gastric aspirate may represent oropharyngeal (swallowed) blood, traumatic insertion, or actual injury to the stomach. If the cribriform plate is fractured or a fracture is suspected, the gastric tube should be inserted orally or through a properly positioned nasopharyngeal airway to prevent intracranial passage of the tube.

E. Monitoring

Adequate resuscitation is best assessed by quantitative improvement of physiologic parameters, ie, ventilatory rate, pulse, blood pressure, pulse pressure, arterial blood gases (ABGs), body temperature, and urinary output, rather than the qualitative assessment done in the primary survey. **Actual values should be obtained as soon as practical after completing the primary survey.**

1. **Ventilatory rate and arterial blood gases** should be used to monitor the patient's airway and breathing. Endotracheal tubes can be dislodged whenever the patient is moved. End-tidal carbon dioxide monitoring is a reliable means of confirming the position of the endotracheal tube in intubated patients. A variety of quantitative devices are available for this purpose. (See Chapter 2, Airway and Ventilatory Management.)

2. **Pulse oximetry** is a valuable adjunct for monitoring injured patients. The pulse oximeter measures the oxygen saturation of hemoglobin colorimetrically, but does **not** measure the PaO_2. A small sensor is placed on the finger, toe, earlobe, or other convenient place. Most devices display pulse rate and oxygen concentration continuously. Appropriate oxygenation is a reflection of proper airway, breathing, and circulatory status.

3. The **blood pressure** should be measured, realizing that it may be a poor measure of actual tissue perfusion.

4. Careful **electrocardiographic (ECG) monitoring** of all trauma patients is recommended.

F. Consider Need for Patient Transfer

Remember: Life-saving measures are initiated when the problem is identified, rather than after the primary survey. During the primary survey and resuscitation phase, the evaluating physician frequently has enough information to indicate the need for transfer of the patient to another facility. This transfer process may be initiated immediately by administrative personnel at the direction of the examining physician, while additional patient care and evaluation are being performed. Once the decision to transfer the patient has been made, referring physician to receiving physician communication is essential.

VI. Roentgenograms

Roentgenograms should be used judiciously and should **not** delay patient resuscitation. In the patient with blunt trauma, three roentgenograms should be obtained—cervical spine, anteroposterior (AP) chest, and AP pelvis. These films can be taken in the resuscitation area, usually with a portable x-ray unit, but should **not** interrupt the resuscitation process. During the secondary survey, open-mouth odontoid and anteroposterior thoracolumbar films may be obtained with a portable x-ray unit if the patient's care is not compromised, and if the mechanism of injury suggests the possibility of spinal injury. After all life-threatening injuries are identified and treated, complete cervical spine, thoracic, and lumbar spine films should be obtained. In the patient with penetrating injuries, an AP chest film and films pertinent to the site(s) of wounding should be obtained. (See Resource Document 5, Roentgenographic Studies.)

VII. Secondary Survey

The secondary survey does not begin until the primary survey (ABCs) is completed, resuscitation is initiated, and the patient's ABCs are reassessed.

The secondary survey is a **head-to-toe evaluation** of the trauma patient, including vital sign assessment—blood pressure, pulse, respirations, and temperature. Each region of the body is completely examined. The potential for missing an injury or to not appreciate the significance of an injury is great, especially in the unresponsive or unstable patient. Examples of these injuries are cited as pitfalls after each anatomic region examined is discussed in this chapter.

In this survey a complete neurologic examination is performed, including a GCS Score, if not done during the primary survey. During this evaluation indicated roentgenograms are obtained. Such examinations can be interspersed into the secondary survey at opportune times.

Special procedures, eg, peritoneal lavage, radiologic evaluation, and laboratory studies, also are obtained during this time. Complete evaluation of the patient requires repeated examination of the patient. The secondary assessment might well be summarized as "tubes and fingers in every orifice."

A. History

Every complete medical assessment should include a good history of the injury-producing mechanism. Many times such a history cannot be obtained from the patient. Prehospital personnel and family must be consulted to obtain present and past information that may shed light on the patient's present physiologic state. The "AMPLE" history is a useful mnemonic to obtain the patient's pertinent history.

A Allergies
M Medications currently taken
P Past illnesses
L Last meal
E Events/environment related to the injury

The patient's present state is greatly influenced by the mechanism of injury. Prehospital personnel can provide valuable insight into such mechanisms and should report pertinent data to the examining physician. Types of injuries can be predicted based on the direction and amount of energy force. Injury usually is classified into two broad categories—blunt and penetrating. (See Resource Document 3, Kinematics of Trauma.)

1. Blunt trauma

Blunt trauma results from automobile collisions, falls, and other transportation-, recreation-, and occupation-related injuries.

Important information to obtain about automobile collisions includes: seat belt usage, steering wheel deformation, direction of impact, damage to the automobile in terms of major deformation or intrusion into the passenger compartment, and ejection of the passenger from the vehicle. Ejection from the vehicle greatly increases the chance of major injury.

Injury patterns may often be predicted by the mechanism of injury which demonstrates the importance of an accurate history. Such injury patterns also are influenced by age groups and activities. (See Table 1, Mechanisms of Injury and Related Suspected Injury Patterns.)

2. Penetrating trauma

Penetrating trauma, injuries from firearms, stabbings, and impaling objects, is increasing rapidly. Factors determining the type and extent of injury and subsequent management include the region of the body injured, the organs in the proximity to the path of the penetrating object, and the velocity of the missile. Therefore, the velocity and caliber of the bullet, the trajectory, and the distance from weapon to wounded may provide important clues to the extent of injury. (See Resource Document 3, Kinematics of Trauma, and related Table 1, Missile Kinetic Energy.)

Table 1
Mechanisms of Injury and Related Suspected
Injury Patterns

Mechanisms of Injury	Suspected Injury Patterns
Frontal impact Bent steering wheel Knee imprint in dashboard Bull's-eye fracture of windshield	Cervical spine fracture Anterior flail chest Myocardial contusion Pneumothorax Transection of aorta (decelerating injury) Fractured spleen or liver Posterior fracture/dislocation of hip and/or knee
Side impact to automobile	Contralateral neck sprain Cervical spine fracture Lateral flail chest Pneumothorax Traumatic aortic rupture Diaphragmatic rupture Fractured spleen or liver (depending on side of impact) Fractured pelvis or acetabulum
Rear impact automobile collision	Cervical spine injury
Ejection from vehicle	Ejection from the vehicle precludes meaningful prediction of injury patterns, but places the patient at a greater risk from virtually all injury mechanisms. Mortality is increased significantly.
Motor vehicle-pedestrian	Head injury Thoracic and abdominal injuries Fractured lower extremities

3. Injuries due to burns and cold

Burns are another significant type of trauma that may occur alone or may be coupled with blunt and penetrating trauma resulting from a burning automobile, explosion, falling debris, the patient's attempt to escape the fire, or an assault with a firearm or knife. Inhalation injury and carbon monoxide intoxication often complicate burn injury. Therefore, it is important to know the circumstances surrounding the burn injury.

Specifically, knowledge of the environment in which the burn injury occurred (open or closed space), as well as substances consumed by the flames (plastics, chemicals, etc), and possible associated injuries sustained is critical in the treatment of the patient.

Acute or chronic hypothermia without adequate protection against heat loss produces either local or generalized cold injuries. Significant heat loss may occur at moderate temperatures (15 to 20 degrees centigrade if wet clothes, decreased activity, or vasodilatation caused by alcohol or drugs compromise the patient's ability to conserve heat. Such historical information can be obtained from prehospital personnel

4. Hazardous environment

History of exposure to chemicals, toxins, and radiation are important to obtain for two reasons. First, these agents can produce a variety of pulmonary, cardiac, or internal organ derangement in the injured patient. Secondly, these same agents also present a hazard to health care providers. Frequently, the physician's only means of preparation is to have knowledge of the general principles of management of such agents and immediate access to the Regional Poison Control Center.

B. Physical Examination

1. Head (See Chapter 6, Head Trauma.)

The secondary survey begins with evaluating the head and identifying all related and significant injuries. The entire scalp and head should be examined for lacerations, contusions, and evidence of fractures. Because edema around the eyes may later preclude an in-depth examination, the eyes should be re-evaluated for

a. Visual acuity

b. Pupillary size

c. Hemorrhages of the conjunctiva and fundi

d. Penetrating injury

e. Contact lenses (remove before edema occurs)

f. Dislocation of the lens

A visual confrontation examination of both eyes can be performed by having the patient read a Snelling Chart or words on an intravenous container or 4 x 4 dressing package. This procedure frequently identifies optic injuries not otherwise apparent. (See Resource Document 13, Ocular Trauma.)

Pitfalls:
1. Hyphema
2. Optic nerve injury
3. Lens dislocation or penetrating injury
4. Head injury
5. Posterior scalp laceration

2. Maxillofacial

Maxillofacial trauma, not associated with airway obstruction or major bleeding, should be treated after the patient is stabilized completely and life-threatening injuries have been addressed. Definitive management may be safely delayed without compromising care at the discretion of appropriate specialists.

Patients with fractures of the midface may have a fracture of the cribriform plate. For these patients, gastric intubation should be performed via the oral route.

Pitfalls:
1. Pending airway obstruction
2. Changes in airway status
3. Cervical spine injuries
4. Exsanguinating midface fracture
5. Lacrimal duct lacerations
6. Facial nerve injuries

3. **Cervical spine and neck** (See Chapter 7, Spine and Spinal Cord Trauma.)

Patients with maxillofacial or head trauma should be presumed to have an unstable cervical spine injury (fracture and/or ligamentous injury), and the neck should be immobilized until all aspects of the cervical spine have been adequately studied and an injury excluded. The absence of neurologic deficit does not exclude injury to the cervical spine, and such injury should be presumed until a complete cervical spine radiographic series is obtained.

Examination of the neck includes both inspection, palpation, and auscultation. Cervical spine tenderness, subcutaneous emphysema, tracheal deviation, and laryngeal fracture may be discovered on a detailed examination. The carotid arteries should be palpated and auscultated for bruits. Evidence of blunt injury over these vessels should be noted and, if present, should arouse a high index of suspicion for carotid artery injury. Occlusion or dissection of the carotid artery may occur late in the injury process without antecedent signs or symptoms.

Protection of a potentially unstable cervical spine injury is imperative for patients wearing any type of protective helmet. Extreme care must be taken when removing the helmet. (See Chapter 2, Airway and Ventilatory Management.)

In penetrating trauma, wounds that extend through the platysma should not be explored manually in the emergency department. This type of injury requires surgical evaluation in the operating room.

Pitfalls:
1. Cervical spine injury
2. Esophageal injury
3. Tracheal or laryngeal injury
4. Carotid injury (penetrating or blunt)

4. **Chest** (See Chapter 4, Thoracic Trauma.)

Visual evaluation of the chest, both anterior and posterior, identifies such conditions as open pneumothorax and large flail segments. A complete evaluation of the chest wall requires palpation of the entire chest cage— feeling each rib and the clavicle. Sternal pressure may be painful if the sternum is fractured or costochondral separations exist. Contusions and hematomas of the chest wall should alert the physician to the possibility of occult injury.

Significant chest injury is manifested by pain and/or shortness of breath. Evaluation of the internal structures is done with the stethoscope, followed by a chest roentgenogram. Breath sounds are auscultated high on the anterior chest wall for pneumothorax and at the posterior bases for hemothorax. Auscultatory findings may be difficult to evaluate in a noisy environment, but may be extremely helpful. Distant heart sounds and narrow pulse pressure may indicate cardiac tamponade. Cardiac tamponade or tension pneumothorax may be suggested by the presence of distended neck veins, although associated hypovolemia may minimize this finding or eliminate it altogether. Decreased breath sounds and shock may be the only indication of tension pneumothorax and the need for immediate chest decompression.

The chest roentgenogram confirms the presence of a hemothorax or pneumothorax. Rib fractures may be present, but they may not be visible on the roentgenograph. A widened mediastinum or deviation of the nasogastric tube to the right may suggest an aortic rupture.

Pitfalls:
1. Tension pneumothorax
2. Open chest wound
3. Flail chest
4. Cardiac tamponade
5. Aortic rupture

5. Abdomen (See Chapter 5, Abdominal Trauma.)

Abdominal injuries must be identified and treated aggressively. The specific diagnosis is not as important as the fact that an injury exists and surgical intervention may be necessary. A normal initial examination of the abdomen does not exclude a significant intra-abdominal injury. Close observation and frequent re-evaluation of the abdomen, preferably by the same observer, is important in managing blunt abdominal trauma. Over time, the patient's abdominal findings may change. Early involvement by a surgeon is essential.

Patients with unexplained hypotension, neurologic injury, impaired sensorium secondary to alcohol and/or other drugs, and equivocal abdominal findings should be considered as candidates for peritoneal lavage. Fractures of the pelvis or the lower rib cage also may hinder adequate diagnostic examination of the abdomen, because pain from these areas may be elicited when palpating the abdomen.

Pitfalls:
1. Liver or splenic rupture
2. Hollow viscus and lumbar spine injuries (seat belts, deceleration)
3. Pancreatic injury
4. Major intra-abdominal vascular injury
5. Renal injury
6. Pelvic fracture(s)

6. Perineum / rectum / vagina (See Chapter 5, Abdominal Trauma.)

The perineum should be examined for contusions, hematomas, lacerations, and urethral bleeding.

A rectal examination is an essential part of the secondary survey. Specifically, the physician should assess for the presence of blood within the bowel lumen, a high-riding prostate, the presence of pelvic fractures, the integrity of the rectal wall, and the quality of the sphincter tone.

For the female patient, a vaginal examination also is an essential part of the secondary survey. The physician should assess for the presence of blood in the vaginal vault and vaginal lacerations. Additionally, pregnancy tests should be performed on all females of childbearing age.

Pitfalls:
1. Urethral injury
2. Rectal injury
3. Bladder injury
4. Vaginal injury

7. Musculoskeletal (See Chapter 7, Spine and Spinal Cord Trauma, and Chapter 8, Extremity Trauma.)

The extremities should be inspected for contusion or deformity. Palpation of the bones, examining for tenderness, crepitation, or abnormal movement, aids in the identification of occult fractures.

Anterior to posterior pressure with the heels of the hands on both anterior iliac spines and the symphysis pubis can identify pelvic fractures. Additionally, assessment of peripheral pulses can identify vascular injuries.

Significant extremity injuries may exist without fractures being evident on examination or roentgenograms. Ligament ruptures produce joint instability. Muscle-tendon unit injuries interfere with active motion of the affected structures. Impaired sensation and/or loss of voluntary muscle contraction strength may be due to nerve injury or to ischemia, including that due to compartment syndrome.

Thoracic and lumbar spinal fractures and/or neurologic injuries must be considered based on physical findings and mechanism of injury. Other injuries may mask the physical findings of spinal injuries, which may go unsuspected unless the physician obtains the appropriate roentgenograms.

Pitfalls:
1. Spine fractures
2. Fractures with vascular compromise
3. Pelvic fractures
4. Digital fractures

8. Neurologic (See Chapter 6, Head Trauma, and Chapter 7, Spine and Spinal Cord Trauma.)

A comprehensive neurologic examination includes not only motor and sensory evaluation of the extremities, but also re-evaluation of the patient's level of consciousness and pupillary size and response. The GCS Score facilitates detection of early changes and trends in the neurologic status.

(See Chart 1, Revised Trauma Score with GCS Score in Chapter 12, Stabilization and Transport.)

Any evidence of paralysis or paresis suggests major injury to the spinal column or peripheral nervous system. Immobilization of the **entire** patient, using short or long spine boards, a semirigid cervical collar, and/or other cervical immobilization devices, must be maintained until spinal injury can be excluded. The common mistake of immobilizing the head and freeing the torso allows the cervical spine to flex with the body as a fulcrum. **Complete immobilization of the entire patient is required at all times until a spine injury is excluded, and especially when a patient is transferred.**

Early consultation with a neurosurgeon is required for patients with neurologic injury. Changes in the level of consciousness should be monitored as these may reflect progression of the intracranial injury. If a patient with a head injury deteriorates neurologically, oxygenation and perfusion of the brain and the adequacy of ventilation (ABCs) must be reassessed. Intracranial surgical intervention may be necessary. The neurosurgeon must make the decision whether such conditions as epidural and subdural hematomas or depressed skull fractures require operative intervention.

Pitfalls:
1. Increased intracranial pressure
2. Subdural or epidural hematoma
3. Depressed skull fracture
4. Spine injury

VIII. Re-evaluation

The trauma patient must be re-evaluated constantly to assure that new findings are not overlooked, and to discover deterioration in previously noted symptoms. As initial life-threatening injuries are managed, other equally life-threatening problems and less severe injuries may become apparent. Underlying medical problems that may severely affect the ultimate prognosis of the patient may become evident. A high index of suspicion and constant alertness facilitate early diagnosis and management.

The relief of severe pain is an important part of the management of the trauma patient. Effective analgesia usually requires the use of intravenous opiates that may adversely affect the surgeon's ability to initially and continuously evaluate the patient accurately. The use of intravenous opiates may cause respiratory depression and mask neurologic signs. Therefore, opiates and other strong analgesics should be withheld until surgical consultation has occurred.

Continuous monitoring of vital signs and urinary output is essential. For the adult patient, maintenance of urinary output of 50 mL/hour is desirable. In the pediatric patient over one year of age, an output of 1 mL/kg/hour should be adequate. Arterial blood gas and cardiac monitoring devices should be employed. Pulse oximetry on critically injured patients and end-tidal carbon dioxide monitoring on intubated patients should be considered.

IX. Definitive Care

The interhospital triage criteria, published by the American College of Surgeons Committee on Trauma, helps determine the level, pace, and intensity of initial management of the multiple-injured patient. It takes into account the patient's physiologic status, obvious and anatomic injury, mechanisms of injury, concurrent diseases, and factors that may alter the patient's prognosis. Emergency department and surgical personnel should use these criteria to determine if the patient requires transfer to a trauma center or closest appropriate hospital capable of providing more specialized care. The closest appropriate hospital should be chosen based on its overall capabilities to care for the injured patient. (See Chapter 12, Stabilization and Transport; Table 1, Triage Decision Scheme in Resource Document 2, Prehospital Triage Criteria; Resource Document 9, Transfer Agreement; and Resource Document 10, Transfer Record.)

X. Disaster

Disasters frequently overwhelm local and regional resources. Plans for management of such conditions must be evaluated and rehearsed frequently to enhance the possibility of significant salvage of injured patients. (See Resource Document 12, Preparations for Disaster.)

XI. Records and Legal Considerations

A. Records

Meticulous record-keeping with time documented for all events is very important. Often more than one physician cares for the patient. Precise records are essential to evaluate the patient's needs and clinical status. Accurate records during the resuscitation can be facilitated by a member of the nursing staff whose sole job is to record and collate all patient information.

Medical-legal problems arise frequently, and precise records are helpful for all concerned. Chronologic reporting with flow sheets helps both the attending physician and consulting physician to quickly assess changes in the patient's condition. (See Resource Document 8, Trauma Flow Sheet; Resource Document 9, Transfer Agreement, and Resource Document 10, Transfer Record.)

B. Consent for Treatment

Consent is sought before treatment if possible. In life-threatening emergencies it is often not possible to obtain such prospective consent. In such cases treatment should be given first and formal consent obtained later. (See Resource Document 14, ATLS and the Law.)

C. Forensic Evidence

If injury due to criminal activity is suspected, the personnel caring for the patient must preserve the evidence. All items, such as clothing and bullets, must be saved for law enforcement personnel. Laboratory determinations of blood alcohol concentrations and other drugs may be particularly pertinent. (See Resource Document 3, Kinematics of Trauma.)

XII. Summary

The injured patient must be evaluated rapidly and thoroughly. The physician must develop treatment priorities for the overall management of the patient, so no steps in the process are omitted. An adequate patient history and accounting of the incident are important in evaluating and managing the trauma patient.

Evaluation and care are divided into four phases.

A. Primary Survey—Assessment of ABCs

1. Airway and cervical spine control

2. Breathing

3. Circulation with hemorrhage control

4. Disability: Brief neurologic evaluation

5. Exposure/Environment: Completely undress the patient, but prevent hypothermia

B. Resuscitation

1. Oxygenation and ventilation

2. Shock management—intravenous lines, Ringer's lactate

3. The management of life-threatening problems identified in the primary survey is continued

4. Monitoring

   a. Arterial blood gases and ventilatory rate

   b. End-tidal carbon dioxide

   c. Electrocardiograph

   d. Pulse oximetry

   e. Blood pressure

C. Secondary Survey—Total Patient Evaluation

1. Head and skull

2. Maxillofacial

3. Neck

4. Chest

5. Abdomen

6. Perineum/rectum/vagina

7. Musculoskeletal

8. Complete neurologic examination

9. Appropriate roentgenograms, laboratory tests, and special studies

10. "Tubes and fingers" in every orifice

D. Definitive Care

After identifying the patient's injuries, managing life-threatening problems, and obtaining special studies, definitive care begins. Definitive care, associated with the major trauma entities, is described in later chapters.

E. Transfer

If the patient's injuries exceed the institution's immediate treatment capabilities, the process of transferring the patient is initiated as soon as the need is identified. Delay in transferring the patient to a facility with a higher level of care may significantly increase the patient's risk of mortality. (See Chapter 12, Stabilization and Transfer.)

Bibliography

1. American College of Surgeons: Technique of helmet removal from injured patients. **ACS Bulletin**, October 1980, pp 19-21.

2. Mackay M: Kinematics of vehicle crashes, in Maull KI, Cleveland HC, Strauch GO et al (ed), **Advances in Trauma**, Volume 2. Chicago, Illinois, Year Book Medical Publishers Inc, 1987.

3. McSwain NE Jr, Kerstein M (ed): **Evaluation and Management of Trauma**. Norwalk, Connecticut, Appleton-Century-Crofts, 1987.

4. McSwain NE Jr, Martinez JA, Timberlake GA: **Cervical Spine Trauma**. New York, New York, Thieme, 1989.

5. Moore, EE (ed): **Early Care of the Injured Patient**, Fourth Edition. Philadelphia, Pennsylvania, BC Decker, 1990.

6. Moore EE: Initial resuscitation and evaluation of the injured patient. In Zuidema GD, Rutherford RB, Ballinger WF (ed): **The Management of Trauma**. Philadelphia, Pennsylvania, WB Saunders and Company, 1985.

7. Moore EE, Mattox KL, Feliciano DV (ed): **Trauma**, Second Edition. Norwalk, Connecticut, Appleton-Lange, 1991.

8. Nahum AM, Melvin J (ed): **The Biomechanics of Trauma**. Norwalk, Connecticut, Appleton-Century-Crofts, 1985.

9. Trunkey DD, Lewis FR Jr (ed): **Current Therapy of Trauma**, Third Edition. Philadelphia, Pennsylvania, BC Decker, 1991.

**Chapter 1:
Initial
Assessment
and
Management**

Skill Station I: Initial Assessment and Management

Chapter 1:
Initial
Assessment
and
Management

Skill
Station I

Resources and Equipment

This list is the recommended equipment to conduct this skill session in accordance with the stated objectives for and intent of the procedures outlined. Additional equipment may be used providing it does not detract from the stated objectives and intent of this skill, or from performing the procedure in a safe method as described and recommended by the ACS Committee on Trauma.

1. Live patient model

2. Nurse assistant

3. Case scenario with related roentgenograms

4. Blanket and sheet (or table padding and covering for patient comfort)

5. Makeup and moulage—see individual scenarios

6. Items needed for **each** scenario:

    a. 4x4s, roller bandage, and tape
    b. Blood pressure cuff and stethoscope
    c. Penlite flashlight (optional)
    d. 1000 mL Ringer's lactate—two or three per patient
    e. Assorted IV catheters and needles, ie, #14- to 16-gauge over-the-needle catheter, #20-gauge Butterfly needle—two to four per patient; and pericardiocentesis kit (optional)
    f. 12- and 50-mL syringes
    g. Spine immobilization devices—long and short (optional)
    h. Semirigid cervical collar
    i. Oxygen mask
    j. Oral airway
    k. Leg traction splint; molded splints
    l. Lighted view box for reviewing roentgenograms
    m. Laryngoscope blade, handle, and ET tube
    n. End-tidal CO_2 monitoring device (optional)
    o. Pulse oximeter (actual or simulated)
    p. #5 tracheostomy tube for cricothyroidotomy
    q. #36 French chest tube and drainage collection device
    r. Scalpel handle
    s. Nasogastric tube
    t. Peritoneal lavage kit
    u. Indwelling urinary catheter and collection bag
    v. Bag-valve mask device and face mask (type that includes a one-way valve preventing back flow of air and secretions)
    w. Soft and rigid suction devices
    x. Portable electrocardiograph monitor (actual or simulated)
    y. Pneumatic antishock garment (optional)
    z. Universal precaution equipment for participants, ie, goggles, gloves, masks, and gowns

Chapter 1:
Initial
Assessment
and
Management

Skill
Station I

Objectives

Performance at this station will allow the participant to practice and demonstrate the following activities in a simulated clinical situation:

1. Using the four phases of patient assessment and management, verbalize to the Instructor while systematically demonstrating the initial management required to stabilize each patient.

2. Using the primary survey assessment techniques, determine and demonstrate:

   a. Airway patency and cervical spine control
   b. Breathing efficacy
   c. Circulatory status with hemorrhage control
   d. Disability: Neurologic status
   e. Exposure/Environment: Undress the patient, but prevent hypothermia

3. Establish resuscitation (management) priorities in the multiple-injured patient based on findings from the primary survey.

4. Integrate appropriate history taking as an invaluable aid in the assessment of the patient situation.

5. Identify the injury-producing mechanism and discuss the injuries that may exist and/or may be anticipated as a result of the mechanism of injury.

6. Using secondary survey techniques, assess the patient from head to toe.

7. Using the primary and secondary survey techniques, re-evaluate the patient's status and response to therapy instituted.

8. Given a series of roentgenograms,

   a. Diagnose fractures
   b. Differentiate associated injuries

9. Outline the definitive care necessary to stabilize each patient in preparation for possible transport to a trauma center or closest appropriate facility.

10. As referring physician, communicate with the receiving physician (Instructor) in a logical, sequential manner:

    a. Patient's history, including mechanism of injury
    b. Physical findings
    c. Management instituted
    d. Patient's response to therapy
    e. Diagnostic tests performed and results
    f. Need for transport
    g. Method of transportation
    h. Anticipated time of arrival

**Chapter 1:
Initial
Assessment
and
Management**

**Skill
Station I**

Skills Procedures

Initial Assessment and Management

Note: Universal precautions are required whenever caring for the trauma patient.

I. Primary Survey and Resuscitation

The student should outline preparations that must be made to facilitate the rapid progression of assessing and resuscitating the patient.

The student should indicate that the patient is to be completely undressed, but that hypothermia should be prevented.

A. Airway with Cervical Spine Control

1. Assessment

   a. Ascertain patency.

   b. Rapidly assess for airway obstruction.

2. Management—Establish a patent airway.

   a. Perform a chin lift or jaw thrust maneuver.

   b. Clear the airway of foreign bodies.

   c. Insert an oropharyngeal or nasopharyngeal airway.

   d. Establish a definitive airway.

   1) Orotracheal or nasotracheal intubation
   2) Jet insufflation of the airway
   3) Surgical cricothyroidotomy

3. Maintain the cervical spine in a neutral position with manual immobilization as necessary when establishing an airway.

B. Breathing: Ventilation and Oxygenation

1. Assessment

   a. Expose the neck and chest—assure immobilization of the head and neck.

   b. Determine the rate and depth of respirations.

   c. Inspect and palpate the neck and chest for tracheal deviation, unilateral and bilateral chest movement, use of accessory muscles, and any signs of injury.

   d. Percuss the chest for presence of dullness or hyperresonance.

   e. Auscultate the chest bilaterally.

**Chapter 1:
Initial
Assessment
and
Management**

**Skill
Station I**

2. Management

    a. Administer high concentrations of oxygen.

    b. Ventilate with a bag-valve-mask or face-mask device.

    c. Alleviate tension pneumothorax.

    d. Seal open pneumothorax.

    e. Attach an end-tidal CO_2 monitoring device (if available) to the endo-tracheal tube.

    f. Attach the patient to a pulse oximeter, if available.

C. Circulation with Hemorrhage Control

1. Assessment

    a. Identify source of external, exsanguinating hemorrhage.

    b. Pulse: Quality, rate, regularity, paradox

    c. Skin color

    d. Blood pressure, time permitting

2. Management

    a. Apply direct pressure to external bleeding site.

    b. Insert two large-caliber intravenous catheters.

    c. Simultaneously obtain blood for hematologic and chemical analyses, type and crossmatch, and arterial blood gases.

    d. Initiate vigorous IV fluid therapy with warmed Ringer's lactate solution and blood replacement.

    e. Apply the pneumatic antishock garment or pneumatic splints as indicated to control hemorrhage.

    f. Attach the patient to an ECG monitor.

    g. Insert urinary and nasogastric catheters unless contraindicated.

    h. Prevent hypothermia.

D. Disability: Brief Neurologic Examination

    1. Determine the level of consciousness using the AVPU method.

    2. Assess the pupils for size, equality, and reaction.

E. Exposure/Environment: Completely undress the patient, but prevent hypothermia.

II. Reassess the Patient—ABCDs and Consider Need for Patient Transfer

III. Secondary Survey and Management

A. AMPLE History and Mechanism of Injury

1. Obtain AMPLE history from patient, family, or prehospital personnel.

2. Obtain history of injury-producing event, identifying injury mechanisms.

B. Head and Maxillofacial

1. Assessment

a. Inspect and palpate entire head and face for lacerations, contusions, fractures, and thermal injury.

b. Re-evaluate pupils.

c. Re-evaluate level of consciousness.

d. Assess eyes for hemorrhage, penetrating injury, visual acuity, dislocation of the lens, and presence of contact lens.

e. Evaluate cranial nerve function.

f. Inspect ears and nose for cerebrospinal fluid leakage.

g. Inspect mouth for evidence of bleeding and cerebrospinal fluid.

2. Management

a. Maintain airway, continue ventilation and oxygenation as indicated.

b. Control hemorrhage.

c. Prevent secondary brain injury.

d. Remove contact lenses.

C. Cervical Spine and Neck

1. Assessment

a. Inspect for signs of blunt and penetrating injury, tracheal deviation, and use of accessory breathing muscles.

b. Palpate for tenderness, deformity, swelling, subcutaneous emphysema, and tracheal deviation.

c. Auscultate the carotid arteries for bruits.

d. Obtain a lateral, crosstable cervical spine roentgenogram.

2. Management: Maintain adequate in-line immobilization and protection of the cervical spine.

D. Chest

1. Assessment

a. Inspect for the anterior, lateral, and posterior chest wall for signs of blunt and penetrating injury, use of accessory breathing muscles, and bilateral respiratory excursions.

b. Auscultate the anterior chest wall and posterior bases for bilateral breath sounds, and heart sounds.

Chapter 1:
Initial
Assessment
and
Management

Skill
Station I

   c. Palpate the entire chest wall for evidence of blunt and penetrating injury, subcutaneous emphysema, tenderness, and crepitation.

   d. Percuss for evidence of hyperresonance or dullness.

   e. Obtain a chest roentgenogram.

2. Management

   a. Tube thoracostomy, as indicated

   b. Attach the chest tube to an underwater seal drainage device.

   c. Correctly dress an open chest wound.

   d. Pericardiocentesis, as indicated

E. Abdomen

1. Assessment

   a. Inspect the anterior and posterior abdomen for signs of blunt and penetrating injury, and internal bleeding.

   b. Auscultate for presence/absence of bowel sounds.

   c. Percuss the abdomen to elicit subtle rebound tenderness.

   d. Palpate the abdomen for tenderness, involuntary muscle guarding, and unequivocal rebound tenderness.

   e. Obtain a roentgenogram of the pelvis.

   f. Perform diagnostic peritoneal lavage, if warranted.

2. Management

   a. Transfer the patient to the operating room, if indicated.

   b. Apply the pneumatic antishock garment, if indicated.

F. Perineum/Rectum/Vagina

1. Perineal assessment

   a. Contusions and hematomas

   b. Lacerations

   c. Urethral bleeding

2. Rectal assessment

   a. Rectal blood

   b. Anal sphincter tone

   c. Bowel wall integrity

   d. Bony fragments

   e. Prostate position

Chapter 1:
Initial
Assessment
and
Management

Skill
Station I

3. Vaginal assessment

    a. Presence of blood in the vaginal vault

    b. Vaginal lacerations

G. Musculoskeletal

1. Assessment

    a. Inspect the upper and lower extremities for evidence of blunt and penetrating injury, including contusions, lacerations, and deformity.

    b. Palpate the upper and lower extremities for tenderness, crepitation, abnormal movement, and sensation.

    c. Palpate all peripheral pulses for presence/absence.

    d. Assess the pelvis for evidence of fracture and associated hemorrhage.

    e. Palpate the thoracic and lumbar spine for evidence of blunt and penetrating injury, including contusions, lacerations, tenderness, deformity, and sensation.

    f. Evaluate roentgenogram of the pelvis for evidence of fracture.

    g. Obtain roentgenograms of suspected fracture sites as indicated.

2. Management

    a. Apply and/or readjust appropriate splinting devices for extremity fractures as indicated.

    b. Maintain immobilization of the patient's thoracic and lumbar spine.

    c. Apply the pneumatic antishock garment if indicated.

    d. Administer tetanus immunization.

    e. Administer medications as indicated or as directed by specialist.

H. Neurologic

1. Assessment

    a. Re-evaluate the pupils and level of consciousness.

    b. Determine the GCS Score.

    c. Evaluate the upper and lower extremities for motor and sensory responses.

    d. Evaluate for evidence of paralysis or paresis.

2. Management

    a. Continue ventilation and oxygenation.

    b. Maintain adequate immobilization of the entire patient.

Chapter 1:
Initial
Assessment
and
Management

Skill
Station I

IV. Patient Re-evaluation

Re-evaluate the patient, noting, reporting, and documenting any changes in the patient's condition and responses to resuscitative efforts. Judicious use of analgesics may be employed **only after** surgical consultation. Continuous monitoring of vital signs and urinary output is essential.

V. Definitive Care: Stabilization and Transport

Outline rationale for patient transfer, transfer procedures, patient's needs during transfer, and indicate need for direct physician-to-physician communication.

Chapter 2:
Airway and Ventilatory Management

Objectives:

Upon completion of this chapter, the physician will be able to identify actual or impending airway obstruction, explain the techniques of establishing and maintaining a patent airway, and confirm the adequacy of ventilation.

Specifically, the physician will be able to:

A. Recognize the signs and symptoms of acute airway obstruction.

B. Identify the clinical settings in which airway compromise is likely to occur.

C. Explain the techniques to establish and maintain a patent airway and confirm the adequacy of ventilation and oxygenation.

    1. Pulse oximetry

    2. End-tidal carbon dioxide measurement

D. Define what is meant by the term definitive airway and the steps needed to maintain oxygenation before, during, and after establishing a definitive airway.

E. Perform definitive airway placement with maintenance of cervical spine alignment during the skill station, and perform percutaneous transtracheal jet insufflation and cricothyroidotomy during the surgical practicum.

F. Demonstrate ventilatory techniques for one and two rescuers.

**Chapter 2:
Airway and
Ventilatory
Management**

American College of Surgeons

I. Introduction

The inability to provide oxygenated blood to the brain and other vital structures is the quickest killer of the injured. Prevention of hypoxemia requires a protected, unobstructed airway and adequate ventilation that must take priority over all other conditions. An airway must be secured, oxygen delivered, and ventilatory support provided. **Supplemental oxygen must be administered to all trauma patients.**

Early preventable deaths from airway problems after trauma include:

1. Failure to recognize the partially obstructed airway and/or patient limitations in providing adequate ventilatory volumes. The combination of partial airway obstruction and impaired ventilatory mechanics can result in life-threatening hypoxemia. This combination can be easily overlooked if more obvious injuries attract the physician's attention. **Remember: Airway and ventilation are the first priorities**

2. Delay in providing an airway when it is needed

3. Delay in providing assisted ventilation when it is needed

4. Technical difficulties in securing a definitive airway and/or providing assisted ventilation. Unintentional intubation of the esophagus can further compromise ventilation and may be rapidly fatal if not recognized promptly and corrected.

5. Aspiration of gastric contents

II. Airway

A. Problem Recognition

Airway compromise may be sudden and complete, insidious and partial, and progressive and/or recurrent. Although often related to pain and/or anxiety, tachypnea may be a subtle but early sign of airway or ventilatory compromise. Therefore, assessment and frequent reassessment of airway patency and adequacy of ventilation are important. The patient with an altered level of consciousness is at particular risk for airway compromise and often requires provision of a definitive airway. The unconscious head-injured patient, the patient obtunded from alcohol and/or other drugs, and the patient with thoracic injuries may have compromised ventilatory effort. In these patients, endotracheal intubation is intended to: (1) provide an airway, (2) deliver supplementary oxygen, (3) support ventilation, and (4) prevent aspiration. **Maintaining oxygenation and preventing hypercarbia are critical in managing the trauma patient, especially if the patient has sustained a head injury.** The physician should anticipate vomiting in all injured patients and be prepared. The presence of gastric contents in the oropharynx confirms a significant risk of aspiration with the patient's very next breath. Immediate suctioning and rotation of the **entire patient** to the lateral position are indicated.

Trauma to the face is another setting that may demand aggressive airway management. The mechanism for this injury is exemplified by the unbelted passenger/driver who is thrown into the windshield and dashboard. Trauma to the midface may produce fractures-dislocations with compromise to the nasopharynx and oropharynx. Facial fractures may be associated with hemorrhage, increased secretions, and dislodged teeth, causing additional problems in maintaining a patent airway. Fractures of the mandible, especially bilateral body fractures, may cause loss of normal muscle support and inability to protrude the tongue. Airway obstruction will result if the patient is in a supine position.

Patients who refuse to lie down may be indicating difficulty in maintaining their airway or handling secretions. Neck injuries may cause airway obstruction by disruption of the larynx and trachea or by compression of the airway from hemorrhage into the soft tissues of the neck.

During initial assessment of the airway, the "talking patient" provides reassurance (at least for the moment) that the airway is patent and not compromised. Therefore, the most important early measure is to talk to the patient and stimulate a verbal response. A positive, appropriate verbal response indicates that the airway is patent, ventilation intact, and brain perfusion adequate. Failure to respond or an inappropriate response suggests an altered level of consciousness or airway/ventilatory compromise.

B. Objective Signs—Airway Obstruction

1. **Look** to see if the patient is agitated or obtunded. Agitation suggests hypoxia, and obtundation suggests hypercarbia. Cyanosis indicates hypoxemia due to inadequate oxygenation and should be sought by inspection of the nail beds and circumoral skin. Look for retractions and the use of accessory muscles of ventilation which, when present, provide additional evidence of airway compromise.

2. **Listen** for abnormal sounds. Noisy breathing is obstructed breathing. Snoring, gurgling, and crowing sounds (stridor) may be associated with partial occlusion of the pharynx or larynx. Hoarseness (dysphonia) implies functional, laryngeal obstruction. The abusive or belligerent patient may be hypoxic and should not be presumed intoxicated.

3. **Feel** for movement of air with the expiratory effort and quickly determine if the trachea is midline.

III. Ventilation

A. Problem Recognition

Assuring a patent airway is an important first step in providing oxygen to the patient—but it is only a first step. An unobstructed airway is not likely to benefit the patient unless the patient also is ventilating adequately. Ventilation may be compromised by airway obstruction but also by altered ventilatory mechanics or central nervous system (CNS) depression. If breathing is not improved by clearing the airway, other etiologies must be sought. Direct trauma to the chest, especially with rib fractures, causes pain with breathing and leads to rapid, shallow ventilation and hypoxemia. Intracranial injury may cause abnormal patterns of breathing and compromise adequacy of ventilation. Cervical spinal cord injury may result in diaphragmatic breathing and interfere with the ability to meet increased oxygen demands. Complete cervical cord transection, which spares the phrenic nerves (C-3,4), results in abdominal breathing and paralysis of the intercostal muscles. Assisted ventilation may be required.

B. Objective Signs

1. **Look** for symmetrical rise and fall of the chest. Asymmetry suggests splinting or a flail chest and any labored breathing should be regarded as an imminent threat to the patient's oxygenation.

2. **Listen** for movement of air on both sides of the chest. Decreased or absent breath sounds over one or both hemithoraces should alert the examiner to the presence of thoracic injury. (See Chapter 4, Thoracic Trauma.) Beware of a rapid respiratory rate—tachypnea may indicate air hunger.

IV. Management

The assessment of airway patency and adequacy of ventilation must be done quickly and accurately. If problems are identified or **suspected**, measures should be instituted immediately to improve oxygenation and reduce the risk of further ventilatory compromise. These include airway maintenance techniques, definitive airway measures (including surgical airway), and methods to provide supplemental ventilation. Because all of these may require some neck motion, protection of the cervical spine must be provided in all patients, especially if the patient has a known, unstable cervical spine injury or is incompletely evaluated and at risk. The neck must be securely immobilized until the possibility of a spinal injury has been excluded with roentgenographic studies or the injury has been recognized and appropriately managed.

Patients wearing a motorcycle or sports helmet who require airway management should have their head and neck held in a neutral position while the helmet is removed. This is a two-person procedure. One person provides in-line manual immobilization from below while the second person expands the helmet laterally and removes it from above. In-line manual immobilization is re-established from above and the patient's head and neck are secured during airway management. Removal of the helmet using a cast cutter while stabilizing the head and neck minimizes cervical spine motion in the patient with a known cervical spine injury.

Supplemental oxygen should be provided before and immediately after airway management measures are instituted. Suction is essential and should be readily available and be of the rigid-type (tonsil suction tip). Patients with facial injuries may have associated cribriform plate fractures and the use of soft suction catheters (or nasogastric tube) inserted through the nose may be complicated by passage of the tube into the cranial vault.

A. Airway Maintenance Techniques

For the patient with an altered sensorium, the tongue prolapses backward and obstructs the hypopharynx. This form of obstruction can be corrected readily by the chin-lift or jaw-thrust maneuver. The airway can then be maintained with an oropharyngeal or nasopharyngeal airway.

1. Chin lift

The fingers of one hand are placed under the mandible, which is gently lifted upward to bring the chin anterior. The thumb of the same hand lightly depresses the lower lip to open the mouth. The thumb may also be placed behind the lower incisors and, simultaneously, the chin gently lifted. The chin-lift maneuver should not hyperextend the neck. This maneuver is useful for the trauma victim because it does not risk compromising a possible cervical spine fracture or converting a fracture without cord injury into one with cord injury.

2. Jaw thrust

The jaw-thrust maneuver is performed by grasping the angles of the lower jaw, one hand on each side, and displacing the mandible forward. When this method is used with the mouth-to-face mask, a good seal and adequate ventilation are achieved.

3. Oropharyngeal airway

The oral airway is inserted into the mouth behind the tongue. The preferred technique is to use a tongue blade to depress the tongue and then insert the airway posteriorly. The airway must not push the tongue backward and block, rather than clear, the airway. This device must not be used in the conscious patient because it may induce gagging, vomiting, and aspiration.

An alternative technique is to insert the oral airway upside-down, so its concavity is directed upward, until the soft palate is encountered. At this point, the airway is rotated 180 degrees, the concavity is directed caudad, and the airway is slipped into place over the tongue. This method should not be used for children, because the rotation of the airway may damage the teeth.

4. Nasopharyngeal airway

The nasopharyngeal airway is inserted in one nostril and passed gently into the posterior oropharynx. The nasopharyngeal airway is preferred to the oropharyngeal airway in the responsive patient because it is better tolerated and less likely to induce vomiting. It should be well lubricated, then inserted into the nostril that appears to be unobstructed. If obstruction is encountered during introduction of the airway, stop and try the other nostril. If the tip of the nasopharyngeal tube is visible in the posterior oropharynx, it may provide safe passage of a nasogastric tube in the patient with facial fractures.

B. Definitive Airway

A definitive airway requires a tube present in the trachea with the cuff inflated, the tube connected to some form of oxygen-enriched assisted ventilation, and the airway secured in place with tape. Definitive airways are of three varieties: orotracheal tube, nasotracheal tube, and surgical airway (cricothyroidotomy or tracheostomy). The decision to provide a definitive airway is based on clinical findings and includes:

a. Apnea

b. Inability to maintain a patent airway by other means

c. Protection of the lower airway from aspiration of blood or vomitus

d. Impending or potential compromise of the airway, eg, following inhalation injury, facial fractures, or sustained seizure activity

e. Closed head injury requiring hyperventilation

f. Failure to maintain adequate oxygenation by face mask oxygen supplementation

The urgency of the situation and circumstances surrounding the need for airway intervention dictate the specific route and method to be used. Continued assisted ventilation is aided by supplemental sedation, analgesics, or muscle relaxants, as indicated. The use of an oximeter may be helpful in determining the need for a definitive airway, the urgency of the need, and, by inference, effectiveness of airway placement. Orotracheal and nasotracheal intubation are the methods used most frequently. The potential for concomitant cervical spine injury is of major concern in the patient requiring an airway. The algorithm appearing at the conclusion of surgical airway in this chapter offers a scheme by which decisions for the appropriate route of airway management can be made.

1. Orotracheal intubation

For the unconscious patient who has sustained blunt trauma and the need for definitive airway is anticipated, determine the urgency for establishing an airway. If there is no immediate need, then a roentgenogram of the cervical spine should be obtained. A normal lateral cervical spine roentgenogram is reassuring and allows for safe orotracheal intubation with midline immobilization of the head and neck. **However, a normal lateral cervical spine film does not exclude a cervical spine injury.** Spinal immobilization should be maintained. If no cervical spine fractures are noted, orotracheal intubation should be performed. If the patient is apneic, the two-person technique for orotracheal intubation with in-line manual cervical immobilization should be attempted.

Following insertion of the orotracheal tube, the cuff should be inflated and assisted ventilation should be instituted. Proper placement of the tube is suggested but not confirmed by hearing equal breath sounds bilaterally and detecting no borborygmi in the epigastrium. The presence of gurgling noises in the epigastrium with inspiration suggests esophageal intubation and warrants repositioning of the tube. If tube position is still in doubt, end-tidal carbon dioxide measurement is a reliable guide to the adequacy of ventilation. Tube position is determined by the colorimetric technique and used primarily to confirm position of the endotracheal tube. It is not used for physiologic monitoring. Absent end-tidal carbon dioxide tension confirms esophageal intubation. When the proper position of the tube is determined, it should be secured in place. If the patient is moved, tube placement should be reassessed.

2. Nasotracheal intubation

Nasotracheal intubation is a useful technique when a cervical spine fracture is confirmed or suspected, or when urgency of airway management precludes a cervical spine roentgenogram. Nasotracheal intubation is contraindicated in the apneic patient and whenever severe midface fractures or suspicion of a basilar skull fracture exist. Precautions regarding cervical spine immobilization should be followed as with orotracheal intubation.

Note: The most important determinant of whether to proceed with orotracheal or nasotracheal intubation is the experience of the physician. Both techniques are safe and effective when performed properly. Esophageal occlusion by cricoid pressure is useful in preventing aspiration and providing better visualization of the airway.

Malpositioning of the endotracheal tube must be considered in all patients who arrive at the hospital with an endotracheal tube in place. This is important because the tube may have been inserted into a mainstem bronchus or dislodged during patient transport from the field or another hospital. Epigastric fullness in a patient already intubated should alert the physician to the possibility of esophageal intubation. Placement must be checked carefully. A chest roentgenogram may be helpful to assess the position of the tube, but it cannot exclude esophageal intubation.

If the patient's condition permits, fiberoptic endoscopy may facilitate difficult orotracheal or nasotracheal intubation. The endoscopic techniques may be used for selected cases of maxillofacial and cervical spine injury and for stocky patients with short necks. If these injuries or conditions preclude orotracheal or nasotracheal intubation, the physician may proceed directly to surgical techniques: needle or surgical cricothyroidotomy.

3. Surgical airway

Inability to intubate the trachea is a clear indication for creating a surgical airway.

When edema of the glottis, fracture of the larynx, or severe oropharyngeal hemorrhage obstructs the airway and an endotracheal tube cannot be placed through the cords, a surgical cricothyroidotomy may be performed to allow air passage. Insertion of a needle through the cricothyroid membrane or into the trachea is a useful technique in emergency situations to provide oxygen on a short-term basis until a definitive airway can be placed. A tracheostomy, done under emergency conditions, is difficult to perform, is often associated with profuse bleeding, and is too time-consuming.

a. Jet insufflation of the airway

Jet insufflation can provide up to 45 minutes of extra time so that intubation can be accomplished on an urgent rather than an emergent basis. The jet insufflation technique is performed by placing a large-caliber plastic cannula, #12- to #14-gauge (#16- to #18-gauge in children), through the cricothyroid membrane into the trachea below the level of the obstruction. The cannula is then connected to wall oxygen at 15 liters/minute (40 to 50 psi) with either a Y-connector or a side hole cut in the tubing attached between the oxygen source and the plastic cannula. Intermittent insufflation, one second on and four seconds off, can then be achieved by placing the thumb over the open end of the Y-connector or the side hole. The patient can be adequately oxygenated for only 30 to 45 minutes using this technique. During the four seconds that the oxygen is not being delivered under pressure, some exhalation occurs. Because of the inadequate exhalation, carbon dioxide slowly accumulates and limits the use of this technique, especially in head-injured patients.

Jet insufflation must be used with caution when complete foreign body obstruction of the glottic area is suspected. Although high pressure may expel the impacted material into the hypopharynx where it can be readily removed, significant barotrauma may occur including pulmonary rupture with tension pneumothorax. Low flow rates (5 to 7 liters per minute) should be used when glottic obstruction is present.

b. Surgical cricothyroidotomy

Surgical cricothyroidotomy is performed by making a skin incision that extends through the cricothyroid membrane. A curved hemostat may be inserted to dilate the opening and a small endotracheal tube or tracheostomy tube (preferably 5 to 7 mm) can be inserted. When the endotracheal tube is used, the cervical collar can be reapplied. One must be alert to the possibility that the endotracheal tube can become malpositioned. Care must be taken, especially with children, to avoid damage to the cricoid cartilage, which is the only circumferential support to the upper trachea. Therefore, surgical cricothyroidotomy is not recommended for children under 12 years of age. (See Chapter 10, Pediatric Trauma.)

4. Airway decision scheme

The airway decision scheme (Figure 1, Airway Algorithm) applies only to the unconscious patient who is in acute respiratory distress (or apneic) and in need of an immediate airway, **and** in whom a cervical spine injury is suspected by mechanism of injury or physical examination. The first priority is to assure continued oxygenation with maintenance of cervical spine immobilization. This is accomplished initially by position (ie, chin lift or jaw thrust) and preliminary airway techniques (ie, oropharyngeal airway or nasopharyngeal airway) already discussed.

In the patient who is still showing some respiratory effort, a nasotracheal tube may be passed if the rescuer is skilled in this technique. Otherwise, an orotracheal tube should be passed while the second rescuer provides in-line immobilization. If neither a nasotracheal or orotracheal tube can be inserted and the patient's respiratory status is in jeopardy, a cricothyroidotomy should be performed.

In the apneic patient, in-line immobilization should be maintained by one rescuer and orotracheal intubation should be performed. If severe maxillofacial injury precludes nasotracheal intubation and orotracheal intubation cannot be achieved for any reason, a cricothyroidotomy is indicated.

It is important that the rescuer maintain oxygenation and ventilation before, during, and immediately upon completion of insertion of the definitive airway. Prolonged periods of inadequate or absent ventilation and oxygenation should be avoided.

C. Ventilation and Oxygenation

The primary goal of ventilation is to achieve maximum cellular oxygenation which is promoted in the trauma patient by providing an environment rich in oxygen and sustained gas exchange at the alveolar capillary membrane through improved ventilatory efforts.

1. Oxygenation

Oxygenated inspired air is best provided via a tight-fitting oxygen reservoir face mask with a flow rate of 10 to 12 liters/minute. Other methods, ie, nasal catheter, nasal cannula, nonrebreather mask, etc can improve inspired oxygen concentration.

Since changes in oxygenation occur rapidly and are impossible to detect clinically, pulse oximetry should be considered when difficulties are anticipated in intubation or ventilation. This includes the transport of the critically injured patient. Pulse oximetry is a noninvasive method to **continuously** measure oxygen saturation (O_2 sat) of arterial blood. It does not measure the partial pressure of oxygen (PaO_2) and depending on the position of the oxyhemoglobin dissociation curve, the PaO_2 may vary widely. (See Table 1, PaO_2 Levels versus O_2 Saturation Levels.) However, a measured saturation of 95% or greater by pulse oximetry is strong corroborating evidence of adequate, peripheral arterial oxygenation (PaO_2 > 70 mm Hg). Pulse oximetry requires intact peripheral perfusion and cannot distinguish oxyhemoglobin from carboxyhemoglobin or methemoglobin, which limits its usefulness in the severely vasoconstricted patient and in the patient with carbon monoxide poisoning. Profound anemia (hemoglobin < 5 gms) and hypothermia (< 30 degrees centigrade) impede the reliability of the technique. However, in most trauma patients pulse oximetry is not only useful, but continuous monitoring of oxygen saturation provides an immediate assessment of therapeutic interventions. (See Skill Station IV, Vascular Access and Monitoring in Chapter 3, Shock.)

2. Ventilation

Effective ventilation can be achieved by mouth-to-face mask or bag-valve-face mask techniques. Frequently, only one person is present to provide ventilation; under these circumstances, mouth-to-face mask ventilation is the preferred method. Studies suggest that one-person ventilation techniques, using a bag-valve mask, are less effective than two-person techniques in which both hands can be used to assure a good seal. Bag-valve-mask ventilation should be considered a two-rescuer technique.

Intubation of the hypoventilated and/or apneic patient may not be successful initially and may require multiple attempts. The patient **must be ventilated periodically** during prolonged efforts to intubate. The physician should practice taking a deep breath when intubation is first attempted. When the physician must breathe, the attempted intubation should be aborted, and the patient should be ventilated.

Table 1
Approximate PaO$_2$ versus O$_2$ Saturation Levels at Sea Level

PaO$_2$ Levels	O$_2$ Saturation Levels
27 mm Hg	50%
30 mm Hg	60%
60 mm Hg	90%
90 mm Hg	100%

Figure 1
Airway Algorithm

**Chapter 2:
Airway and
Ventilatory
Management**

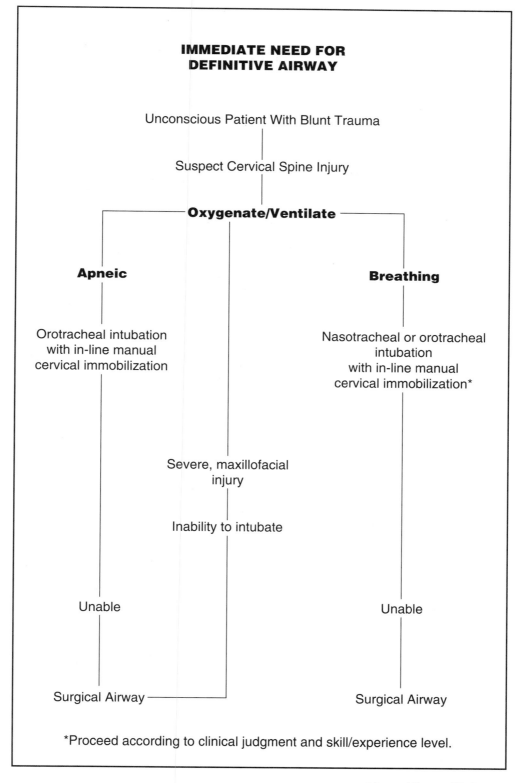

**IMMEDIATE NEED FOR
DEFINITIVE AIRWAY**

Unconscious Patient With Blunt Trauma

Suspect Cervical Spine Injury

Oxygenate/Ventilate

Apneic

Breathing

Orotracheal intubation
with in-line manual
cervical immobilization

Nasotracheal or orotracheal
intubation
with in-line manual
cervical immobilization*

Severe, maxillofacial
injury

Inability to intubate

Unable

Unable

Surgical Airway

Surgical Airway

*Proceed according to clinical judgment and skill/experience level.

With intubation of the trachea accomplished, assisted ventilation should follow, using positive-pressure breathing techniques. A volume- or pressure-regulated respirator can be employed, depending on availability of the equipment. The physician should be alert for the complications secondary to changes in intrathoracic pressure, which can convert a simple pneumothorax to a tension pneumothorax, or even create a pneumothorax secondary to barotrauma.

V. Summary

A. Actual or impending airway obstruction should be suspected in all injured patients.

B. With all airway maneuvers, the cervical spine must be protected by in-line immobilization.

C. Clinical signs suggesting airway compromise should be managed by securing a patent airway and providing adequate oxygen-enriched ventilation.

D. A definitive airway should be inserted if there is any doubt on the part of the physician as to the integrity of the patient's airway.

E. A definitive airway should be placed early after the patient has been ventilated with oxygen-enriched air and prolonged periods of apnea must be avoided.

F. Airway management requires assessment and reassessment of airway patency, tube position, and ventilatory effectiveness.

G. The selection of orotracheal or nasotracheal routes for intubation is based on the experience and skill level of the physician.

H. Surgical airway is indicated whenever an airway is needed and intubation is unsuccessful.

Bibliography

1. Aprahamian C, Thompson BM, Finger WA, et al: Experimental cervical spine injury model: evaluation of airway management and splinting techniques. **Annals of Emergency Medicine** 1984;13(8):584-587.

2. Brantigan CO, Grow JB Sr: Cricothyroidotomy: elective use in respiratory problems requiring tracheotomy. **The Journal of Thoracic and Cardiovascular Surgery** 1976;71:72-81.

3. Emergency percutaneous and transtracheal ventilation. **Journal of American College of Emergency Physicians/Annals of Emergency Medicine** October 1979;8(10):396.

4. Frame SB, Simon JM, Kerstein MD, et al: Percutaneous transtracheal catheter ventilation (PTCV) in complete airway obstruction—a canine model. **Journal of Trauma** 1989;29(6):774-781.

5. Fremstad JD, Martin SH: Lethal complication from insertion of nasogastric tube after severe basilar skull fracture. **Journal of Trauma** 1978;18:820-822.

6. Guildner CV: Resuscitation—opening the airway. A comparative study of techniques for opening an airway obstructed by the tongue. **Journal of American College of Emergency Physicians** 1976;5:588-590.

7. Harrison RR, Maul KI, Keenan RL, et al: Mouth-to-mask ventilation: a superior method of rescue breathing. **Annals of Emergency Medicine** 1982;11:74-76.

8. Iserson KV: Blind nasotracheal intubation. **Annals of Emergency Medicine** 1981;10:468.

9. Jorden RC, Moore EE, Marx JA, et al: A comparison of PTV and endotracheal ventilation in an acute trauma model. **Journal of Trauma** 1985;25(10):978-983.

10. Kress TD et al: Cricothyroidotomy. **Annals of Emergency Medicine** 1982;11:197.

11. Majernick TG, Bieniek R, Houston JB, et al: Cervical spine movement during orotracheal intubation. **Annals of Emergency Medicine** 1986;15(4):417-420.

12. Nasotracheal intubation in the emergency department. **Critical Care Medicine** 1980;8:667-682.

13. Seshul MB Sr, Sinn DP, Gerlock AJ Jr: The Andy Gump fracture of the mandible: a cause of respiratory obstruction or distress. **Journal of Trauma** 1978;18:611-612.

14. Walter J, Doris PE, Shaffer MA: Clinical presentation of patients with acute cervical spine injury. **Annals of Emergency Medicine** 1984;13(7):512-515.

15. Yeston NS: Noninvasive measurement of blood gases. **Infections in Surgery** 1990;9(2):18-24.

Chapter 2:
Airway and
Ventilatory
Management

Skill Station II:
Airway and Ventilatory Management

Chapter 2:
Airway and
Ventilatory
Management

Skill
Station II

Resources and Equipment

This list is the recommended equipment to conduct this skill session in accordance with the stated objectives for and intent of the procedures outlined. Additional equipment may be used providing it does not detract from the stated objectives and intent of this skill, or from performing the procedure in a safe method as described and recommended by the ACS Committee on Trauma.

1. Adult intubation manikins—two or three

2. Infant intubation manikin—one or two

3. Adult orotracheal tubes—one of each size

4. Adult nasotracheal tubes—two

5. Infant endotracheal tubes—one of each size, uncuffed

6. Laryngoscope handles—one for each manikin

7. Laryngoscope blades—infant and adult sizes, straight and curved

8. Extra batteries for laryngoscope handles

9. Extra laryngoscope bulbs

10. Stethoscopes—two

11. Soapy water to lubricate endotracheal tubes

12. Nasal anesthetic spray (simulation purposes only) (optional)

13. Semirigid cervical collar, applied to one adult intubation manikin

14. Magill forcep—one

15. Malleable endotracheal tube stylet—one or two

16. Oropharyngeal airway—assorted sizes

17. Nasopharyngeal airway—assorted sizes

18. Bag-valve-mask device—one or two

19. Pocket face mask—one or two. (**Note:** Type that includes a one-way valve preventing the back flow of air and secretions)

20. Rigid suction device—one (tonsil suction device)

21. End-tidal CO_2 colorimetric device (optional)

22. Tongue blades—several

Chapter 2:
Airway and
Ventilatory
Management

Skill
Station II

Objectives

Performance at this station will allow the participant to practice and demonstrate the following skills on adult and infant intubation manikins.

1. Ventilate the patient, comparing ventilatory volumes delivered via the rescuer's lungs and a face mask versus the bag-valve-mask device.

2. Insert oral and nasal pharyngeal airways.

3. Using both oral and nasal routes, intubate the trachea of an adult intubation manikin, within the guidelines listed, and provide effective ventilation.

4. Intubate the trachea of an infant intubation manikin with an endotracheal tube within the guidelines listed, and provide effective ventilation.

5. Relate the indications and complications of trauma to airway management when performing oral endotracheal intubation and nasotracheal intubation.

Procedures

Six procedures for acute airway management are outlined in Skill Station II:

1. Oropharyngeal airway insertion
2. Nasopharyngeal airway insertion
3. Ventilation without intubation
4. Orotracheal intubation
5. Nasotracheal intubation
6. Infant endotracheal intubation

Chapter 2:
Airway and
Ventilatory
Management

Skill
Station II

Skills Procedures

Airway and Ventilatory Management

Note: Universal precautions are required whenever caring for the trauma patient.

I. Oropharyngeal Airway Insertion

A. Select the proper-sized airway. (Place the airway against the patient's face. The correctly sized airway will extend from the center of the patient's mouth to the angle of the jaw.)

B. Open the patient's mouth with either the chin lift maneuver or the crossed-finger technique (scissors technique).

C. Insert a tongue blade on top of the patient's tongue far enough back to depress the tongue adequately, being careful not to gag the patient.

D. Insert the airway posteriorly, gently sliding the airway over the curvature of the tongue until the device's flange rests on top of the patient's lips. The airway must not push the tongue backward and block the airway.

E. Remove the tongue blade.

F. Ventilate the patient with a pocket face mask or bag-valve-mask device.

II. Nasopharyngeal Airway Insertion

A. Assess the nasal passages for any apparent obstruction (polyps, fractures, hemorrhage, etc).

B. Select the appropriately sized airway.

C. Lubricate the nasal pharyngeal airway with a water-soluble lubricant or tap water.

D. Insert the tip of the airway into the nostril and direct it posteriorly and toward the ear.

E. Gently pass the nasal pharyngeal airway through the nostril into the hypopharynx with a slight rotating motion, until the flange rests against the nostril.

F. Ventilate the patient with a pocket face mask or bag-valve-mask device.

III. Ventilation Without Intubation

A. Mouth-to-Pocket Face Mask (One-person Technique)

Remember: In accordance with universal precautions, only use the type of pocket face mask that includes a one-way valve to prevent back flow of air and secretions.

**Chapter 2:
Airway and
Ventilatory
Management**

**Skill
Station II**

1. Attach oxygen tubing to the face mask. Oxygen flow rate should be 12 L/minute.

2. Apply the face mask to the patient, using both hands.

3. Assure an adequate seal of the mask to the face.

4. Secure an open airway by using the jaw-thrust or chin-lift maneuver.

5. Taking a deep breath, place your mouth over the mouth port and blow.

6. Assess the ventilatory efforts by observing the patient's chest movement.

7. Ventilate the patient in this manner every five seconds.

B. Bag-Valve-Mask Ventilation (Two-person Technique)

1. Select the appropriately sized mask to fit the patient's face.

2. Connect the oxygen tubing to the bag-valve device, and adjust the flow of oxygen to 12 L/minute.

3. Assure that the patient's airway is patent and secured by previously described techniques.

4. The **first person** applies the mask to the patient's face, ascertaining a tight seal with both hands.

5. The **second person** ventilates the patient by squeezing the bag with both hands.

6. The adequacy of ventilation is assessed by observing the patient's chest movement.

7. The patient should be ventilated in this manner every five seconds.

IV. Adult Orotracheal Intubation

A. Assure that adequate ventilation and oxygenation are in progress, and that suctioning equipment is immediately available in the event the patient vomits.

B. Inflate the cuff of the endotracheal tube to ascertain that the balloon does not leak, then deflate the cuff.

C. Connect the laryngoscope blade to the handle, and check the bulb for brightness.

D. Have an assistant manually immobilize the head and neck. The patient's neck must not be hyperextended or hyperflexed during this procedure.

E. Hold the laryngoscope in the left hand.

F. Insert the laryngoscope into the right side of the patient's mouth, displacing the tongue to the left.

G. Visually examine the epiglottis and then the vocal cords.

H. Gently insert the endotracheal tube into the trachea without applying pressure on the teeth or oral tissues.

I. Inflate the cuff with enough air to provide an adequate seal. **Do not overinflate the cuff.**

J. Check the placement of the endotracheal tube by bag-valve-to-tube ventilation.

K. Visually observe lung expansion with ventilation.

L. Auscultate the chest and abdomen with a stethoscope to ascertain tube position.

M. Secure the tube. If the patient is moved, the tube placement should be reassessed.

N. If endotracheal intubation is not accomplished within seconds or in the same time required to hold your breath before exhaling, discontinue attempts, ventilate the patient with a bag-valve-mask device, and try again.

O. Placement of the tube must be checked carefully. A chest roentgenogram may be helpful to assess the position of the tube, but it cannot exclude esophageal intubation.

P. **Optional procedure:** Attach an end-tidal CO_2 colorimetric device (if available) to the endotracheal tube, between the adapter and the ventilating device. Use of the colorimetric device provides a reliable means of confirming the position of the endotracheal tube in the trachea.

Q. **Optional procedure:** Attach a pulse oximeter device to one of the patient's fingers (intact peripheral perfusion must exist) to measure and monitor the patient's oxygen saturation levels. Pulse oximetry is useful to monitor oxygen saturation levels continuously, and provides an immediate assessment of therapeutic interventions.

**Chapter 2:
Airway and
Ventilatory
Management**

**Skill
Station II**

V. Adult Nasotracheal Intubation

Remember: Blind nasotracheal intubation is contraindicated in the apneic patient and whenever severe midface fractures or suspicion of basilar skull fracture exist.

A. If a cervical spine fracture is suspected, leave the cervical collar in place to assist in maintaining immobilization of the neck.

B. Assure that adequate ventilation and oxygenation are in progress.

C. Inflate the cuff of the endotracheal tube to ascertain that the balloon does not leak, then deflate the cuff.

D. If the patient is **conscious**, spray the nasal passage with an anesthetic and vasoconstrictor to anesthetize and constrict the mucosa. If the patient is **unconscious**, it is adequate to spray the nasal passage only with a vasoconstrictor.

E. Have an assistant maintain manual immobilization of the head and neck.

F. Lubricate the nasotracheal tube with a local anesthetic jelly and insert the tube (with or without a stylet) into the nostril.

G. Guide the tube slowly but firmly into the nasal passage, going up from the nostril (to avoid the large inferior turbinate) and then backward and down

**Chapter 2:
Airway and
Ventilatory
Management**

**Skill
Station II**

into the nasopharynx. The curve of the tube should be aligned to facilitate passage along this curved course.

H. As the tube passes through the nose and into the nasopharynx, it must turn downward to pass through the pharynx.

I. Once the tube has entered the pharynx, listen to the airflow emanating from the endotracheal tube. Advance the tube until the sound of the moving air is maximal, suggesting location of the tip at the opening of the trachea. While listening to air movement, determine the point of inhalation and advance the tube quickly. If tube placement is unsuccessful, repeat the procedure by applying gentle pressure on the thyroid cartilage. **Remember, intermittently ventilate and oxygenate the patient.**

J. **Optional method:** If an endotracheal stylet is utilized, bend the lower end of the tube and stylet (approximately the last one-fourth) to a near 90-degree angle. As the tube is inserted, the end of the tube should point to the ipsilateral ear. Be sure that the stylet is recessed approximately one-half inch from the end of the tube to prevent trauma during insertion. Gently, yet firmly, guide the tube into the pharynx, and through the glottis and vocal cords. Continue to advance the tube with gentle pressure as you withdraw the stylet.

K. Inflate the cuff with enough air to provide an adequate seal. Avoid over-inflation.

L. Check the placement of the endotracheal tube by bag-valve-to-tube ventilation.

M. Visually observe lung expansion with ventilation.

N. Auscultate the chest and abdomen with a stethoscope to ascertain tube position.

O. Secure the tube. If the patient is moved, the tube placement should be reassessed.

P. If endotracheal intubation is not accomplished within 30 seconds or in the same time required to hold your breath before exhaling, discontinue attempts, ventilate the patient with a bag-valve-mask device, and try again.

Q. Placement of the tube must be checked carefully. A chest roentgenogram may be helpful to assess the position of the tube, but it cannot exclude esophageal intubation.

R. **Optional procedure:** Attach an end-tidal CO_2 colorimetric device (if available) to the endotracheal tube, between the adapter and the ventilating device. The use of this device provides a reliable means of confirming the position of the endotracheal tube in the trachea.

S. **Optional procedure:** Attach a pulse oximeter device to one of the patient's fingers (intact peripheral perfusion must exist) to measure and monitor the patient's oxygen saturation levels. Pulse oximetry is useful to monitor oxygen saturation levels continuously, and provides an immediate assessment of therapeutic interventions.

Complications of Orotracheal and Nasotracheal Intubation

**Chapter 2:
Airway and
Ventilatory
Management**

**Skill
Station II**

1. Esophageal intubation, leading to hypoxia and death

2. Right mainstem bronchus intubation, resulting in ventilation of the right lung only, collapse of the left lung, and pneumothorax

3. Inability to intubate, leading to hypoxia and death

4. Induction of vomiting, leading to aspiration, hypoxia, and death

5. Dislocation of the mandible

6. Laceration of the soft tissues of the airway, posterior pharynx, epiglottis, and/or larynx

7. Trauma to the airway resulting in hemorrhage and potential aspiration

8. Chipping or loosening of the teeth (caused by levering of the laryngoscope blade against the teeth)

9. Rupture/leak of the endotracheal tube cuff, resulting in loss of seal during ventilation, and necessitating reintubation

10. Cervical spine injury

11. Conversion of a cervical vertebral injury without neurologic deficit to a cervical cord injury with neurologic deficit

VI. Infant Orotracheal Intubation

A. Ensure that adequate ventilation and oxygenation are in progress.

B. Connect the laryngoscope blade and handle; check the light bulb for brilliance.

C. Hold the laryngoscope in the left hand.

D. Insert the laryngoscope blade in the right side of the mouth, moving the tongue to the left.

E. Observe the epiglottis, then the vocal cords.

F. Insert the endotracheal tube.

G. Check the placement of the tube by bag-valve-to-tube ventilation.

H. Check the placement of the endotracheal tube by observing lung inflations and auscultating the chest and abdomen with a stethoscope.

I. Secure the tube. If the patient is moved, the tube placement should be reassessed.

J. If endotracheal intubation is not accomplished within 30 seconds or in the same time required to hold your breath before exhaling, discontinue attempts, ventilate the patient with a bag-valve-mask device, and try again.

K. Placement of the tube must be checked carefully. A chest roentgenogram may be helpful to assess the position of the tube, but it cannot exclude esophageal intubation.

Chapter 2:
Airway and
Ventilatory
Management

Skill
Station II

L. **Optional procedure:** Attach an end-tidal CO_2 colorimetric device to the endotracheal tube, between the adapter and the ventilating device. The use of this device provides a reliable means of confirming the position of the endotracheal tube in the trachea.

M. **Optional procedure:** Attach a pulse oximeter device to one of the patient's fingers (intact peripheral perfusion must exist) to measure and monitor the patient's oxygen saturation levels. Pulse oximetry is useful to monitor oxygen saturation levels continuously, and provides an immediate assessment of therapeutic interventions.

Skill Station III: Cricothyroidotomy

Chapter 2:
Airway and
Ventilatory
Management

Skill
Station III

This surgical procedure, if performed on a live, anesthetized animal, must be conducted in a USDA-Registered Animal Laboratory Facility. (See *ATLS® Instructor Manual,* Section II, Chapter 9—Policies, Procedures, and Protocols for Surgical Skills Practicum.)

Resources and Equipment

This list is the recommended equipment to conduct this skill session in accordance with the stated objectives for and intent of the procedures outlined. Additional equipment may be used providing it does not detract from the stated objectives and intent of this skill, or from performing the procedure in a safe method as described and recommended by the ACS Committee on Trauma.

1. Live, anesthetized animals

2. Licensed veterinarian (see reference to guidelines above)

3. Animal trough, ropes (sandbags optional)

4. Electric shears with #40 blade

5. Animal intubation equipment

    a. Endotracheal tubes
    b. Laryngoscope blade and handle
    c. Respirator with 15-mm adapter

6. Tables or instrument stands

7. #12- to #14-gauge over-the-needle catheters (8.5 cm in length)

8. Antiseptic swabs

9. Jet insufflation equipment

    a. Oxygen tubing with a hole cut in one side of the tubing.
    b. Unregulated oxygen source of 50 psi or greater (or wall outlet) with oxygen flow meter attached

10. Pediatric 3.0-mm endotracheal tube adapter

11. 6- and 12-mL syringes

12. Strips of 1/2-inch (1.25 cm) tape

13. Surgical instruments

    a. Scalpel handles with #10 and #11 blades
    b. Hemostats
    c. Tracheal hook (optional)
    d. Tracheal spreader (optional)
    e. Small rake retractors

Chapter 2:
Airway and
Ventilatory
Management

Skill
Station III

14. Endotracheal tubes or #5 tracheostomy tubes

15. Twill-tape

16. 4x4 sponges

17. Surgical garb (gloves, shoe covers, and scrub suits or cover gowns)

Objectives

1. Performance at this station will allow the participant to practice and demonstrate the technique of needle cricothyroidotomy and surgical cricothyroidotomy on a live, anesthetized animal.

2. Upon completion of this station, the participant will be able to identify the surface markings and structures to be noted while performing a needle cricothyroidotomy and surgical cricothyroidotomy.

3. Upon completion of this station, the participant will be able to discuss the indications of needle cricothyroidotomy and surgical cricothyroidotomy.

4. Upon completion of this station, the participant will be able to discuss complications of these procedures.

Procedures

1. Needle cricothyroidotomy
2. Surgical cricothyroidotomy

Skills Procedures

Cricothyroidotomy

Chapter 2:
Airway and
Ventilatory
Management

Skill
Station III

Note: Universal precautions are required whenever caring for the trauma patient.

I. Needle Cricothyroidotomy

A. Assemble and prepare oxygen tubing by cutting a hole toward one end of the tubing. Connect the other end of the oxygen tubing to an oxygen source, capable of delivering 50 psi or greater at the nipple, and assure free flow of oxygen through the tubing.

B. Place the patient in a supine position.

C. Assemble a #12- or #14-gauge, 8.5-cm, over-the-needle catheter to a 6- to 12-mL syringe.

D. Surgically prepare the neck, using antiseptic swabs.

E. Palpate the cricothyroid membrane, anteriorly, between the thyroid cartilage and cricoid cartilage. Stabilize the trachea with the thumb and forefinger of one hand to prevent lateral movement of the trachea during the procedure.

F. Puncture the skin midline with the needle attached to a syringe, directly over the cricothyroid membrane (ie, midsaggital). A small incision with a #11 blade facilitates passage of the needle through the skin.

G. Direct the needle at a 45-degree angle caudally, while applying negative pressure to the syringe.

H. Carefully insert the needle through the lower half of the cricothyroid membrane, aspirating as the needle is advanced.

I. Aspiration of air signifies entry into the tracheal lumen.

J. Remove the syringe and withdraw the stylet while gently advancing the catheter downward into position, being careful not to perforate the posterior wall of the trachea.

K. Attach the oxygen tubing over the catheter needle hub, and secure the catheter to the patient's neck.

L. Intermittent ventilation can be achieved by occluding the open hole cut into the oxygen tubing with your thumb for one second and releasing it for four seconds. After releasing your thumb from the hole in the tubing, passive exhalation occurs. **Note:** Adequate PaO_2 can be maintained for only 30 to 45 minutes.

M. Continue to observe lung inflations and auscultate the chest for adequate ventilation.

Chapter 2:
Airway and
Ventilatory
Management

Skill
Station III

Complications of Needle Cricothyroidotomy

1. Asphyxia

2. Aspiration

3. Cellulitis

4. Esophageal perforation

5. Exsanguinating hematoma

6. Hematoma

7. Posterior tracheal wall perforation

8. Subcutaneous and/or mediastinal emphysema

9. Thyroid perforation

10. Inadequate ventilations leading to hypoxia and death

II. Surgical Cricothyroidotomy

A. Place the patient in a supine position with the neck in a neutral position. Palpate the thyroid notch, cricothyroid interval, and the sternal notch for orientation. Assemble the necessary equipment.

B. Surgically prepare and anesthetize the area locally, if the patient is conscious.

C. Stabilize the thyroid cartilage with the left hand.

D. Make a transverse skin incision over the cricothyroid membrane. Carefully incise through the membrane.

E. Insert the scalpel handle into the incision and rotate it 90 degrees to open the airway. (A hemostat or tracheal spreader also may be used instead of the scalpel handle.)

F. Insert an appropriately sized, cuffed endotracheal tube or tracheostomy tube into the cricothyroid membrane incision, directing the tube distally into the trachea.

G. Inflate the cuff and ventilate the patient.

H. Observe lung inflations and auscultate the chest for adequate ventilation.

I. Secure the endotracheal or tracheostomy tube to the patient to prevent dislodging.

J. **Caution:** Do not cut or remove the cricothyroid cartilage.

Complications of Surgical Cricothyroidotomy

1. Asphyxia
2. Aspiration (eg, blood)
3. Cellulitis
4. Creation of a false passage into the tissues
5. Subglottic stenosis/edema
6. Laryngeal stenosis
7. Hemorrhage or hematoma formation
8. Laceration of the esophagus
9. Laceration of the trachea
10. Mediastinal emphysema
11. Vocal cord paralysis, hoarseness

**Chapter 2:
Airway and
Ventilatory
Management**

**Skill
Station III**

Figure 1
Surgical Cricothyroidotomy

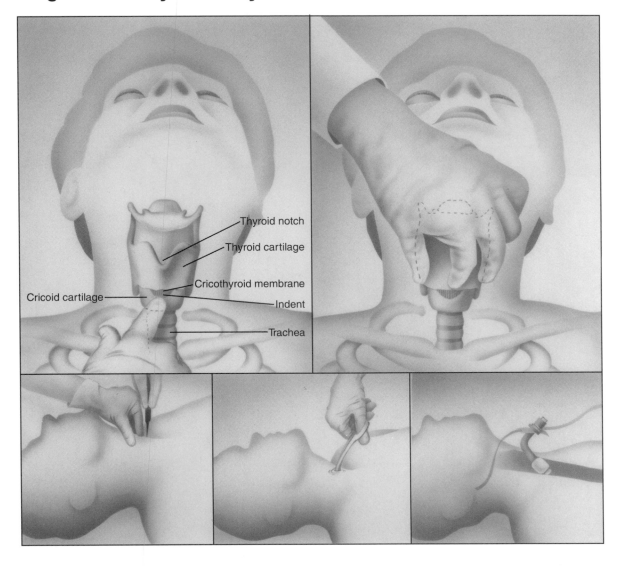

**Chapter 2:
Airway and
Ventilatory
Management**

**Skill
Station III**

Chapter 3:
Shock

Objectives:

Upon completion of this topic, the physician will be able to identify and apply principles of management related to the initial diagnosis and treatment of shock in the injured patient. Specifically, the physician will be able to:

A. Define shock.

B. Discuss the similarities and differences in the various etiologies and presentations of shock.

C. Recognize the clinical shock syndrome and correlate the patient's acute clinical signs with the degree of volume deficit.

D. Discuss the basic principles of emergency treatment of hemorrhagic shock and their application based on the patient's clinical response to therapy.

E. Discuss fluid management problems unique to the trauma patient.

F. Demonstrate various techniques of central and peripheral vascular access, including cutdowns and intraosseous insertion.

Chapter 3:
Shock

American College of Surgeons

I. Introduction

The initial step in managing shock in the injured patient is to **recognize its presence.** No laboratory tests immediately diagnose shock. The initial diagnosis is based on clinical appreciation of the presence of **inadequate organ perfusion and tissue oxygenation.** Thus, the definition of shock as an abnormality of the circulatory system that results in inadequate organ perfusion and tissue oxygenation also becomes an operative tool for diagnosis and treatment.

The second step in the initial management of shock is to **identify the probable cause** of the shock state. For the trauma patient this identification process is directly related to the mechanism of injury. All types of shock may be present in the trauma patient. Most injured patients in shock are hypovolemic, but cardiogenic shock or tension pneumothorax may be the cause and must be considered in patients with specific injuries above the diaphragm. The clinical situations that make this problem more likely are discussed later in this chapter. Neurogenic shock results from extensive injury to the central nervous system or the spinal cord. For all practical purposes, **shock does not result from isolated head injuries.** Spinal cord injury victims may initially present in shock from both vasodilatation and relative hypovolemia. Septic shock is unusual but must be considered for patients whose arrival at the emergency facility has been greatly delayed.

The physician's management responsibilities begin first with recognizing the presence of the shock state. Initiating treatment should be simultaneous with the identification of a probable cause of the shock state. The response to initial treatment, coupled with the findings on initial and secondary patient survey, usually provides enough information to determine the cause of the shock state. **Hemorrhage is the most common cause of the shock state in the injured patient.**

Three components of cardiac physiology are classically defined in shock as: (1) preload, (2) pump, and (3) afterload. Preload is equated with venous capacitance and volume status. Myocardial contractility is the pump that drives the system. Afterload is systemic (peripheral) vascular resistance. The initial treatment of shock is directed toward restoring cellular and organ perfusion with adequately oxygenated blood. In hemorrhagic shock this means **increasing preload** or restoring adequate circulating blood volume rather than merely restoring the patient's blood pressure and pulse rate. Therefore, **vasopressors are contraindicated** for the treatment of hemorrhagic shock.

A significant percentage of injured patients who are in hypovolemic shock require surgical intervention, and many of these require early intervention to relieve the shock. **Therefore, the presence of shock in an injured patient demands the immediate involvement of a qualified surgeon.**

II. Initial Patient Assessment

A. Recognition of Shock

Full-blown circulatory shock, evidenced by inadequate perfusion of the skin, kidneys, and central nervous system, is easy to recognize. However, after the airway and breathing are evaluated, careful evaluation of the patient's circulatory status is important to identify earlier stages of shock. Sole reliance on systolic blood pressure as an indicator of shock results in a delayed recognition of the shock state. **Remember**, compensatory mechanisms may preclude a measurable fall in systolic pressure until the patient has lost up to 30% of his blood volume. Specific attention should be directed to pulse rate, respiratory rate, skin circulation, and pulse pressure (the difference between systolic and diastolic pressure). The earliest signs of shock are tachycardia and cutaneous vasoconstriction. **Accordingly, any injured patient who is cool and tachycardic is in shock until proven otherwise.** The normal heart rate varies with age. Tachycardia is present when the heart rate is greater than 160 in an infant, 140 in a preschool age child, 120 from school age to puberty, and 100 in an adult. The elderly patient may not exhibit tachycardia because of the limited cardiac response to catecholamine stimulation or certain medications such as propranolol. **A narrowed pulse pressure** suggests significant blood loss and involvement of compensatory mechanisms.

Use of the hematocrit (or hemoglobin concentration) is unreliable and inappropriate for estimating acute blood loss or diagnosing shock. Massive blood loss may produce a minimal acute decrease in hematocrit. Thus, a very low hematocrit suggests significant blood loss or pre-existing anemia, while a normal hematocrit does not rule out significant blood loss.

B. Clinical Differentiation of Etiology of Shock

1. Hemorrhagic shock

Hemorrhage is the most common cause of shock after injury, and virtually all multiply injured patients have an element of hypovolemia. In addition, most nonhemorrhagic shock states respond partially or briefly to volume resuscitation. Therefore, once the shock state is identified, treatment usually is begun as if the patient were hypovolemic. However, as treatment is instituted, it is important to identify the small number of patients whose shock has been caused by some other etiology, and the larger group of patients for whom a secondary factor complicates their hypovolemic/hemorrhagic shock. The specifics of treatment of hemorrhagic shock are covered in greater detail in the next section of this chapter. This section focuses on differentiating other potential etiologies of shock.

The major differentiating factor in identifying the cause of shock in a trauma patient is whether the condition is hemorrhagic or nonhemorrhagic. This is especially true for a patient with injuries above the diaphragm, when cardiogenic shock and tension pneumothorax may be a potential cause of the shock state. A high index of suspicion and careful observation of the patient's response to initial treatment should enable the physician to recognize and manage all forms of shock. The initial determination of the etiology depends on an appropriate history, a careful physical examination, and selected additional tests.

2. Nonhemorrhagic shock

a. Cardiogenic shock

Myocardial dysfunction may occur from myocardial contusion, cardiac tamponade, air embolus, or rarely a myocardial infarction associated with the patient's injury. Cardiac contusion is not uncommon in rapid deceleration blunt trauma to the thorax. All patients with blunt thoracic trauma need constant ECG monitoring to detect injury patterns and dysrhythmias. Blood CPK-isoenzymes and specific isotope studies of the myocardium rarely have any value in diagnosing or managing the patient in the emergency department. Ultrasound can be useful in the diagnosis of tamponade or valvular rupture, but it is often not practical or immediately available in the emergency department. Myocardial contusion may be an indication for early central venous pressure monitoring of fluid resuscitation in the emergency department.

Cardiac tamponade is most common in penetrating thoracic trauma. It can occur rarely in blunt trauma to the thorax. Tachycardia, muffled heart sounds, and dilated, engorged neck veins with hypotension resistant to fluid therapy suggest cardiac tamponade. Tension pneumothorax may mimic cardiac tamponade. Appropriate placement of a needle temporarily relieves these two life-threatening conditions.

b. Tension pneumothorax

Tension pneumothorax develops when a flap valve leak allows air to enter the pleural space but prevents its escape. Intrapleural pressure rises, causing total lung collapse and a shift of the mediastinum to the opposite side, with subsequent impairment of venous return and fall in cardiac output. Tension pneumothorax is a true surgical emergency, requiring immediate diagnosis and treatment. The presence of subcutaneous emphysema, absent breath sounds, hyperresonance to percussion, tracheal shift, and acute respiratory distress make the diagnosis and warrant thoracic decompression without waiting for roentgenographic confirmation.

c. Neurogenic shock

Isolated head injuries do not cause shock. The presence of shock in a patient with a head injury necessitates a search for another cause of shock. Spinal cord injury may produce hypotension due to loss of sympathetic tone. **Remember,** loss of sympathetic tone compounds the physiologic effects of hypovolemia, and hypovolemia compounds the physiologic effects of sympathetic denervation. The classic picture of neurogenic shock is hypotension without tachycardia or cutaneous vasoconstriction. A narrowed pulse pressure is not seen in neurogenic shock. Patients sustaining a spinal injury often have concurrent torso trauma. Therefore, patients with known or suspected neurogenic shock should be treated initially for hypovolemia. Failure to restore perfusion or blood pressure with fluid resuscitation may indicate either continuing hemorrhage or neurogenic shock. Central venous pressure monitoring may be helpful in managing this sometimes complex problem. (See Chapter 7, Spine and Spinal Cord Trauma.)

d. Septic shock

Shock due to infection immediately after injury is uncommon. However, if the patient's arrival at the emergency facility is delayed for several hours, this problem may occur. Septic shock is particularly likely to occur in patients with penetrating abdominal injuries and contamination of the peritoneal cavity with intestinal contents. The volume status of the patient in septic shock is clinically significant. Septic patients who are hypovolemic are difficult to distinguish clinically from those in hypovolemic shock (tachycardia, cutaneous vasoconstriction, impaired urinary output, decreased systolic pressure, narrow pulse pressure). Patients with sepsis and normal or nearly normal circulating volume may have a modest tachycardia, warm pink skin, a systolic pressure near normal, and wide pulse pressure.

III. Hemorrhagic Shock in the Injured Patient

Hemorrhage is the most common cause of shock in the trauma patient. However, the trauma patient's response to blood loss is made more complex by changes in the body fluids (particularly in the extracellular fluid) that impact on the circulating blood volume and cellular function. The classic response to blood loss must be considered in the context of the fluid changes associated with soft-tissue injury and the changes associated with severe, prolonged shock, and the pathophysiologic results of resuscitation and reperfusion.

A. Pathophysiology

Early circulatory responses to blood loss are compensatory, ie, **progressive vasoconstriction** of cutaneous, muscle, and visceral circulation to preserve blood flow to the kidneys, heart, and brain. **Tachycardia** is the earliest measurable circulatory sign.

At the cellular level, inadequately perfused and oxygenated cells initially compensate by shifting to anaerobic metabolism, which further results in the formation of lactic acid and the development of metabolic acidosis. If shock is prolonged, the cellular membrane loses its ability to maintain the normal electrical gradient, and cellular swelling occurs, leading to cellular damage and death, and tissue swelling. This process compounds the overall impact on blood loss and hypoperfusion. The administration of isotonic electrolyte solutions helps combat this process. Therefore, management is directed toward reversing this phenomenon with adequate oxygenation, ventilation, and appropriate fluid resuscitation. Resuscitation may be accompanied by a marked increase in interstitial edema, the result of the "reperfusion injury" to the capillary-interstitial membrane. This may result in larger volumes of resuscitation fluid than initially anticipated.

B. Definition of Hemorrhage

Hemorrhage is defined as an **acute loss of circulating blood**. Although there is considerable variability, the normal adult blood volume is approximately 7% of body weight. For example: a 70-kilogram male has approximately five liters of circulating blood volume. The blood volume of obese adults is estimated based on their ideal body weight, because calculation based on actual weight can result in significant overestimation. For children, the blood volume is calculated at 8% to 9% of the body weight (80 to 90 mL/kg). (See Chapter 10, Pediatric Trauma.)

C. Direct Effects of Hemorrhage

Classes of hemorrhage, based on percentage of acute blood volume loss, are outlined individually in this chapter for the **purposes of teaching and comprehending** the physiologic and clinical manifestations of hemorrhagic shock. The distinction between classes is not always so apparent in any single trauma patient, and **treatment should be directed more by the response to initial therapy than relying solely on the initial classification.** Nevertheless, this classification system is useful in emphasizing the early signs and physiology of the shock state. **Class I** is exemplified by the condition of the blood donor. **Class II** is uncomplicated shock, but crystalloid fluid resuscitation is required. **Class III** is a complicated state in which at least crystalloid and perhaps blood replacement are required. **Class IV** can be considered as a preterminal event, and unless very aggressive measures are taken, the patient dies within minutes. (See Table 1, Estimated Fluid and Blood Losses.)

All medical personnel involved in the initial assessment and resuscitation of the patient in hemorrhagic shock must quickly recognize important factors that may accentuate or diminish the patient's physiologic response. Important factors that may profoundly alter the classic vascular dynamics include: (1) the patient's age; (2) severity of injury with special attention to type and anatomical location of injury; (3) time lapse between injury concurrence and initiation of treatment; and (4) prehospital fluid therapy and application of the pneumatic antishock garment (PASG).

It is dangerous to wait until the trauma patient fits a precise physiologic classification of shock before initiating aggressive therapy. Aggressive fluid resuscitation must be initiated when early signs and symptoms of blood loss are apparent or suspected, not when the blood pressure is falling or absent.

1. Loss of up to 15%—Class I Hemorrhage

The clinical symptoms of this volume loss are minimal. In uncomplicated situations, minimal tachycardia occurs. No measurable changes occur in blood pressure, pulse pressure, or respiratory rate. For otherwise healthy patients, this amount of blood loss does not require replacement. Transcapillary refill and other compensatory mechanisms restore blood volume within 24 hours. However, in the presence of other fluid changes, this amount of blood loss can produce clinical symptoms. Replacement of the primary fluid losses corrects the circulatory state.

2. 15% to 30% blood volume loss—Class II Hemorrhage

In a 70-kilogram male, this volume loss represents 750 to 1500 mL of blood. Clinical symptoms include tachycardia (heart rate above 100 in an adult), tachypnea, and a decrease in pulse pressure (the difference between the systolic and diastolic pressures). This decrease in pulse pressure is primarily related to a rise in the diastolic component. (The main reason for the rise in diastolic pressure is an elevation in catecholamines which produces an increase in peripheral resistance.) Because the systolic pressure changes minimally in early hemorrhagic shock, it is important to evaluate the pulse pressure rather than the systolic pressure. Other pertinent clinical findings with this degree of blood loss include subtle central nervous system changes (anxiety, which may be expressed as fright or hostility). Notably, despite the significant blood loss and cardiovascular changes, urinary output is only mildly affected (the measured flow is usually 20 to 30 mL per hour).

Again, accompanying fluid losses can compound the clinical expression of this amount of blood loss. The majority of such patients may eventually require blood transfusion, but can be stabilized initially with other replacement fluids.

3. 30% to 40% blood volume loss—Class III Hemorrhage

This amount of blood loss (approximately 2000 mL in an adult) can be devastating. Patients almost always present with the classic signs of inadequate perfusion, including marked tachycardia and tachypnea, significant changes in mental status, and a measurable fall in systolic pressure. Note that in an uncomplicated case, this is the smallest amount of blood loss that consistently causes a drop in systolic pressure. Although patients with this degree of blood loss almost always require transfusion, remember that these symptoms can result from lesser degrees of blood loss combined with other fluid losses. Thus, the decision to transfuse is based on the patient's response to initial fluid resuscitation and evidence of end-organ perfusion and oxygenation, as described later in this chapter.

4. More than 40% blood volume loss—Class IV Hemorrhage

This degree of exsanguination is immediately life-threatening. Symptoms include marked tachycardia, a significant depression in systolic blood pressure, and a very narrow pulse pressure (or an unobtainable diastolic pressure). Urinary output is negligible, and mental status is markedly depressed. The skin is cold and pale. Such patients frequently require rapid transfusion and immediate surgical intervention. These decisions are based on the patient's response to the initial management techniques described in this chapter. Loss of more than 50% of the patient's blood volume results in loss of consciousness, pulse, and blood pressure.

D. Fluid Changes Secondary to Soft-Tissue Injury

Major soft-tissue injuries and fractures compound the circulatory status of the injured patient in two ways. First, blood is frequently lost into the site of injury, particularly in cases of major fractures. For instance, a fractured tibia or humerus may be associated with as much as a unit and a half (750 mL) blood loss. Twice that amount (up to 1500 mL) is commonly associated with femur fractures, and **several liters of blood may accumulate in a retroperitoneal hematoma associated with a pelvic fracture**.

The second factor to be considered is the obligatory edema that occurs in injured soft tissues. This condition is related to the magnitude of soft-tissue injury and consists of extracellular fluid. Because the plasma is part of the extracellular fluid, these changes have a significant impact on circulating blood volume. For instance, the two liters of edema that may be associated with a massive femur fracture may consist of 1500 mL of interstitial fluid and only 500 mL of plasma volume. In general, roughly 25% of such fluid translocation is evidenced by a decrease in the plasma volume. The impact of these changes on circulating blood volume and the reason they compound fluid loss then becomes obvious.

IV. Initial Management of Hemorrhagic Shock

As in many emergency situations, diagnosis and treatment must be performed in rapid succession. For most trauma patients, treatment is instituted as if the patient had hypovolemic shock, unless evidence to the contrary is clear.

A. Physical Examination

The physical examination is directed at the immediate diagnosis of life-threatening injuries and includes assessment of the ABCs. Baseline recordings are important to the subsequent monitoring of the patient. Vital signs, urinary output, and level of consciousness are important. A more detailed examination of the patient follows as the situation permits.

1. Airway and breathing

Establishing a patent airway with adequate ventilatory exchange and oxygenation is the first priority. Supplementary oxygen via a bag-valve-mask reservoir system is delivered to maintain arterial oxygen tension between 80 and 100 mm Hg.

2. Circulation—Hemorrhage control

Priorities include: Control obvious hemorrhage; obtain adequate intravenous access; and assess tissue perfusion. Bleeding from external wounds usually can be controlled by direct pressure to the bleeding site, eg, scalp, neck, and upper and lower extremities. The pneumatic antishock trouser may be used to control bleeding from pelvic or lower extremity fractures, but the device should **not** interfere with rapid re-establishment of intravascular volume by the intravenous route. The adequacy of tissue perfusion dictates the amount of fluid resuscitation required.

3. Disability—Neurologic examination

A brief neurologic examination determining the level of consciousness, eye motion and pupillary response, motor function, and degree of sensation is performed. These data are useful in assessing cerebral perfusion, following the evolution of neurologic disability, and prognosticating future recovery. (See Chapter 6, Head Trauma.)

4. Exposure—Complete examination

After addressing the life-saving priorities, the patient must be completely undressed and carefully examined from "head to toe" as part of the search for associated injuries. The performance of other diagnostic and therapeutic maneuvers is part of this secondary survey. **Remember**, when undressing the patient, preventing iatrogenic hypothermia is essential.

5. Gastric dilatation—Decompression

Gastric dilatation often occurs in the trauma patient and may cause unexplained hypotension. **This condition makes shock difficult to treat, and in the unconscious patient, it represents a significant risk of aspiration—a potentially fatal complication.** The physician's responsibility does not end with the passage of the gastric tube. The tube must be properly positioned, attached to appropriate suction, and be functioning.

6. Urinary catheter insertion

Bladder decompression allows for the assessment of urine for hematuria and constant monitoring of renal perfusion via the urinary output. Blood at the urethral meatus or a nonpalpable prostate in the male is a contraindication to inserting a transurethral catheter. (See Chapter 5, Abdominal Trauma.)

B. Vascular Access Lines

Access to the vascular system must be obtained promptly. This is best done by establishing two large-caliber (minimum of 16-gauge) peripheral intravenous catheters before any consideration is given to a central line. Poiseuille's Law states that flow is proportional to the fourth power of the radius of the cannula, and inversely related to its length. Hence, short, large-caliber peripheral IVs are preferred to infuse large volumes of fluid rapidly. The most desirable sites for peripheral intravenous lines in adults are: (1) percutaneous peripheral access via the forearm or antecubital veins, and (2) cutdown on the saphenous or arm veins. If circumstances prevent the use of peripheral veins, large-caliber, central venous access is indicated, using the Seldinger technique. In children younger than six years, intraosseous needle access should be attempted before central line insertion. The important determinant for selecting a procedure and route for establishing vascular access is the level of the physician's skill and experience.

As intravenous lines are started, blood samples are drawn for appropriate laboratory analyses, including type and crossmatch, toxicology studies, and pregnancy testing of all females of childbearing age. It also may be useful to obtain arterial blood gases at this time. A chest roentgenogram should be obtained after attempts at inserting a subclavian or internal jugular central venous pressure monitoring line to document its position and evaluate for pneumothorax.

C. Initial Fluid Therapy

Isotonic electrolyte solutions are used for initial resuscitation. This type of fluid provides transient intravascular expansion and further stabilizes the vascular volume by replacing accompanying fluid losses into the interstitial and intracellular spaces. Ringer's lactate solution is the initial fluid of choice. Normal saline is the second choice. Although normal saline is a satisfactory replacement fluid in the volumes administered to injured patients, it has the potential to cause hyperchloremic acidosis. This potential is enhanced if renal function is impaired.

An initial fluid bolus is given as rapidly as possible. The usual dose is one to two liters for an adult and 20 mL/kilogram for a pediatric patient. The patient's response is observed during this initial fluid administration, and further therapeutic and diagnostic decisions are based on this response.

The amount of fluid and blood required for resuscitation is difficult to predict on initial evaluation of the patient. Table 1, Estimated Fluid and Blood Losses, outlines general guidelines for establishing the amount and type of fluid and blood the patient probably requires. A rough guideline for the total amount of crystalloid volume acutely required is to replace each one milliliter of blood loss with three milliliters of crystalloid fluid, thus allowing for restitution of plasma volume lost into the interstitial and intracellular spaces. However, it is more important to assess the patient's response to fluid resuscitation and evidence of adequate end-organ perfusion and oxygenation. If, during resuscitation, the amount of fluid administered deviates widely from these estimates, a careful reassessment of the situation and a search for unrecognized injuries or other causes of shock are necessary.

V. Evaluation of Fluid Resuscitation and Organ Perfusion

A. General

The same signs and symptoms of inadequate perfusion that are used to diagnose shock are useful determinants of patient response. The return of normal blood pressure, pulse pressure, and pulse rate are positive signs and indicate that circulation is normalizing. However, these observations give no information regarding organ perfusion. Improvements in the central nervous system status and skin circulation are important evidence of enhanced perfusion, but are difficult to quantitate. The urinary output can be quantitated and the renal response to restoration of perfusion is reasonably sensitive (if not modified by diuretics). For this reason urinary output is one of the prime monitors of resuscitation and patient response. Changes in central venous pressure can provide useful information, and the risk of a central venous pressure line is justified for complex cases. Measurements of left heart function (obtained with a Swan-Ganz catheter) are rarely indicated for the management of the injured patient in the emergency department.

B. Urinary Output

Within certain limits, urinary output can be used as a monitor of renal blood flow. Adequate volume replacement should produce a urinary output of approximately **50 mL/hour in the adult. One mL/kg/hour** is an adequate urinary output for the **pediatric patient.** For children **under one year of age, two mL/kg/hour** should be maintained. Inability to obtain urinary output at these levels (or decreasing urinary output with an increasing specific gravity) suggests inadequate resuscitation. This situation should stimulate further volume replacement and diagnostic endeavors.

C. Acid/Base Balance

Patients in early hypovolemic shock have respiratory alkalosis due to tachypnea. Respiratory alkalosis gives way to mild metabolic acidosis in the early phases of shock and does not require treatment. Severe metabolic acidosis may develop from long-standing or severe shock. Metabolic acidosis is due to anaerobic metabolism resulting from inadequate tissue perfusion, and persistence is usually due to inadequate fluid resuscitation. Persistent acidosis in the normothermic shock patient should be treated with increased fluids and **not** intravenous sodium bicarbonate, unless the pH is less than 7.2.

Table 1
Estimated Fluid and Blood Losses[1]
Based on Patient's Initial Presentation

	Class I	Class II	Class III	Class IV
Blood Loss (mL)	Up to 750	750-1500	1500-2000	> 2000
Blood Loss (%BV)	Up to 15%	15-30%	30-40%	> 40%
Pulse Rate	< 100	> 100	> 120	> 140
Blood Pressure	Normal	Normal	Decreased	Decreased
Pulse Pressure (mm Hg)	Normal or increased	Decreased	Decreased	Decreased
Respiratory Rate	14-20	20-30	30-40	> 35
Urine Output (mL/hr)	> 30	20-30	5-15	Negligible
CNS/Mental Status	Slightly anxious	Mildly anxious	Anxious and confused	Confused and lethargic
Fluid Replacement (3:1 Rule)	Crystalloid	Crystalloid	Crystalloid and blood	Crystalloid and blood

[1] For a 70-kg male.

The guidelines in Table 1 are based on the "three-for-one" rule. This rule derives from the empiric observation that most patients in hemorrhagic shock require as much as 300 mL of electrolyte solution for each 100 mL of blood loss. Applied blindly, these guidelines can result in excessive or inadequate fluid administration. For example, a patient with a crush injury to the extremity may have hypotension out of proportion to his blood loss and require fluids in excess of the 3:1 guideline. In contrast, a patient whose ongoing blood loss is being replaced requires less than 3:1. The use of bolus therapy with careful monitoring of the patient's response can moderate these extremes.

VI. Therapeutic Decisions Based on Response to Initial Fluid Resuscitation

The patient's response to initial fluid resuscitation is the key to determining subsequent therapy. (See Table 2, Responses to Initial Fluid Resuscitation.) Having established a preliminary diagnosis and plan based on the initial evaluation of the patient, the physician can now modify management based on the patient's response to the initial fluid resuscitation. Observing the response to the initial resuscitation identifies those patients whose blood loss was greater than estimated and those with ongoing bleeding. In addition, it limits the probability of over-transfusion or unneeded transfusion of blood in those whose initial status was disproportionate to the amount of blood loss. It is particularly important to distinguish the patient who is "hemodynamically stable" from one who is "hemodynamically normal." A hemodynamically stable patient may be persistently tachycardic, tachypneic, and oliguric, clearly remaining underperfused and underresuscitated. In contrast, the hemodynamically normal patient is one who exhibits no signs of inadequate tissue perfusion. The potential response patterns can be discussed in three groups.

A. Rapid Response to Initial Fluid Administration

A small group of patients respond rapidly to the initial fluid bolus and remain stable and hemodynamically normal when the initial fluid bolus has been completed and the fluids are slowed to maintenance rates. Such patients usually have lost minimal (less than 20%) blood volume. No further fluid bolus or immediate blood administration is indicated for this small group of patients. Type and crossmatched blood should be kept available. **Surgical consultation and evaluation are necessary during initial assessment and treatment.**

B. Transient Response to Initial Fluid Administration

The largest group of patients responds to the initial fluid bolus. However, in some patients, as the initial fluids are slowed, the circulatory perfusion indices may begin to show deterioration, indicating either an ongoing blood loss or inadequate resuscitation. Most of these patients initially have lost an estimated 20% to 40% of their blood volume. Continued fluid administration and initiation of blood administration are indicated. The response to blood administration should identify patients who are still bleeding and require rapid surgical intervention.

C. Minimal or No Response to Initial Fluid Administration

This response is seen in a small but significant percentage of injured patients. For most of these patients, failure to respond to adequate crystalloid and blood administration in the emergency department dictates the need for immediate surgical intervention to control exsanguinating hemorrhage. On very rare occasions, failure to respond may be due to pump failure as a result of myocardial contusion or cardiac tamponade. The possible diagnosis of non-hemorrhagic shock always should be entertained in this group of patients. Central venous pressure monitoring helps differentiate between the various shock etiologies.

VII. Blood Replacement

The decision to begin transfusion is based on the patient's response, as described in the previous section.

A. Packed Red Blood Cells versus Whole Blood Therapy

Either whole blood or packed red blood cells can be used to resuscitate the trauma patient. However, in an effort to maximize blood product availability, most blood centers currently provide component therapy (packed cells, platelets, fresh frozen plasma, etc). The main purpose in transfusing blood is to restore the oxygen-carrying capacity of the intravascular volume. Volume resuscitation itself can be accomplished with crystalloids, with the added advantage of contributing to interstitial and intracellular volume restitution.

Table 2
Responses to Initial Fluid Resuscitation*

	Rapid Response	Transient Response	No Response
Vital Signs	Return to normal	Transient improvement; recurrence of ↓BP and ↑HR	Remain abnormal
Estimated Blood Loss	Minimal (10% - 20%)	Moderate and ongoing (20% - 40%)	Severe (> 40%)
Need for More Crystalloid	Low	High	High
Need for Blood	Low	Moderate - high	Immediate
Blood Preparation	Type and crossmatch	Type-specific	Emergency blood release
Need for Operative Intervention	Possibly	Likely	Highly likely
Surgical Consultation	Yes	Yes	Yes

*2000 mL Ringer's lactate in adults, 20 mL/kg Ringer's lactate in children, over 10 to 15 minutes.

B. Crossmatched, Type-specific and Type O Blood

1. Fully crossmatched blood is preferable. However, the complete cross-matching procedure requires approximately one hour in most blood banks. For patients who stabilize rapidly, crossmatched blood should be obtained and should be available for transfusion when indicated.

2. Type-specific or "saline crossmatched" blood can be provided by most blood banks within ten minutes. Such blood is compatible with ABO and Rh blood types. Incompatibilities of minor antibodies may exist. Such blood is of first choice for patients with life-threatening shock situations, such as transient responders described in the previous section.

3. If type-specific blood is unavailable, type O packed cells are indicated for patients with exsanguinating hemorrhage. For life-threatening blood loss, the use of unmatched, type-specific blood is preferred over type O blood, unless multiple unidentified casualties are being treated simultaneously. To avoid sensitization and future complications, Rh-negative cells are preferable, particularly for females of childbearing age.

C. Blood Filters

Macropore (160 microns) intravenous filtering devices are used when whole blood transfusions are given. These filters remove microscopic clots and debris. The use of micropore blood filters has not been demonstrated to be of significant value.

D. Warming Fluids–Plasma and Crystalloid

Iatrogenic hypothermia in the resuscitation phase of trauma patients can and must be prevented. The use of blood warmers is cumbersome yet most desirable in the emergency department. The most efficient and easiest way to prevent hypothermia in any patient receiving massive volumes of crystalloid is to heat the fluid to 39 degrees centigrade before using it. Blood, plasma, and glucose-containing solutions cannot be warmed in the microwave oven.

E. Autotransfusion

Adaptation of standard tube thoracostomy collection devices are commercially available to allow for the sterile collection, anticoagulation (generally with sodium-citrate solutions, not heparin), and retransfusion of shed blood. Collection of shed blood for autotransfusion should be considered for any major hemothorax. Equipment to collect, wash, and retransfuse blood lost during operative procedures also is commercially available. Bacterial contamination may limit the usefulness of such devices during many operations.

F. Coagulopathy

Coagulopathy is a rare problem in the first hour of treatment of the multiply injured patient. Hypothermia and massive transfusion with resultant dilution of platelets and clotting factors are the usual causes of coagulopathies in the injured patient. Prothrombin time, partial thromboplastin time, and platelet count are valuable baseline studies to obtain in the first hour, especially if the patient has a history of coagulation disorders or takes medications that alter coagulation. Transfusion of platelets, cryoprecipitate, and fresh frozen plasma should be guided by these coagulation parameters, including fibrinogen. Routine use of such products is generally not warranted.

G. Calcium Administration

Most patients receiving blood transfusions do not need calcium supplements. Excessive, supplemental calcium may be harmful.

VIII. Pneumatic Antishock Garment (PASG)

The application of the PASG can raise systolic pressure by increasing peripheral vascular resistance and myocardial afterload. The efficacy of PASG inhospital or in the rural setting remains unproven, and in the urban prehospital setting, controversial.

A. Indications

Current indications for use of the PASG are:

1. Splinting and control of pelvic fractures with **continuing hemorrhage and hypotension**

2. Intra-abdominal trauma with severe hypovolemia in patients who are en route to the operating room or another facility

B. Contraindications

1. Pulmonary edema

2. Known diaphragmatic rupture

3. Uncontrolled hemorrhage outside the confines of the garment (ie, thoracic, upper extremity, scalp, face, or neck injury)

C. Dangers

The use of the PASG **must not delay volume replacement or rapid transport.** Prolonged inflation of the leg components of the PASG can result in compartment syndrome, particularly in the patient in shock with extremity trauma. Precise time of garment inflation must be recorded. **If inflation of the abdominal component of the PASG causes an increase in the patient's respiratory rate or respiratory distress, it must be deflated immediately, regardless of the patient's blood pressure. Diaphragmatic rupture is assumed until proven otherwise.**

D. Deflation and Removal of the PASG

Several specific points bear emphasis in deflation procedures. The PASG should not be an impediment to IV access and volume resuscitation. Individual segments may be carefully deflated for IV access, examination of extremities, angiography, etc. In general, if the patient requires transfer to another facility, the garment is left in situ, inflated as indicated. For patients transferred by air, effective inflation pressures may increase due to changes in atmospheric pressure. A similar change may occur when the PASG is applied in a cold environment, and the patient is then brought into a warm emergency department.

The deflation process is gradual, beginning with the abdominal segment. Air is allowed to escape slowly, while blood pressure is closely monitored. A fall in systolic blood pressure of more than 5 mm Hg is an indication for more fluid resuscitation prior to continued deflation.

IX. Pitfalls in the Diagnosis and Treatment of Shock

A. Equating Blood Pressure with Cardiac Output

Treatment of hypovolemic (hemorrhagic) shock requires correcting inadequate organ perfusion, which means increasing organ blood flow and tissue oxygenation. Increasing blood flow means increasing cardiac output. Ohm's Law ($V = I \times R$) applied to cardiovascular physiology states that blood pressure (V) is proportional to cardiac output (I) and systemic vascular resistance (R) (afterload). It is a mistake to necessarily equate an increase in blood pressure with a concomitant increase in cardiac output. An increase in peripheral resistance (ie, vasopressor therapy) with no change in cardiac output results in increased blood pressure, but no improvement in tissue perfusion or oxygenation.

B. Age

Hypotension from hemorrhage due to trauma is poorly tolerated by the older patient. Aggressive therapy with fluids and early surgery are often warranted to save the patient and prevent serious complications, such as myocardial infarction or a cerebrovascular accident.

C. Athletes

Rigorous training routines change the cardiovascular dynamics of this group of patients. Blood volume can increase 15% to 20%, cardiac output can increase six-fold, stroke volume can increase 50%, and resting pulse is generally at 50. This group's ability to compensate for blood loss is truly remarkable. The usual responses to hypovolemia may not be manifested in athletes, even though significant blood loss may have occurred.

D. Medications

Beta-adrenergic receptor blockers and calcium antagonists can significantly alter the patient's hemodynamic response to hemorrhage.

E. Hypothermia

Patients suffering from hypothermia and hemorrhagic shock are resistant to appropriate blood and fluid resuscitative measures and often develop a coagulopathy. Therefore, body temperature is an important vital sign to record during the initial assessment phase. Theoretically, esophageal or bladder recording is an accurate clinical measurement of the core temperature. Although not ideal, a rectal temperature alerts the treating physician to the problem. A trauma victim under the influence of alcohol and exposed to cold temperature extremes may become hypothermic. Rapid rewarming in a warmed environment with appropriate external warming devices, heated respiratory gases, and warmed intravenous fluids generally correct the patient's hypotension and hypothermia. Core rewarming (peritoneal or thoracic cavity irrigation with warmed—39 degrees centigrade—crystalloid solutions, or extracorporeal bypass) may occasionally be indicated. (See Chapter 9, Injury Due to Burn and Cold.) Hypothermia is best treated by prevention.

F. Pacemaker

Patients with pacemakers are unable to respond to blood loss in the expected fashion. Considering the significant number of patients with myocardial conduction defects who have such devices in place, central venous pressure monitoring is invaluable in these patients to guide fluid therapy.

X. Reassessing Patient Response and Avoiding Complications

Inadequate volume replacement with subsequent organ failure is the most common complication of hemorrhagic shock. Immediate, appropriate, and aggressive therapy that restores organ perfusion minimizes these untoward events. Three specific concerns are outlined in the succeeding paragraphs.

A. Continued Hemorrhage

Obscure hemorrhage is the most common cause of poor patient response to fluid therapy. These patients are generally included in the Transient Response category as defined previously. Under this circumstance, consider immediate surgical intervention.

B. Fluid Overload and CVP Monitoring

After the patient's initial assessment and management have been completed, the risk of fluid overload is minimized by monitoring the patient carefully. **Remember**, the goal of therapy is restoration of organ perfusion and adequate tissue oxygenation, signified by appropriate urinary output, central nervous system function, skin color, and return of pulse and blood pressure toward normal.

Central venous pressure (CVP) monitoring is a relatively simple procedure and is used as a standard guide for assessing the ability of the right side of the heart to accept a fluid load. Properly interpreted, the response of the CVP to fluid administration helps evaluate volume replacement. Several points to remember are:

1. The precise measure of cardiac function is the relationship between ventricular-end diastolic volume and stroke volume. It is apparent that comparison of right atrial pressure (CVP) to cardiac output (as reflected by evidence of perfusion or blood pressure, or even by direct measurement) is an indirect and, at best, an insensitive estimate of this relationship. Remembering these facts is important to avoid over dependence on CVP monitoring.

2. The initial CVP level and the actual blood volume are not necessarily related. The initial CVP is sometimes high even with a significant volume deficit, especially in patients with chronic obstructive pulmonary disease, generalized vasoconstriction, and rapid fluid replacement. The initial venous pressure also may be high secondary to the application of the PASG or the inappropriate use of exogenous vasopressors.

3. A minimal rise in the initial, low CVP with fluid therapy suggests the need for further volume expansion (minimal or no response to fluid resuscitation category).

4. A declining CVP suggests ongoing fluid loss and the need for additional fluid or blood replacement (transient response to fluid resuscitation category).

5. An abrupt or persistent elevation in the CVP suggests volume replacement is adequate, is too rapid, or that cardiac function is compromised.

6. **Remember**, the CVP line is **not** a primary intravenous fluid resuscitation route. It should be inserted on an elective rather than emergent basis.

7. Pronounced elevations of the CVP may be caused by hypervolemia as a result of overtransfusion, cardiac dysfunction, cardiac tamponade, or increased intrathoracic pressure from a pneumothorax. Catheter malposition may produce an erroneously measured high CVP.

Access for a central venous pressure line can be obtained via a variety of routes. Appropriate antiseptic techniques are used when central lines are placed. Ideal placement of an intravenous catheter is in the superior vena cava, just proximal to the right atrium. Techniques are discussed in detail in Skill Station IV, Vascular Access and Monitoring.

Central venous lines are not without complications. Infections, vascular injury, embolization, thrombosis, and pneumothorax are encountered. Central venous pressure monitoring reflects right heart function. It may not be representative of the left heart function in patients with primary myocardial dysfunction or abnormal pulmonary circulation.

C. Recognition of Other Problems

When the patient fails to respond to therapy, consider ventilatory problems, unrecognized fluid loss, acute gastric distention, cardiac tamponade, myocardial infarction, diabetic acidosis, hypoadrenalism, and neurogenic shock. **Constant re-evaluation**, especially when patients deviate from expected patterns, is the key to recognizing such problems as early as possible.

XI. Summary

Shock therapy, based on sound physiologic principles, is usually successful. Hypovolemia is the cause of shock in most trauma patients. Management of these patients requires immediate hemorrhage control and fluid replacement. Other possible causes of the shock state must be considered. The patient's response to initial fluid therapy determines further therapeutic and diagnostic procedures. The goal of therapy is restoration of organ perfusion. In hypovolemic shock, vasopressors are rarely, if ever, needed. Central venous pressure measurement is a valuable tool for confirming the volume status and monitoring the rate of fluid administration.

Bibliography

1. American Heart Association and American Academy of Pediatrics: Intraosseous infusion. In: Chameides, L (ed): **Textbook of Pediatric Advanced Life Support.** Dallas, American Heart Association 1988, pp 43-44.

2. Canizaro PC, Prager MD, Shires GT: The infusion of Ringer's lactate solution during shock. **American Journal of Surgery** 1971;122:494.

3. Cary LC, Lowery BD, Cloutier CT: Hemorrhagic shock. In: Ravitch MM (ed): **Current Problems in Surgery**. Chicago, Yearbook Medical Publishers, Jan 1971, pp 1-48.

4. Carrico CJ, Canizaro PC, Shires GT: Fluid resuscitation following injury: rationale for the use of balanced salt solutions. **Critical Care Medicine** 1976;4(2):46-54.

5. Cloutier CT: Pathophysiology and treatment of shock. In Moylan JA (ed): **Trauma Surgery**. Philadelphia, JB Lippincott, 1988, pp 27-44.

6. Cogbill TH, Blintz M, Johnson JA, et al: Acute gastric dilatation after trauma. **The Journal of Trauma** 1987;27(10):1113-1117.

7. Counts RB, Haisch C, Simon TL, et al: Hemostasis in massively transfused trauma patients. **Annals of Surgery** 1979;190(1):91-99.

8. Glover JL, Broadie TA: Intraoperative autotransfusion. **World Journal of Surgery** 1987; 11:60-64.

9. Granger DN: Role of xanthine oxidase and granulocytes in ischemia-reperfusion injury. **American Journal of Physiology** 1988; 255:H1269-1275.

10. Harrigan C, Lucas CE, Ledgerwood AM, et al: Serial changes in primary hemostasis after massive transfusion. **Surgery** 1985;98:836-840.

11. Hogman CF, Bagge L, Thoren L: The use of blood components in surgical transfusion therapy. **World Journal of Surgery** 1987;11:2-13.

12. Jurkovich GJ: Hypothermia in the trauma patient. In: Maull KI (ed): **Advances in Trauma.** Chicago, Yearbook Medical Publishers, 1989, pp 111-140.

13. Martin DJ, Lucas CE, Ledgerwood AM, et al: Fresh frozen plasma supplement to massive red blood cell transfusion. **Annals of Surgery** 1985;202:505.

14. Peck KR and Altieri M: Intraosseous infusions: anold technique with modern applications. **Orthopedic Nursing** 1989;8(3):46-48.

15. Poole GV, Meredith JW, Pennell T, et al: Comparison of colloids and crystalloids in resuscitation from hemorrhagic shock. **Surgery, Gynecology and Obstetrics** 1982;154:577-586.

16. Roberts JR and Hedges JR: Assessment of oxygenation. In **Clinical Procedures in Emergency Medicine** Second Edition. Philadelphia, WB Saunders Company, 1991, pp 67-83.

17. Schwartz SI: Hemostasis, surgical bleeding and transfusion. In: Schwartz S (ed): **Principles of Surgery, 5th Edition.** New York, McGraw-Hill, 1989, pp 105-135.

18. Shires GT: Principles and management of hemorrhagic shock. In: Shires GT (ed): **Principles of Trauma Care, 3rd Edition.** New York, McGraw-Hill, 1985, pp 3-42.

19. Velanovich V: Crystalloid versus colloid fluid resuscitation: a meta analysis of mortality. **Surgery** 1990; 105:65-71.

20. Virgilio RW, Rice CL, Smith DE, et al: Crystalloid vs colloid resuscitation: is one better? A randomized clinical study. **Surgery** February 1979;85(2):129-139.

21. Werwath DL, Schwab CW, Scholter JR, et al: Microwave oven: a safe new method of warming crystalloids. **American Journal of Surgery** 1984;12:656-659.

Skill Station IV:
Vascular Access and Monitoring

Resources and Equipment

This list is the recommended equipment to conduct this skill session in accordance with the stated objectives for and intent of the procedures outlined. Additional equipment may be used providing it does not detract from the stated objectives and intent of this skill, or from performing the procedures in a safe method as described and recommended by the ACS Committee on Trauma.

1. Live patient model

2. Jugular and subclavian IV manikin (optional)

3. Fresh chicken or turkey legs

4. Subclavian intravenous set-up

5. Central venous pressure set-up

6. Needles and intravenous catheters

   a. Assorted intravenous over-the-needle catheters (#14-, #16-, and #18-gauge, 15-20 cm or 6-8 inches in length)
   b. #18-gauge needle (3.75 cm or 1.5 inches in length)
   c. #19-gauge needle (3.75 cm or 1.5 inches in length)
   d. #16- or #18-gauge bone aspiration/transfusion needle (1.25 cm or 0.5 inch in length)

7. 7.0-8.5 Fr rapid infuser catheter kit with guidewire

8. Methylene-blue dye (optional)

9. Antiseptic swabs

10. 12- and 20-mL syringes

11. Lidocaine 1% (demonstration purposes only)

12. 1000 mL Ringer's lactate with macrodrip

13. Large-caliber intravenous and extension tubings

14. Portable intravenous stand (optional)

15. 3x3 gauze sponges

16. Vial of sterile saline

17. Pulse oximetry monitoring device, power cord, sensors, and operator's manual

18. Broselow Pediatric Resuscitation Measuring Tape

Objectives

1. Performance at this station will allow the participant to practice and demonstrate the techniques of subclavian, internal jugular, and femoral intravenous, as well as intraosseous line insertions.

2. Upon completion of this station, the participant will be able to describe the surface markings for percutaneous access into a:

    a. Subclavian vein
    b. Internal jugular vein
    c. Femoral vein
    d. Proximal tibia or distal femur

3. Upon completion of this station, the participant will be able to identify the intravenous fluid used for the following types of shock and associated trauma:

    a. Hemorrhagic (hypovolemic) shock
    b. Nonhemorrhagic shock

4. Upon completion of this station, the participant will be able to:

    a. Discuss the purpose of pulse oximetry monitoring.
    b. Demonstrate the proper method of activating the device, setting alarm limits, and applying the optical sensors to appropriate body parts.
    c. Discuss the indications for using a pulse oximetry monitoring device, its functional limits of accuracy, and reasons for malfunction or inaccuracy.
    d. Accurately interpret the pulse oximeter monitor readings and relate their significance to the care of the trauma patient.

Procedures

1. Subclavian venipuncture: Infraclavicular approach

2. Internal jugular venipuncture

3. Femoral venipuncture

4. Intraosseous puncture/infusion

5. Pulse oximetry monitoring

Note: The Broselow Pediatric Resuscitation Measuring Tape is included on the equipment list for this station. A specific skill is not outlined for its use; however, participants need to be aware of its availability and its use when managing pediatric trauma. By measuring the height of the child, the child's estimated weight can be determined readily. One side of the tape provides drugs and their recommended doses for the pediatric patient based on weight. The other side provides equipment needs for the pediatric patient based on size. Therefore, participation at this station should include an orientation to the tape and its use.

Skills Procedures

Vascular Access and Monitoring

Note: Universal precautions are required whenever caring for the trauma patient.

I. Subclavian Venipuncture: Infraclavicular Approach

(See Figure 1)

A. Place the patient in a supine position, at least 15 degrees head-down to distend the neck veins and prevent an air embolism. Only if the cervical spine has been cleared radiographically can the patient's head be turned away from the venipuncture site.

B. Cleanse the skin well around the venipuncture site and drape the area. Sterile gloves should be worn when performing this procedure.

C. If the patient is awake, use a local anesthetic at the venipuncture site.

D. Introduce a large-caliber needle, attached to a 12-mL syringe with 0.5 to 1 mL saline, 1 cm below the junction of the middle and medial thirds of the clavicle.

E. After the skin has been punctured, with the bevel of the needle upward, expel the skin plug that may occlude the needle.

F. The needle and syringe are held parallel to the frontal plane.

G. Direct the needle medially, slightly cephalad, and posteriorly behind the clavicle toward the posterior, superior angle to the sternal end of the clavicle (toward finger placed in the suprasternal notch).

H. Slowly advance the needle while gently withdrawing the plunger of the syringe.

I. When a free flow of blood appears in the syringe, rotate the bevel of the needle caudally, remove the syringe, and occlude the needle with a finger to prevent an air embolism.

J. Quickly insert the catheter to a predetermined depth (tip of catheter should be above the right atrium for fluid administration).

K. Remove the needle and connect the catheter to the intravenous tubing.

L. Affix the catheter (eg, with suture), apply antibiotic ointment, and dress the area.

M. Tape the intravenous tubing in place.

N. Attach the central venous pressure set-up to the intravenous tubing and adjust the manometer (level at zero) with the level of the patient's right atrium.

O. Obtain a chest film to identify the position of the intravenous line and a possible pneumothorax.

P. **Optional Method:** Seldinger technique as outlined in III. Femoral Venipuncture: Seldinger Technique.

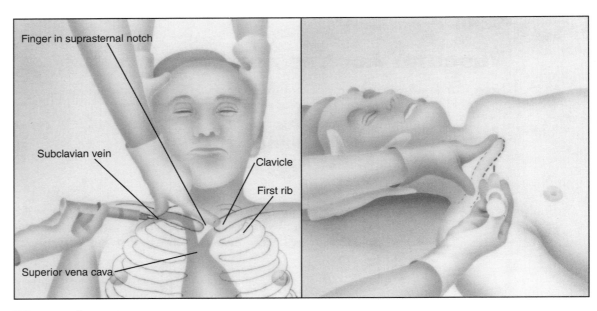

Figure 1
Subclavian Venipuncture: Infraclavicular Approach

II. Internal Jugular Venipuncture: Middle or Central Route

(See Figure 2)

A. Place the patient in a supine position, at least 15 degrees head-down to distend the neck veins and to prevent an air embolism. Only if the cervical spine has been cleared radiographically, can the patient's head be turned away from the venipuncture site.

B. Cleanse the skin well around the venipuncture site and drape the area. Sterile gloves should be worn when performing this procedure.

C. If the patient is awake, use a local anesthetic at the venipuncture site.

D. Introduce a large-caliber needle, attached to a 12-mL syringe with 0.5 to 1 mL of saline, into the center of the triangle formed by the two lower heads of the sternomastoid and the clavicle.

E. After the skin has been punctured, with the bevel of the needle upward, expel the skin plug that may occlude the needle.

F. Direct the needle caudally, parallel to the sagittal plane, at a 30-degree posterior angle with the frontal plane.

G. Slowly advance the needle while gently withdrawing the plunger of the syringe.

H. When a free flow of blood appears in the syringe, remove the syringe and occlude the needle with a finger to prevent an air embolism. If the vein is not entered, withdraw the needle and redirect it 5 to 10 degrees laterally.

I. Quickly insert the catheter to a predetermined depth (tip of catheter should be above the right atrium for fluid administration).

J. Remove the needle and connect the catheter to the intravenous tubing.

K. Affix the catheter in place (eg, with suture), apply antibiotic ointment, and dress the area.

L. Tape the intravenous tubing in place.

M. Attach the central venous pressure set-up to the intravenous tubing and adjust the manometer (level at zero) with the level of the patient's right atrium.

N. Obtain a chest film to identify the position of the intravenous line and a possible pneumothorax.

O. **Optional Method:** Seldinger technique as outlined in III. Femoral Venipuncture: Seldinger Technique.

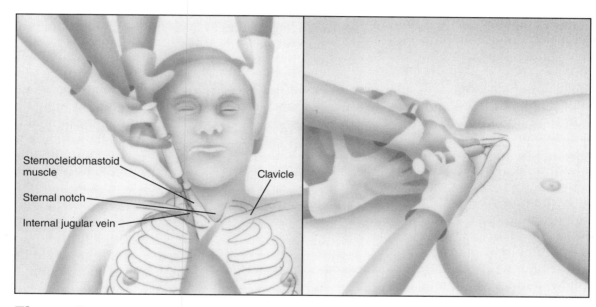

Sternocleidomastoid muscle
Clavicle
Sternal notch
Internal jugular vein

Figure 2
Internal Jugular Venipuncture: Middle or Central Route

Complications of Central Intravenous Venipuncture

1. Hematoma formation
2. Cellulitis
3. Thrombosis
4. Phlebitis
5. Nerve transection
6. Arterial puncture
7. Pneumothorax
8. Hemopneumothorax (eg, with subclavian venipuncture)
9. Nerve puncture
10. Chylothorax (eg, with internal jugular venipuncture)
11. Arteriovenous fistula
12. Peripheral neuropathy
13. Lost catheters
14. Inaccurate monitoring techniques
15. Improperly placed catheters

III. Femoral Venipuncture: Seldinger Technique

(See Figure 3)

A. Place the patient in a supine position.

B. Cleanse the skin well around the venipuncture site and drape the area. Sterile gloves should be worn when performing this procedure.

C. Locate the femoral vein by palpating the femoral artery. The vein lies directly medial to the femoral artery (nerve, artery, vein, empty space). A finger should remain on the artery to facilitate anatomical location and to avoid insertion of the catheter into the artery.

D. If the patient is awake, use a local anesthetic at the venipuncture site.

E. Introduce a large-caliber needle attached to a 12-mL syringe with 0.5 to 1 mL of saline. The needle, directed toward the patient's head, should enter the skin directly over the femoral vein.

F. The needle and syringe are held parallel to the frontal plane.

G. Directing the needle cephalad and posteriorly, slowly advance the needle while gently withdrawing the plunger of the syringe.

H. When a free flow of blood appears in the syringe, remove the syringe and occlude the needle with a finger to prevent an air embolism.

I. Insert the guidewire and remove the needle. Then insert the catheter over the guidewire.

J. Remove the guidewire and connect the catheter to the intravenous tubing.

K. Affix the catheter in place (ie, with suture), apply antibiotic ointment, and dress the area.

L. Tape the intravenous tubing in place.

M. Attach the central venous pressure set-up to the intravenous tubing and adjust the manometer (level at zero) with the level of the patient's right atrium.

N. Obtain chest and abdominal roentgenograms to identify the position and placement of the intravenous catheter.

Complications of Femoral Venipuncture

1. Hematoma formation
2. Cellulitis
3. Thrombosis
4. Phlebitis
5. Nerve transection and/or puncture
6. Arterial puncture
7. Arteriovenous fistula
8. Peripheral neuropathy
9. Lost catheters
10. Inaccurate monitoring techniques
11. Improperly placed catheter

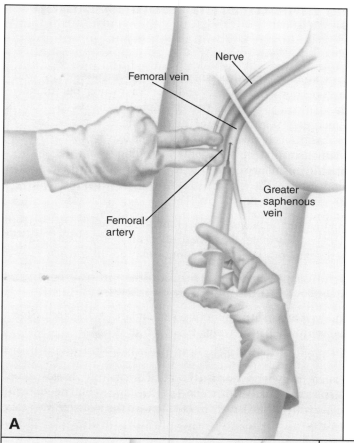

Femoral vein

Nerve

Greater
saphenous
vein

Femoral
artery

A

**Figure 3
Femoral
Venipuncture**

**Chapter 3:
Shock**

**Skill
Station IV**

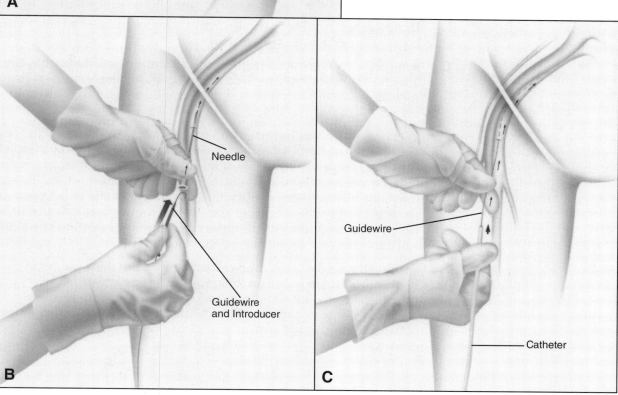

Needle

Guidewire
and Introducer

B

Guidewire

Catheter

C

IV. Intraosseous Puncture/Infusion: Proximal Tibial Route

(See Figure 4)

Note: This procedure is limited to children six years of age or younger, for whom venous access is impossible due to circulatory collapse or for whom percutaneous peripheral venous cannulation has failed on two attempts. Intraosseous infusions should be limited to emergency resuscitation of the child and discontinued as soon as other venous access has been obtained. (Methylene-blue dye may be mixed with the sterile saline for demonstration purposes only. Providing the needle has been properly placed within the medullary canal, the methylene-blue dye/saline solution seeps from the upper end of the chicken or turkey bone when the solution is injected. See item H.)

A. Place the patient in a supine position. Selecting an uninjured lower extremity, place sufficient padding under the knee to effect an approximate 30-degree angle and allow the patient's heel to rest comfortably on the gurney.

B. Identify the puncture site—anteromedial surface of the proximal tibia, approximately one finger-breadth (1 to 3 cm) below the tubercle.

C. Cleanse the skin well around the puncture site and drape the area. Sterile gloves should be worn when performing this procedure.

D. If the patient is awake, use a local anesthetic at the puncture site.

E. At a 90-degree angle, introduce a short (threaded or smooth), large-caliber, bone-marrow aspiration needle (or a short, #18-gauge spinal needle with stylet) into the skin with needle bevel directed toward the foot and away from the epiphyseal plate.

F. Using a gentle twisting or boring motion, advance the needle through the bone cortex and into the bone marrow.

G. Remove the stylet and attach to the needle a 12-mL syringe filled with approximately 6 mL of sterile saline. Gently withdraw on the plunger of the syringe. Aspiration of bone marrow into the syringe signifies entrance into the medullary cavity.

H. Inject the saline into the needle to expel any clot that may occlude the needle. If the saline flushes through the needle easily and there is no evidence of swelling, the needle should be in the appropriate place. If bone marrow was not aspirated as outlined in G., but the needle flushes easily when injecting the saline without evidence of swelling, the needle should be in the appropriate place. Additionally, proper placement of the needle is indicated if the needle remains upright without support and intravenous solution flows freely without evidence of subcutaneous infiltration.

I. Connect the needle to the large-caliber intravenous tubing and begin fluid infusion. The needle is then carefully screwed further into the medullary cavity until the needle hub rests on the patient's skin. If a smooth needle is used, it should be stabilized at a 45 to 60 degree angle to the anteromedial surface of the child's leg.

J. Apply antibiotic ointment and a 3x3 sterile dressing. Secure the needle and tubing in place.

K. Routinely re-evaluate the placement of the intraosseous needle, assuring that it remains through the bone cortex and in the medullary canal. **Remember**, intraosseous infusion should be limited to emergency resuscitation of the child and discontinued as soon as other venous access has been obtained.

Complications of Intraosseous Puncture

1. Local abscess and cellulitis
2. Osteomyelitis
3. Sepsis
4. Through and through penetration of the bone
5. Subcutaneous or subperiosteal infiltration
6. Pressure necrosis of the skin
7. Transient bone marrow hypocellularity
8. Physeal plate injury
9. Hematoma

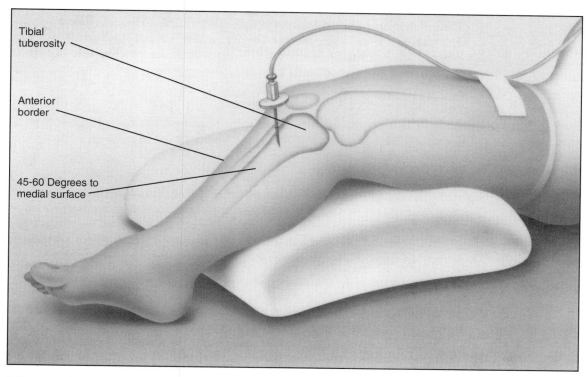

**Figure 4
Intraosseous Puncture**

V. Pulse Oximetry Monitoring

The pulse oximeter provides continuous, noninvasive measurements of oxygen saturation of functional hemoglobin and pulse rate that are updated with each heart beat. The device combines the principles of spectrophotometric oximetry and plethysmography. It consists of an electro-optical sensor that is applied to the patient, and a monitor that processes and displays the measurements. The sensor contains low-voltage, low-intensity light-emitting diodes (LEDs) as light sources and a photodiode as a light receiver. (An oximeter is a photoelectric instrument that measures the oxygen saturation of blood. A spectrophotometer is a tool that estimates the quantity of colored material in a light path by determining the amount of light absorbed. A plethysmograph is a device that measures variations in the volume of an organ, part, or limb caused by pulsatile variations in the amount of blood present or passing through it.)

When the light from the LEDs is transmitted through blood and other body tissues, a portion of the light is absorbed by the blood and by each tissue component. The photodiode in the sensor measures the light that passes through without being absorbed, and this measurement is used to determine how much light is absorbed. The results of these measurements are conveyed both audibly and visually into pulse rate and percent arterial hemoglobin oxygen saturation displays on the device.

With each heart beat, a pulse of oxygenated arterial blood flows to the sensor site. The relative amount of light absorbed by oxygenated hemoglobin differs from deoxygenated hemoglobin. The pulse oximeter uses these measurements to determine the percentage of hemoglobin that is saturated with oxygen.

Initially, light absorption is determined when the pulsatile blood is not present, serving as the "reference" or "baseline" absorption of tissue and nonpulsatile blood. Absorption is then measured after the next heart beat when pulsatile blood enters the tissue. Subsequently, the light absorption is changed by the presence of the pulse of arterial blood.

The microprocessor in the monitor then corrects the measurements during the pulsatile flow for the amount of light absorbed during the initial (no pulsatile flow) measurements. The ratio of the corrected absorption is then used to determine functional oxygen saturation (oxygenated hemoglobin conveyed as a percentage of only the hemoglobin capable of transporting oxygen—oxyhemoglobin and reduced hemoglobin; dysfunctional hemoglobin is excluded from this calculation).

The pulse oximeter is calibrated to read oxyhemoglobin saturation (%SAO_2) of functional hemoglobin as compared to a CO-oximeter. Significant levels of dysfunctional hemoglobin (hemoglobin incapable of reversibly binding oxygen, eg, carboxyhemoglobin, methemoglobin), may affect the accuracy of the instrument. Indocyanine green, methylene-blue, and other intravascular dyes, depending on their concentrations, may interfere with the accuracy of the instrument. Instrument performance also may be affected by excessive patient movement, electrocautery interference, intense surrounding light, severe anemia, severe vasoconstriction, and hypothermia. (See Chapter 2, Airway and Ventilatory Management.)

A. Assemble the necessary equipment and set up the device.

   1. Plug one end of the power cord into the device's AC power inlet and the other end into a properly grounded AC outlet.

   2. Connect the patient sensor module to the device.

   3. If ECG synchronization is to be used, provide an ECG signal to the device.

B. Select an appropriate sensor and apply it to the patient's ear lobe, finger tip, toe tip, nose bridge, or foot band (neonates). **Remember,** the sensor should not be applied to an ischemic or injured body part.

C. Turn the device to "On," review the "Start Up" displays (pulse search, oxygen saturation, pulse rate, ECG in use), and confirm effective operation of the device.

D. Identify the "Oxygen Saturation" and "Pulse Rate" readings, test the alarms, and reset the alarm limits as necessary.

E. Evaluate the "Oxygen Saturation" and "Pulse Rate" findings.

   1. Are they appropriate?

   2. What do they indicate?

   3. What might affect these results?

   4. What is the estimated arterial oxygen partial pressure?

F. Turn the device to "Off" and disconnect the sensors from the patient.

G. Discuss the following potential problems and causes:

   1. No indication of pulse, saturation, and/or pulse rate were displayed.

   2. The perfusion indicator tracks the pulse, but there is no oxygen saturation or pulse rate display.

   3. Saturation and/or pulse rate displays are changing rapidly, and the perfusion indicator is erratic.

   4. The pulse rate does not correlate with other monitors or monitoring methods.

   5. The oxygen saturation measurement does not correlate with blood gas determinations.

Hemoglobin Oxygen Saturation versus Arterial Oxygen Pressure

The relationship between partial pressure of oxygen in arterial blood (PaO_2) and percent arterial hemoglobin oxygen saturation ($\%SaO_2$) is displayed in Figure 5. The sigmoid shape of this curve indicates that the relationship between saturation and arterial oxygen partial pressure is nonlinear. This is particularly important in the middle range of this curve, where small changes in PaO_2 will effect large changes in saturation. **Remember,** the pulse oximeter measures arterial oxygen saturation, not arterial oxygen partial pressure. (See Table 1, PaO_2 versus O_2 Saturation Levels, Chapter 2, Airway and Ventilatory Management.)

Standard blood gas measurements report both arterial oxygen pressure (PaO_2) and a calculated hemoglobin saturation (%SaO_2). When oxygen saturation is calculated from blood gas PaO_2, the calculated value may differ from the oxygen saturation measured by the pulse oximeter. This is because an oxygen saturation value that has been calculated from the blood gas PaO_2 has not necessarily been correctly adjusted for the effects of variables that shift the relationship between PaO_2 and saturation. These variables include temperature, pH, $PaCO_2$, 2,3-DPG, and the concentration of fetal hemoglobin.

Figure 5
PaO_2 (mm Hg) and %SaO_2 Relationship

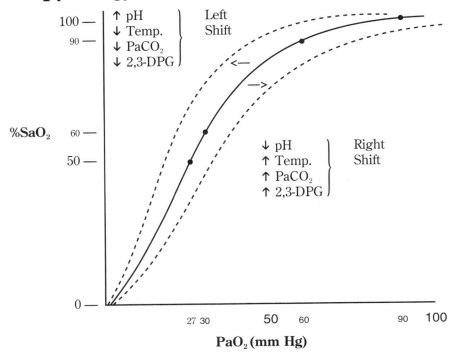

Skill Station V: Venous Cutdown

This surgical procedure, if performed on a live-anesthetized animal, must be conducted in a USDA-Registered Animal Laboratory. (See *ATLS® Instructor Manual*, Section II, Chapter 9—Policies, Procedures, and Protocols for Surgical Skills Practicum.)

Resources and Equipment

This list is the recommended equipment to conduct this skill session in accordance with the stated objectives for and intent of the procedures outlined. Additional equipment may be used providing it does not detract from the stated objectives and intent of this skill, or from performing the procedures in a safe method as described and recommended by the ACS Committee on Trauma.

1. Live, anesthetized animals

2. Licensed veterinarian (see guidelines referenced above)

3. Animal troughs, ropes (sandbags optional)

4. Animal intubation equipment

   a. Endotracheal tubes
   b. Laryngoscope blade and handle
   c. Respirator with 15-mm adapter

5. Electric shears with #40 blade

6. Local anesthetic set, including antiseptic

7. Tables or instrument stands

8. #14- to #20-gauge cutdown catheters

9. Suture

   a. 3-0 ties
   b. 4-0 suture with swaged needle

10. Surgical instruments

    a. Scalpel handles with #10 and #11 blades
    b. Small hemostats
    c. Needle holders
    d. Single-toothed spring retractors

11. 4x4 gauze sponges

12. Surgical drapes

13. 500-mL Ringer's lactate with macrodrip tubing

14. Vein introducer (optional)

15. Surgical garb (gloves, shoe covers, and scrub suits or cover gowns)

Objectives

1. Performance at this station will allow the participant to practice and demonstrate on a live anesthetized animal the technique of peripheral venous cutdown.

2. Upon completion of this station, the participant will be able to identify the surface markings and structures to be noted in performing a peripheral venous cutdown.

3. Upon completion of this station, the participant will be able to discuss the indications and contraindications for a peripheral venous cutdown.

Anatomic Considerations for Venous Cutdown

1. The primary site for a peripheral venous cutdown is the greater saphenous vein at the ankle, which is located at a point approximately 2 cm anterior and superior to the medial malleolus. (See Figure 1, Saphenous Venous Cutdown.)

2. A secondary site is the antecubital medial basilic vein, located 2.5 cm lateral to the medial epicondyle of the humerus at the flexion crease of the elbow.

Skills Procedure

Venous Cutdown

Note: Universal precautions are required whenever caring for the trauma patient.

I. Venous Cutdown

A. Prepare the skin of the ankle with antiseptic solution and drape the area.

B. Infiltrate the skin over the vein with 0.5% lidocaine.

C. A full-thickness transverse skin incision is made through the area of anesthesia to a length of 2.5 cm.

D. By blunt dissection, using a curved hemostat, the vein is identified and dissected free from any accompanying structures.

E. Elevate and dissect the vein for a distance of approximately 2 cm, to free it from its bed.

F. Ligate the distal, mobilized vein, leaving the suture in place for traction.

G. Pass a tie about the vein, cephalad.

H. Make a small transverse venotomy and gently dilate the venotomy with the tip of a closed hemostat.

I. Introduce a plastic cannula through the venotomy and secure it in place by tying the upper ligature about the vein and cannula. The cannula should be inserted an adequate distance to prevent dislodging.

J. Attach the intravenous tubing to the cannula and close the incision with interrupted sutures.

K. Apply a sterile dressing with a topical antibiotic ointment.

Complications of Peripheral Venous Cutdown

1. Cellulitis

2. Hematoma

3. Phlebitis

4. Perforation of the posterior wall of the vein

5. Venous thrombosis

6. Nerve transection

7. Arterial transection

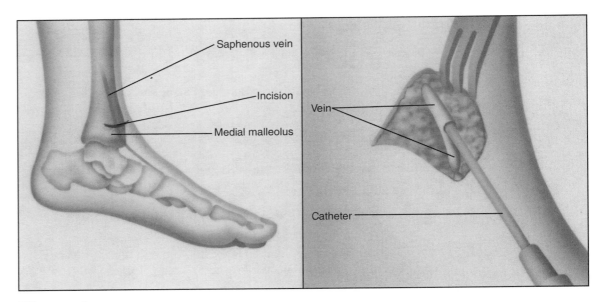

Figure 1
Saphenous Venous Cutdown

Chapter 4:
Thoracic Trauma

Objectives:

Upon completion of this topic, the physician will be able to identify and initiate treatment of life-threatening thoracic injuries.

Specifically, the physician will be able to:

A. Identify and manage the following **immediately** life-threatening chest injuries evidenced in the **primary survey:**

   1. Airway obstruction

   2. Tension pneumothorax

   3. Open pneumothorax

   4. Massive hemothorax

   5. Flail chest

   6. Cardiac tamponade

B. Identify and initiate treatment of the following **potentially** life-threatening injuries assessed during the **secondary survey**:

   1. Pulmonary contusion

   2. Myocardial contusion

   3. Aortic disruption

   4. Traumatic diaphragmatic rupture

   5. Tracheobronchial disruption

   6. Esophageal disruption

C. Explain the purpose of, define the complications of, and demonstrate the ability to perform needle thoracentesis, chest tube insertion, and pericardiocentesis in a surgical skill practicum.

Chapter 4:
Thoracic
Trauma

I. Introduction

A. Incidence

Chest injuries cause one of every four trauma deaths in North America. Many of these patients die after reaching the hospital. Many of these deaths can be prevented by prompt diagnosis and treatment coupled with an understanding of pathophysiologic factors associated with thoracic trauma.

Because most injuries occur at a distance from a trauma center, recognition of the features of thoracic injuries that require early intervention and influence transport is very important. Less than 10% of blunt chest injuries require an operation, and 15% to 30% of penetrating chest injuries require open thoracotomy. Most patients sustaining thoracic trauma may be managed by simple procedures within the capabilities of any physician taking this course. Therefore, the responsibility for the initial management of most chest-injury patients rests with the physician who first examines the patient, and not the trauma surgeon to whom the patient may be transferred.

B. Pathophysiology

Tissue hypoxia, hypercarbia, and acidosis often result from chest injuries. Tissue hypoxia results from inadequate delivery of oxygen to the tissues because of hypovolemia (blood loss), pulmonary ventilation/perfusion mismatch (contusion, hematoma, aveolar collapse, etc), and changes in intrathoracic pressure relationships (tension pneumothorax, open pneumothorax, etc). Hypercarbia implies hypoventilation. Acutely, hypoxia is more important. Respiratory acidosis is caused by inadequate ventilation, changes in intrathoracic pressure relationships, depressed level of consciousness, etc. Metabolic acidosis is caused by hypoperfusion of the tissues (shock).

C. Initial Assessment and Management

1. Patient management must consist of:

   a. Primary survey

   b. Resuscitation of vital functions

   c. Detailed secondary survey

   d. Definitive care

2. Because hypoxia is the most serious feature of chest injury, early interventions are designed to ensure that an adequate amount of oxygen is delivered from the lung to the tissues.

3. Immediately life-threatening injuries are treated as quickly and as simply as possible.

4. Most life-threatening thoracic injuries are treated with an appropriately placed chest tube or needle.

5. The secondary survey is guided by a high index of suspicion for specific injuries.

II. Primary Survey of Life-threatening Injuries

A. Airway

1. Assess for airway patency and air exchange by listening for airway movement at the patient's nose and mouth.

2. Assess for intercostal and supraclavicular muscle retractions.

3. Assess the oropharynx for foreign body obstruction, particularly in the unconscious patient.

B. Breathing

Expose the patient's chest completely and evaluate breathing. Assess respiratory movement and quality of respiration by observing, palpating, and listening.

The signs of chest injury or hypoxia that are particularly important and often subtle include an increased rate of breathing and a change in the breathing pattern, especially toward progressively more shallow respirations. Cyanosis is a late sign of hypoxia in the trauma patient. However, the absence of cyanosis does not indicate adequate tissue oxygenation or an adequate airway.

C. Circulation

1. Assess the patient's pulse for quality, rate, and regularity. **Remember**, the radial and dorsalis pedis pulses may be absent in the hypovolemic patient.

2. Assess the blood pressure for pulse pressure.

3. Observe and palpate the skin for color and temperature to assess the peripheral circulation.

4. Check to see if the neck veins are distended. **Remember**, neck veins may not be distended in hypovolemic patients with cardiac tamponade.

5. A cardiac monitor should be attached to the patient. Patients sustaining thoracic trauma—especially in the area of the sternum or from a rapid deceleration injury—are susceptible to myocardial contusion and/or coronary artery spasm, which may lead to dysrhythmias. Hypoxia and/or acidosis enhance this possibility. Premature ventricular contractions, a common dysrhythmia, may require treatment with an immediate lidocaine bolus (1 mg/kg) followed by a lidocaine drip (2 to 4 mg/minute). Electromechanical dissociation (EMD) is manifest by an electrocardiogram (ECG) showing a rhythm while the patient has no identifiable pulse. EMD may be present in cardiac tamponade, tension pneumothorax, profound hypovolemia, or even worse, cardiac rupture.

D. Thoracotomy

Closed heart massage for cardiac arrest or EMD is ineffective for a hypovolemic patient. Patients with exsanguinating, penetrating precordial injuries who arrive pulseless but with myocardial electrical activity may be candidates for emergency department thoracotomy. Assuming a surgeon is present, a left anterior thoracotomy, cross-clamping of the descending thoracic aorta, pericardiotomy, and open chest massage in conjunction with intravas-

cular volume restoration may be initiated. Emergency department thoracotomy for patients with blunt thoracic injuries, in whom there is no electrical
cardiac activity, is rarely effective.

III. Life-threatening Chest Injuries Identified in the Primary Survey

A. Airway Obstruction

Airway obstruction at the alveolar level is a potentially life-threatening injury
that is assessed and managed during the secondary survey and definitive
care phases. Chapter 2 deals with the management of life-threatening situations of the upper airway.

B. Tension Pneumothorax

A tension pneumothorax develops when a "one-way-valve" air leak occurs
either from the lung or through the chest wall. Air is forced into the thoracic
cavity without any means of escape, completely collapsing the affected lung.
The mediastinum and trachea are displaced to the opposite side, decreasing
venous return and compressing the opposite lung.

The most common causes of tension pneumothorax are mechanical ventilation with positive end-expiratory pressure, spontaneous pneumothorax in
which ruptured emphysematous bullae have failed to seal, and blunt chest
trauma in which a parenchymal lung injury has failed to seal. Occasionally
traumatic defects in the chest wall may cause a tension pneumothorax. A significant incidence of pneumothorax is associated with subclavian or internal
jugular venous catheter insertion.

**Tension pneumothorax is a clinical diagnosis and should not be made
radiologically.** A tension pneumothorax is characterized by respiratory distress, tachycardia, hypotension, tracheal deviation, unilateral absence of
breath sounds, neck vein distention, and cyanosis as a late manifestation.
Because of the similarity in their symptomology, a tension pneumothorax initially may be confused with cardiac tamponade. However, a tension pneumothorax is more common. Differentiation may be made by a hyperresonant
percussion note over the ipsilateral chest.

Tension pneumothorax requires **immediate decompression** and is managed initially by rapidly inserting a needle into the second intercostal space
in the midclavicular line of the affected hemithorax. This maneuver converts
the injury to a simple pneumothorax. (Note: The possibility of subsequent
pneumothorax as a result of the needle stick now exists.) Repeated reassessment is necessary. Definitive treatment usually requires only the insertion
of a chest tube into the fifth intercostal space (nipple level), anterior to the
midaxillary line.

C. Open Pneumothorax ("Sucking Chest Wound")

Large defects of the chest wall, which remain open, result in an open pneumothorax or sucking chest wound. Equilibration between intrathoracic pressure and atmospheric pressure is immediate. If the opening in the chest wall
is approximately two thirds the diameter of the trachea, air passes preferen-

tially through the chest defect with each respiratory effort, because air tends to follow the path of least resistance through the large chest-wall defect. Effective ventilation is thereby impaired, leading to hypoxia.

Manage an open pneumothorax by promptly closing the defect with a sterile occlusive dressing, large enough to overlap the wound's edges, and taped securely on three sides. Taping the occlusive dressing on three sides provides a flutter-type valve effect. As the patient breathes in, the dressing is occlusively sucked over the wound, preventing air from entering. When the patient exhales, the open end of the dressing allows air to escape. A chest tube should be placed remote from the wound as soon as possible. Securely taping all edges of the dressing can cause air to accumulate in the thoracic cavity resulting in a tension pneumothorax unless a chest tube is in place. Any occlusive dressing (plastic wrap, petrolatum gauze, etc) may be used as a stopgap so rapid assessment can continue. Definitive surgical closure of the defect is usually required.

D. Massive Hemothorax

Massive hemothorax results from a rapid accumulation of more than 1500 mL of blood in the chest cavity. It is most commonly caused by a penetrating wound that disrupts the systemic or hilar vessels. It may also be the result of blunt trauma. The blood loss is complicated by hypoxia. The neck veins may be flat secondary to severe hypovolemia or may be distended because of the mechanical effects of intrathoracic blood. This condition is discovered when shock is associated with the absence of breath sounds and/or dullness to percussion on one side of the chest.

Massive hemothorax is initially managed by the simultaneous restoration of blood volume and decompression of the chest cavity. Large-caliber intravenous lines and rapid crystalloid infusion are begun and type-specific blood is administered as soon as possible. If an auto-transfusion device is available, it may be used. A single chest tube (#38 French) is inserted at the nipple level, anterior to the midaxillary line, and rapid restoration of volume continues as decompression of the chest cavity is completed. When massive hemothorax is suspected, prepare for autotransfusion. If 1500 mL is immediately evacuated, it is highly likely that the patient will require an early thoracotomy.

Some patients who have an initial volume output of less than 1500 mL, but continue to bleed, may require a thoracotomy. This decision is based on the rate of continuing blood loss (200 mL/hour). During patient resuscitation, the volume of blood initially drained from the chest tube and the rate of continuing blood loss must be factored into the amount of intravenous fluid replacement. The color of the blood (arterial or venous) is a poor indicator of the necessity for thoracotomy.

Penetrating anterior chest wounds medial to the nipple line and posterior wounds medial to the scapula should alert the physician to the possible need for thoracotomy, because of possible damage to the great vessels, hilar structures, and the heart, with the associated potential for cardiac tamponade. **Thoracotomy is not indicated unless a surgeon is present and the procedure is performed by a physician qualified by training and experience.**

E. Flail Chest

A flail chest occurs when a segment of the chest wall does not have bony continuity with the rest of the thoracic cage. This condition usually results from trauma associated with multiple rib fractures. The presence of a flail chest segment results in severe disruption of normal chest wall movement. If the injury to the underlying lung is significant, serious hypoxia may result. The major difficulty in flail chest stems from the injury to the underlying lung. Although chest wall instability leads to paradoxical motion of the chest wall with inspiration and expiration, this defect alone does not cause hypoxia. Associated pain with restricted chest wall movement and underlying lung injury contribute to the patient's hypoxia.

Flail chest may not be apparent initially because of splinting of the chest wall. The patient moves air poorly, and movement of the thorax is asymmetrical and uncoordinated. Palpation of abnormal respiratory motion and crepitus of rib or cartilage fractures aids diagnosis. A satisfactory chest roentgenogram may suggest multiple rib fractures, but may not show costochondral separation. Arterial blood gases, suggesting respiratory failure with hypoxia, also may aid in diagnosing a flail chest.

Initial therapy includes adequate ventilation, administration of humidified oxygen, and fluid resuscitation. **In the absence of systemic hypotension**, the administration of crystalloid intravenous solutions should be carefully controlled to prevent overhydration. The injured lung in a flail chest is sensitive to both underresuscitation of shock and fluid overload. Specific measures to optimize fluid measurement must be taken for the patient with flail chest.

The definitive treatment is to re-expand the lung, ensure oxygenation as completely as possible, administer fluids judiciously, and provide analgesia to improve ventilation. Some patients can be managed without the use of a ventilator. However, prevention of hypoxia is of paramount importance for the trauma patient, and a short period of intubation and ventilation may be necessary until the diagnosis of the entire injury pattern is complete. A careful assessment of the respiratory rate, arterial oxygen tension, and an estimate of the work of breathing will indicate appropriate timing for intubation and ventilation. Not all patients with a flail chest require immediate endotracheal intubation.

F. Cardiac Tamponade

Cardiac tamponade most commonly results from penetrating injuries. Blunt injury also may cause the pericardium to fill with blood from the heart, great vessels, or pericardial vessels. The human pericardial sac is a fixed fibrous structure, and only a relatively small amount of blood is required to restrict cardiac activity and interfere with cardiac filling. Removal of small amounts of blood or fluid, often as little as 15 mL to 20 mL, by pericardiocentesis may result in immediate hemodynamic improvement.

The classic Beck's triad consists of venous pressure elevation, decline in arterial pressure, and muffled heart tones. However, muffled heart tones are difficult to assess in the noisy emergency department. Distended neck veins, caused by the elevated central venous pressure, may be absent due to hypovolemia. Pulsus paradoxus, a decrease in systolic pressure during inspiration in excess of 10 mm Hg, also may be absent in some patients or difficult to detect in some emergency settings. In addition, tension pneumothorax—particularly on the left side—may mimic cardiac tamponade. Kussmaul's sign (a rise in venous pressure with inspiration when breathing spontaneously) is a true paradoxical venous pressure abnormality associated with tamponade. Electromechanical dissociation in the absence of hypovolemia and tension pneumothorax suggests cardiac tamponade.

Pericardiocentesis is indicated for patients who do not respond to the usual measures of resuscitation for hemorrhagic shock and who have the potential for cardiac tamponade. Insertion of a central venous line may aid diagnosis. Life-saving pericardiocentesis should not be delayed for this diagnostic adjunct. A high index of suspicion coupled with a patient who is unresponsive to resuscitative efforts are all that is necessary to initiate pericardiocentesis by the subxyphoid method.

Even though cardiac tamponade is strongly suspected, the initial administration of intravenous fluid will raise the venous pressure and improve cardiac output transiently while preparations are made for pericardiocentesis via the subxyphoid route. The use of a plastic-sheathed needle is preferable, but the urgent priority is to aspirate blood from the pericardial sac. Electrocardiographic monitoring may identify current of injury and needle-induced dysrhythmias. Because of the self-sealing qualities of the myocardium, aspiration of pericardial blood alone may relieve symptoms temporarily. However, all patients with positive pericardiocentesis due to trauma will require open thoracotomy and inspection of the heart. Pericardiocentesis may not be diagnostic or therapeutic because the blood in the pericardial sac is clotted. Preparations for transfer of these patients to the appropriate facility is necessary. Open pericardiotomy may be life-saving but is indicated **only** when a qualified surgeon is available.

Once these injuries and other immediate, life-threatening injuries have been treated, attention may be directed to the secondary survey and definitive care phase of potential, life-threatening thoracic injuries.

IV. Potentially Lethal Chest Injuries Identified in the Secondary Survey

The secondary survey requires further in-depth physical examination, an upright chest roentgenogram if the patient's condition permits, arterial blood gases, and an electrocardiogram. In addition to lung expansion and the presence of fluid, the chest film should be examined for widening of the mediastinum, a shift of the midline, or loss of anatomic detail. Multiple rib fractures and fractures of the first and/or second rib(s) are evidence of severe force delivered to the chest and underlying tissues.

Six potentially lethal injuries are considered herein:

1. Pulmonary contusion
2. Myocardial contusion
3. Aortic disruption
4. Traumatic diaphragmatic rupture

5. Tracheobronchial disruption

6. Esophageal disruption

Unlike immediately life-threatening conditions, these injuries are not obvious on initial physical examination. Diagnosis requires a **high index of suspicion**. All are more often missed than diagnosed during the initial posttraumatic period. However, if these injuries are overlooked, lives may be lost.

A. Pulmonary Contusion With or Without Flail Chest

Pulmonary contusion is the most common potentially lethal chest injury seen in North America. The respiratory failure may be subtle and develops over time rather than occurring instantaneously. The plan for definitive management may change with time warranting careful monitoring and re-evaluation of the patient.

Some patients with stable conditions may be managed selectively without endotracheal intubation or mechanical ventilation. Patients with significant hypoxia should be intubated and ventilated within the first hour after injury. Associated medical conditions, eg, chronic pulmonary disease and renal failure, predispose to the need for early intubation and mechanical ventilation.

If the patient cannot maintain satisfactory oxygenation or has any of the above complicating features, intubation and mechanical ventilation should be considered. Pulse oximetry, ABG determinations, ECG monitoring, and appropriate ventilatory equipment are necessary for optimal management. Any patient with the aforementioned pre-existing conditions and who is to be transferred should be intubated and ventilated.

B. Myocardial Contusion

Myocardial contusion, although difficult to diagnose, is another potentially lethal injury from blunt chest trauma. The patient's reported complaints of discomfort are often bypassed as being associated with chest wall contusion or fractures of the sternum and/or ribs. The diagnosis of myocardial contusion is established by abnormalities on the electrocardiogram, two-dimensional echocardiography, and associated history of injury. The electrocardiographic changes are variable and may even indicate frank myocardial infarction. Multiple premature ventricular contractions, unexplained sinus tachycardia, atrial fibrillation, bundle branch block (usually right), and ST segment changes are the most common electrocardiographic findings. Elevated central venous pressure in the absence of obvious cause may indicate right ventricular dysfunction secondary to contusion.

Patients with myocardial contusion are at risk for sudden dysrhythmias. They should be admitted to the critical care unit for close observation and cardiac monitoring.

C. Traumatic Aortic Rupture

Traumatic aortic rupture is a common cause of sudden death after an automobile collision or a fall from a great height. Tears of the aorta and major pulmonary arteries, most of which result from blunt trauma, are usually fatal at the scene. For survivors, salvage is frequently possible, if aortic rupture is identified and treated early.

Patients with aortic rupture, who are potentially salvageable, tend to have a laceration near the ligamentum arteriosum of the aorta. Continuity maintained by an intact adventitial layer prevents immediate death. Many of the surviving patients die in the hospital if left untreated. Some blood may escape into the mediastinum, but one characteristic shared by all survivors is that this is a **contained** hematoma. Other than the initial pressure drop associated with the loss of 500 mL to 1000 mL of blood, hypotension responds to intravascular infusion. Persistent or recurrent hypotension is usually due to an unidentified bleeding site. Although free rupture of a transected aorta into the left chest does occur and causes hypotension, it is usually fatal unless the patient is operated on within a few minutes.

Specific signs and symptoms are frequently absent. A high index of suspicion triggered by a history of decelerating force and characteristic radiologic findings, followed by arteriography, are the means of making the diagnosis. Angiography should be performed liberally because the findings of the chest roentgenogram, especially the supine view, are unreliable. Approximately 10% of the aortograms will be positive for aortic rupture if liberal indications for using angiography are employed for all patients with widened mediastinum. Adjunctive radiologic signs, which may or may not be present, indicate the likelihood of major vascular injury in the chest. They include:

1. **Widened mediastinum**

2. Fractures of the first and second ribs

3. Obliteration of the aortic knob

4. Deviation of the trachea to the right

5. Presence of a pleural cap

6. Elevation and rightward shift of the right mainstem bronchus

7. Depression of the left mainstem bronchus

8. Obliteration of space between the pulmonary artery and the aorta

9. Deviation of the esophagus (nasogastric tube) to the right

False-positive and false-negative findings occur with each roentgenographic sign. Therefore, no single finding reliably predicts or excludes significant injury. A widened mediastinum is the most consistent finding. The slightest suspicion of aortic injury should be evaluated angiographically, which is considered the gold standard. Transesophageal ultrasonography may be a useful diagnostic tool. Computed tomography (CT) is time consuming and may not provide a definitive diagnosis.

The treatment is either direct repair of the aorta or resection of the injured area and grafting. A qualified surgeon should treat such a patient.

D. Traumatic Diaphragmatic Rupture

A traumatic diaphragmatic rupture is more commonly diagnosed on the left side because the liver obliterates the defect on the right side, while the appearance of bowel, stomach, or nasogastric tube is more easily detected in the left chest. Blunt trauma produces large radial tears that lead to herniation. Penetrating trauma produces small perforations that often take some time, even years, to develop into diaphragmatic hernias.

These injuries are missed initially if the chest film is misinterpreted as showing an elevated left diaphragm, acute gastric dilatation, a loculated pneumohemothorax, or subpulmonary hematoma. If a laceration of the left diaphragm is suspected, a gastric tube should be inserted. When the gastric tube appears in the thoracic cavity on the chest film, the need for special contrast studies is eliminated. Occasionally, the diagnosis is not identified on the initial roentgenogram or after chest tube evacuation of the left thorax. An upper gastrointestinal contrast study should be performed if the diagnosis is not clear. The appearance of peritoneal lavage fluid in the chest tube drainage also confirms the diagnosis.

Right diaphragmatic ruptures are rarely diagnosed in the early postinjury period. The liver often prevents herniation of other abdominal organs into the chest. The appearance of an elevated right diaphragm on chest roentgenogram may be the only finding. Operation for other abdominal injuries often reveals diaphragmatic tears. The treatment is direct repair.

E. Tracheobronchial Tree Injuries

1. Larynx

Fracture of the larynx is a rare injury, and is indicated by the following triad:

a. Hoarseness

b. Subcutaneous emphysema

c. Palpable fracture crepitus

If the patient's airway is totally obstructed or the patient is in severe respiratory distress, an attempt at intubation is warranted. If intubation is unsuccessful, a tracheostomy (not surgical cricothyroidotomy) is indicated, followed by operative repair. If the patient has sustained blunt trauma to the larynx, exhibits subtle symptoms, and a fracture is suspected, computed tomography may be helpful in identifying a fracture of the larynx.

2. Trachea

Direct trauma to the trachea, including the larynx, can be either penetrating or blunt. Blunt injuries may be subtle, and history is all-important.

Penetrating trauma is overt and requires immediate surgical repair. Penetrating injuries are often associated with esophageal, carotid artery, and jugular vein trauma. Because of the blast effect, penetrating injuries caused by missiles are often associated with extensive tissue destruction surrounding the area of penetration.

Noisy breathing indicates partial airway obstruction that suddenly may become complete. Absence of breathing suggests that complete obstruction already exists. When the level of consciousness is depressed, detection of significant airway obstruction is more subtle. Observations of labored respiratory effort may be the only clue to airway obstruction and tracheobronchial injury. Endoscopic procedures and CT scanning aid the diagnosis.

3. Bronchus

Injury to a major bronchus is an unusual and fatal injury that is frequently overlooked. The majority of such injuries result from blunt trauma and occur within one inch of the carina. Although most patients with this injury die at the scene, those who reach the hospital alive have a 30% mortality, often due to associated injuries.

If suspicion of a bronchial injury exists, immediate surgical consultation is warranted. A patient with a bronchial injury frequently presents with hemoptysis, subcutaneous emphysema, or tension pneumothorax with a mediastinal shift. A pneumothorax associated with a persistent large air leak after tube thoracotomy suggests a bronchial injury. More than one chest tube may be necessary to overcome a very large leak. Bronchoscopy confirms the diagnosis of the injury.

Treatment of tracheobronchial injuries may require only airway maintenance until the acute inflammatory and edema processes resolve. Major deviation or compression of the trachea by extrinsic masses, ie, hematomas, must be treated. Intubation frequently may be unsuccessful because of the anatomic distortion from paratracheal hematoma, major laryngotracheal injury, and associated injuries. For such patients, operative intervention is indicated. Patients surviving with bronchial injuries may require direct surgical intervention by thoracotomy.

F. Esophageal Trauma

Esophageal trauma is most commonly penetrating. Blunt esophageal trauma, although very rare, may be lethal if unrecognized. Blunt injury of the esophagus is caused by a forceful expulsion of gastric contents into the esophagus from a severe blow to the upper abdomen. This forceful ejection produces a linear tear in the lower esophagus, allowing leakage into the mediastinum. The resulting mediastinitis and immediate or delayed rupture into the pleural space cause empyema. Esophageal trauma may be caused by mishaps of instrumentation (nasogastric tubes, endoscopes, dilators, etc).

The clinical picture is identical to that of postemetic esophageal rupture. Esophageal injury should be considered for any patient who (1) has a left pneumothorax or hemothorax without a rib fracture, (2) has received a severe blow to the lower sternum or epigastrium and is in pain or shock out of proportion to the apparent injury, or (3) has particulate matter in their chest tube after the blood begins to clear. Presence of mediastinal air also suggests the diagnosis, which often can be confirmed by contrast studies and/or esophagoscopy.

Wide drainage of the pleural space and mediastinum with direct repair of the injury via thoracotomy is the treatment if feasible. If the repair is tenuous or not feasible, esophageal diversion in the neck and gastrostomy of the lower and upper gastric segments usually is carried out, thereby avoiding continued soiling of the mediastinum and pleura by gastric and esophageal contents.

V. Other Manifestations of Chest Injuries

A. Subcutaneous Emphysema

Subcutaneous emphysema may result from airway injury, lung injury, or rarely, blast injury. Although it does not require treatment, the underlying injury must be addressed.

B. Crushing Injury to the Chest (Traumatic Asphyxia)

Findings associated with a crush injury to the chest include upper torso, facial, and arm plethora with petechiae secondary to superior vena cava compression. Massive swelling and even cerebral edema may be present. Underlying injuries must be treated.

C. Simple Pneumothorax

Pneumothorax results from air entering the potential space between the visceral and parietal pleura. Both penetrating and nonpenetrating trauma may cause this injury. Lung laceration with air leakage is the most common cause of pneumothorax resulting from blunt trauma.

The thorax is normally completely filled by the lung, held to the chest wall by surface tension between the pleural surfaces. Air in the pleural space collapses lung tissue. This collapsed lung does not participate in oxygen exchange. A ventilation/perfusion defect occurs because the blood circulated to the nonventilated area is not oxygenated.

When a pneumothorax is present, breath sounds are decreased on the affected side. Percussion demonstrates hyperresonance. An upright, expiratory roentgenogram of the chest aids the diagnosis.

A pneumothorax is best treated with a chest tube in the fourth or fifth intercostal space, anterior to the midaxillary line. Observation and/or aspiration of any pneumothorax is risky. Once a chest tube has been inserted and connected to an underwater seal apparatus with or without suction, a chest roentgenogram is necessary to confirm re-expansion of the lung. General anesthesia should never be administered for definitive care of injuries in patients who have sustained traumatic pneumothorax or who are at risk for unexpected intraoperative pneumothorax, until a chest tube has been inserted. The chest also should be decompressed before transporting the patient with a pneumothorax via air ambulance.

D. Hemothorax

The primary cause of hemothorax is lung laceration or laceration of an intercostal vessel or internal mammary artery due to either penetrating or blunt trauma. In the vast majority of cases this bleeding is self-limiting and does not require operative intervention.

Hemothorax, sufficient to appear on chest roentgenogram, is usually treated with a large-caliber chest tube. The chest tube evacuates blood, reduces the risk of a clotted hemothorax, and provides a method for monitoring blood loss. Although many factors are involved in the decision to operate on a patient with a hemothorax, the amount of blood drainage from the chest tube is a major factor. If a liter of blood is obtained through the chest tube, surgical consultation is warranted. Persistent drainage of more than 200 mL per hour for four hours may indicate the need for thoracotomy.

E. Scapular and Rib Fractures

The ribs are the most commonly injured component of the thoracic cage. Injuries to the ribs are often significant. Pain on motion results in splinting of the thorax, which impairs ventilation. Tracheobronchial secretions cannot be eliminated easily. The incidence of atelectasis and pneumonia rises strongly with pre-existing lung disease.

The upper ribs (1 to 3) are protected by the bony framework of the upper limb. The scapula, humerus, and clavicle, along with their muscular attachments, provide a barrier to rib and scapular injury. Fractures of the scapula, and first or second ribs often indicate major injury to the head, neck, spinal cord, lungs, and the great vessels. Because of the severity of the associated injuries, mortality can be as high as 50%. Surgical consultation is warranted.

The middle ribs (4 to 9) sustain the majority of blunt trauma. Anteroposterior compression of the thoracic cage will bow the ribs outward with a fracture in the midshaft. Direct force applied to the ribs tends to fracture them and drive the ends of the bones into the thorax with more potential for intrathoracic injury, such as a pneumothorax. As a general rule, a young patient with a more flexible chest wall is less likely to sustain rib fractures. Therefore, the presence of multiple rib fractures in young patients implies a greater transfer of force than in older patients. Fractures of the lower ribs (10 to 12) should increase suspicion for hepatosplenic injury.

Localized pain, tenderness on palpation, and crepitus are present in rib injury patients. A palpable or visible deformity suggests rib fractures. A chest roentgenogram should be obtained primarily to exclude other intrathoracic injuries and not just to identify rib fractures. Fractures of anterior cartilages or separation of costochondral junctions have the same implications as rib fractures, but will not be seen on the roentgenographic examinations. Special rib technique roentgenograms are expensive, may not detect all rib injuries, add nothing to treatment, require painful positioning of the patient, and are not useful. Taping, rib belts, and external splints are contraindicated. Relief of pain is important to enable adequate ventilation. Intercostal block, epidural anesthesia, and systemic analgesics may be necessary.

F. Other Indications for Chest Tube Insertion

1. Selected patients with suspected severe lung injury, especially those being transferred by air or ground vehicle

2. Individuals undergoing general anesthesia for treatment of other injuries (eg, cranial or extremity), who have suspected significant lung injury

3. Individuals requiring positive pressure ventilation who are suspected of having substantial chest injury

VI. Summary

Thoracic trauma is common in the multiple-injured patient and can be associated with life-threatening problems. These patients can usually be treated or their conditions temporarily relieved by relatively simple measures such as intubation, ventilation, tube thoracostomy, and needle pericardiocentesis. The ability to recognize these important injuries and the skill to perform the necessary procedures can be life-saving.

Bibliography

1. Blair E, Topuzulu C, Deane RS: Major chest trauma. **Current Problems in Surgery** May 1969;2-69.

2. DelRossi AJ (ed): Blunt thoracic trauma. **Trauma Quarterly** 1990;6(3):1-74.

3. Eddy AL, Rusch VW, Marchioro T, et al: Treatment of traumatic rupture of the thoracic aorta: a 15-year experience. **Archives of Surgery** 1990;125:1351-1356.

4. Evans J, Gray LA Jr, Rayner A, et al: Principles for management of penetrating cardiac wounds. **Annals of Surgery** 1970;189(6):777-784.

5. Graham JG, Mattox KL, Beall AC Jr: Penetrating trauma of the lung. **Journal of Trauma** 1979;19:665.

6. Hiatt JR, Yeatman LA Jr, Child JS: The value of echocardiography in blunt chest trauma. **Journal of Trauma** 1988;28:914-920.

7. Jones KW: Thoracic trauma. **Surgical Clinics of North America** 1980;60-957.

8. Liedtke AJ, DeMuth WE: Nonpenetrating cardiac injuries: a collective review. **American Heart Journal** 1973;86:687.

9. Marnocha KE, Maglinte DDT, Woods J, et al: Blunt chest trauma and suspected aortic rupture: reliability of chest radiograph findings. **Annals of Emergency Medicine** 1985;14(7):644-649.

10. Mulder DS, Schennid H, Angood P: Thoracic injuries. In Maull KI, Cleveland HC, Strauch GO, et al (eds): **Trauma Volume 1**, Chicago, Illinois, Yearbook, 1986.

11. Ramzy AI, Rodriguez A, Turney SZ: Management of major tracheobronchial ruptures in patients with multiple system trauma. **Journal of Trauma** 1988;28:914-920.

12. Richardson JD, Adams L, Flint LM: Selective management of flail chest and pulmonary contusion. **Annals of Surgery** 1982;196

13. Shannon FL, Moore EE, Moore JB: Emergency department thoracotomy. In Moore EE, Mattox KL, Feliciano DV (eds): **Trauma**, East Norwalk, Connecticut, Appleton-Lange, 1988.

14. Snow N, Lucas AE, Richardson JD: Intra-aortic balloon counterpulsation for cardiogenic shock from cardiac contusion. **Journal of Trauma** 1982;22(5):426-429.

Chapter 4:
Thoracic
Trauma

American College of Surgeons

Skill Station VI:
Roentgenographic Identification of Thoracic Injuries

Resources and Equipment

This list is the recommended equipment to conduct this skill session in accordance with the stated objectives for and intent of the procedures outlined. Additional equipment may be used providing it does not detract from the stated objectives and intent of this skill or from performing the procedure in a safe method as described and recommended by the ACS Committee on Trauma.

1. Thoracic roentgenograms (available from the ACS, ATLS Division)

2. Identification key to roentgenograms

3. View boxes to display films

Objectives

1. Upon completion of this station, the participant will be able to identify various thoracic injuries by using six specific anatomic guidelines for examining a series of chest roentgenograms.

    a. Soft tissues of the chest wall

    b. Bony thorax

    c. Pleural spaces and lung parenchyma

    d. Trachea and bronchi

    e. Diaphragm

    f. Mediastinum

2. Given a series of roentgenograms, the participant will be able to:

    a. Diagnose fractures.

    b. Delineate associated injuries.

    c. Define other areas of possible injury.

**Chapter 4:
Thoracic
Trauma**

**Skill
Station VI**

American College of Surgeons

Skill Procedure

Roentgenographic Identification of Thoracic Injuries

Note: Chest roentgenograms are obtained during the primary survey/resuscitation phase or the secondary survey, based on the urgency of the patient's condition. Six-foot, upright films provide better anatomic detail of the chest; however, practicality and safety dictate that anterioposterior (AP), supine films are adequate for identifying injuries in the potentially or obviously unstable patient. For example, when the patient's torso or neck has been injured or when the unconscious patient is at risk of aspirating, an AP supine roentgenogram should be obtained. A lateral thoracic film may be necessary to identify a suspected sternal fracture.

A systematic review of the roentgenogram must be performed, preferably using a view box. The anatomic guidelines outlined herein identify areas in the thorax that should be assessed when examining a chest film. Each of these areas should be assessed for potential injury when viewing the specific roentgenograms associated with this skill station. (See Resource Document 5, Roentgenographic Studies.)

I. Soft Tissues

Assess for:

1. Displacement or disruption of tissue planes

2. Evidence of subcutaneous air

II. Bony Thorax

A. Clavicle

Assess for evidence of:

1. Fracture

2. Associated injury, eg, great vessel injury

B. Scapula

Assess for evidence of:

1. Fracture

2. Associated injury, eg, airway or great vessel injury, pulmonary contusion

C. Ribs

1. Ribs 1 through 3: Assess for evidence of:

    a. Fracture

    b. Associated injury, eg, pneumothorax, major airway or great vessel injury

2. Ribs 4 through 9: Assess for evidence of:

   a. Fracture, especially in two or more contiguous ribs in two places (flail chest)

   b. Associated injury, eg, pneumothorax, hemothorax, pulmonary contusion

3. Ribs 9 through 12: Assess for evidence of:

   a. Fracture, especially in two or more places (flail chest)

   b. Associated injury, eg, pneumothorax, pulmonary contusion, spleen, liver, and/or kidney

D. Sternum

1. Assess the sternomandibular junction and sternal body for evidence of fracture. (Sternal fractures may be confused on the AP film as a mediastinal hematoma. After the patient is stabilized, a coned-down view, over-penetrated film, lateral view, or CT may be obtained to better illuminate a suspected sternal fracture.)

2. Assess for associated injuries, eg, myocardial contusion, great vessel injury (widened mediastinum).

III. Pleural Space and Lung Parenchyma

A. Pleural Space

1. Assess for abnormal collections of fluid that may represent a hemothorax.

2. Assess for abnormal collections of air that may represent a pneumotho-rax—usually seen as an apical lucent area absent of bronchial or vascu-lar markings.

B. Lung Parenchyma

1. Assess the lung fields for infiltrates that may suggest pulmonary contu-sion, hematoma, aspiration, etc. Pulmonary contusion appears as air space consolidation that can be irregular and patchy or homogenous, dif-fuse, or extensive.

2. Assess the parenchyma for evidence of laceration. Lacerations appear as a hematoma, vary according to the magnitude of injury, and appear as areas of consolidation.

IV. Trachea and Bronchi

A. Assess for the presence of interstitial or pleural air that may represent a large airway injury.

B. Assess for tracheal lacerations that may present as pneumomediastinum, pneumothorax, subcutaneous and interstitial emphysema of the neck, or pneumoperitoneum.

C. Assess for bronchial disruption that may present as a free pleural communication producing a massive pneumothorax with a persistent air leak that is unresponsive to tube thoracostomy.

V. Diaphragm

Diaphragmatic rupture requires a high index of suspicion, based on the mechanism of injury, the patient's signs and symptoms, and roentgenographic findings. Initial chest roentgenograms may not clearly identify a diaphragmatic injury. Sequential films or additional studies may be required.

A. Carefully evaluate the diaphragm for:

1. Elevation (may rise to fourth intercostal space with full expiration)

2. Disruption (stomach or bowel gas above the diaphragm)

3. Poor identification (irregular or obscure) due to overlying fluid or soft tissue masses

B. Roentgenographic changes suggesting injury include:

1. Elevation, irregularity, or obliteration of the diaphragm—segmental or total

2. Mass-like density above the diaphragm may be due to a fluid-filled bowel, omentum, liver, kidney, spleen, or pancreas (may appear as a "loculated pneumothorax")

3. Air or contrast-containing stomach or bowel above the diaphragm

4. Contralateral mediastinal shift

5. Widening of the cardiac silhouette if the peritoneal contents herniate into the pericardial sac

6. Pleural effusion

7. The inferior border of the liver may appear higher than expected; lower rib fractures, pulmonary contusions, and the appearance of foreign bodies in the chest cavity may be associated with diaphragmatic injury; eg, a nasogastric tube coiled in the chest may represent a stomach herniated into the thorax or a hole in the esophagus

C. Assess for associated injuries, eg, splenic, pancreatic, renal, and liver.

VI. Mediastinum

A. Assess for air or blood that may either displace mediastinal structures, blur the demarcation between tissue planes, or outline them with radiolucency.

B. Assess for radiologic signs associated with cardiac or major vascular injury.

    1. Air or blood in the pericardium may result in an enlarged cardiac silhouette. Progressive changes in the cardiac size may represent an expanding pneumopericardium or hemopericardium.

    2. Aortic rupture may be suggested by:

        a. Widened mediastinum—most reliable finding

        b. Fractures of the first and second ribs

        c. Obliteration of the aortic knob

        d. Deviation of the trachea to the right

        e. Presence of a pleural cap

        f. Elevation and rightward shift of the right mainstem bronchus

        g. Depression of the left mainstem bronchus

        h. Obliteration of the space between the pulmonary artery and the aorta

        i. Deviation of the esophagus (nasogastric tube) to the right

VII. Roentgenographic Reassessment

After careful, systematic evaluation of the initial chest film, additional roentgenograms or radiographic studies may be necessary as historical facts or physical findings dictate. For example, repeat chest films may be indicated if significant changes in the patient's status develop. Computed tomography and arteriography may be indicated for specificity of diagnosis.

Table 1
Chest Roentgenographic Suggestions

Abnormal Findings	Diagnoses to Consider
Any rib fracture	Pneumothorax
Fracture, first 3 ribs	Airway or great vessel injury
Lower ribs, 9 to 12	Abdominal injury
Two or more rib fractures in two or more places	Flail chest, pulmonary contusion
GI gas pattern in the chest (loculated air)	Diaphragmatic rupture
NG tube in the chest	Diaphragmatic rupture or ruptured esophagus
Air fluid level in the chest	Hemothorax or diaphragmatic rupture
Sternal fracture	Myocardial contusion, head injury, c-spine injury
Mediastinal hematoma	Great vessel injury, sternal fracture
Disrupted diaphragm	Abdominal visceral injury
Respiratory distress without roentgenographic findings	CNS injury, aspiration
Persistent large pneumothorax after chest tube insertion	Bronchial tear, esophageal disruption
Mediastinal air	Esophageal disruption, pneumoperitoneum, tracheal injury
Scapular fracture	Airway or great vessel injury, or pulmonary contusion
Free air under the diaphragm	Ruptured hollow abdominal viscus

**Chapter 4:
Thoracic
Trauma**

**Skill
Station VI**

American College of Surgeons

Skill Station VII:
Chest Trauma Management

These surgical procedures, if performed on a live, anesthetized animal, must be conducted in a USDA-Registered Animal Laboratory Facility. (See *ATLS*® *Instructor Manual*, Section II, Chapter 9—Policies, Procedures, and Protocols for Surgical Skills Practicum.)

Resources and Equipment

This list is the recommended equipment to conduct this skill session in accordance with the stated objectives for and intent of the procedures outlined. Additional equipment may be used providing it does not detract from the stated objectives and intent of this skill, or from performing the procedure in a safe method as described and recommended by the ACS Committee on Trauma.

1. Live, anesthetized animals

2. Licensed veterinarian (see guidelines referenced above)

3. Animal troughs, ropes (sandbags optional)

4. Animal intubation equipment

    a. Endotracheal tubes
    b. Laryngoscope blade and handle
    c. Respirator with 15-mm adapter

5. Electric shears with #40 blade

6. Tables or instrument stands

7. Needles and catheters

    a. Assorted #14-gauge over-the-needle catheters (3 to 6 cm in length)
    b. #18-gauge spinal needles (5 to 6 inches or 12.7 to 15.2 cm in length)
    c. #22-gauge spinal needles (5 to 6 inches or 12.7 to 15.2 cm in length)
    d. Pericardiocentesis catheter kit (optional)

8. Syringes

    a. 6-mL syringes
    b. 12-mL syringes
    c. 35-mL syringes, plastic and glass

9. Suture

    a. 2-0 and 3-0 silk with cutting needle
    b. 2-0 and 3-0 silk with taper needle
    c. 4-0 Monofilament/noncutting needle (optional)

10. Drugs

    a. Lidocaine 1% (optional)
    b. Heparin 1:1000 (optional)

11. Chest tubes without trocars—#32-French (for animal use); #36-40 French (for patient use)

12. 3x3 or 4x4 gauze sponges

13. One-inch (2.5 cm) adhesive tape

14. Underwater seal device

15. Small basin for water to inject into the pericardial sac (methylene-blue dye may be added to the water for a more dramatic appearance when performing pericardiocentesis)

16. Flutter-type valve

17. Three-way stopcocks

18. Surgical instruments

    a.   Scalpel handles with #10 and #11 blades
    b.   Needle holders
    c.   Small Finochetti chest retractors or small self-retaining chest retractors
    d.   Mosquitoes
    e.   Heavy curved scissors
    f.   Suture scissors
    g.   Metsenbaum curved dissecting scissors
    h.   Tissue forceps—with and without teeth

19. Antiseptic swabs

20. Surgical drapes (optional)

21. Electrocardiographic monitor (optional)

22. Surgical garb (gloves, shoe covers, and scrub suits or cover gowns)

Objectives

1. Performance at this station will allow the participant to practice and demonstrate on a live, anesthetized animal the techniques of inserting a chest needle and chest tube for the emergency care of hemothoraces and/or pneumothoraces.

2. Upon completion of this station, the participant will be able to describe the surface markings and technique for pleural decompression with needle thoracentesis and chest tube insertion.

3. Upon completion of this station, the participant will be able to discuss the underlying pathophysiology of cardiac tamponade as a result of trauma.

4. Upon completion of this station, the participant will be able to describe the surface markings and technique for pericardiocentesis.

5. Performance at this station will allow the participant to practice and demonstrate on a live, anesthetized animal the technique of inserting a needle into the pericardium (peri-cardiocentesis) for the emergency treatment of cardiac tamponade or hemopericardium.

6. Upon completion of this station, the participant will be able to discuss the complications of needle thoracentesis, chest tube insertion, and pericardiocentesis.

Procedures

1. Needle thoracentesis
2. Chest tube insertion
3. Pericardiocentesis

Skills Procedures
Chest Trauma Management

Note: Universal precautions are required whenever caring for the trauma patient.

I.   Needle Thoracentesis

Note: This procedure is for the rapidly deteriorating critical patient who has a life-threatening tension pneumothorax. If this technique is used and the patient does not have a tension pneumothorax, a pneumothorax and/or damage to the lung may occur.

A. Assess the patient's chest and respiratory status.

B. Administer high-flow oxygen and ventilate as necessary.

C. Identify the second intercostal space, in the midclavicular line on the side of the tension pneumothorax.

D. Surgically prepare the chest.

E. Locally anesthetize the area if the patient is conscious or if time permits.

F. Place the patient in an upright position if a cervical spine injury has been excluded.

G. Keeping the Luer-Lok in the distal end of the catheter, insert an over-the-needle catheter (3 to 6 cm long) into the skin and direct the needle just over (ie, superior to) the rib into the intercostal space.

H. Puncture the parietal pleura.

I. Remove the Luer-Lok from the catheter and listen for a sudden escape of air when the needle enters the parietal pleura, indicating that the tension pneumothorax has been relieved.

J. Remove the needle and replace the Luer-Lok in the distal end of the catheter. Leave the plastic catheter in place and apply a bandage or small dressing over the insertion site.

K. Prepare for a chest-tube insertion, if necessary. The chest tube should be inserted at the nipple level anterior to the midaxillary line of the affected hemothorax.

L. Connect the chest tube to an underwater seal device or a flutter-type-valve apparatus and remove the catheter used to relieve the tension pneumothorax initially.

M. Obtain a chest roentgenogram.

Complications of Needle Thoracentesis

1. Local cellulitis
2. Local hematoma
3. Pleural infection, empyema
4. Pneumothorax

II. Chest Tube Insertion

A. Fluid resuscitation via at least one, large-caliber intravenous catheter, and monitoring of vital signs should be in process.

B. Determine the insertion site—usually the nipple level (5th intercostal space) anterior to the midaxillary line on the affected side. A second chest tube may be used for a hemothorax.

C. Surgically prepare and drape the chest at the predetermined site of the tube insertion.

D. Locally anesthetize the skin and rib periosteum.

E. Make a 2- to 3-cm transverse (horizontal) incision at the predetermined site and bluntly dissect through the subcutaneous tissues, just over the top of the rib.

F. Puncture the parietal pleura with the tip of a clamp and put a gloved finger into the incision to avoid injury to other organs and to clear any adhesions, clots, etc.

G. Clamp the proximal end of the thoracostomy tube and advance the thoracostomy tube into the pleural space to the desired length.

H. Look for "fogging" of the chest tube with expiration or listen for air movement.

I. Connect the end of the thoracostomy tube to an underwater-seal apparatus.

J. Suture the tube in place.

K. Apply a dressing, and tape the tube to the chest.

L. Obtain a chest roentgenogram.

M. Obtain arterial blood gas values as necessary.

Complications of Chest Tube Insertion

1. Anaphylactic or allergic reaction to surgical preparation or anesthetic

2. Chest tube dislodgment from the chest wall or disconnection from the underwater-seal apparatus

3. Chest bottle elevated above the level of the chest, and fluid flows into the chest cavity

4. Chest tube kinking or clogging

5. Damage to the intercostal nerve, artery, or vein

   a. Converting a pneumothorax to a hemopneumothorax
   b. Resulting in intercostal neuritis/neuralgia

6. Damage to internal mammary vessels if puncture is too medial, resulting in hemopneumothorax

7. Incorrect tube position, extrathoracic or intrathoracic

8. Intercostal myalgia

9. Introduction of pleural infection (eg, thoracic empyema)

10. Laceration or puncture of intrathoracic and/or abdominal organs, all of which can be prevented by using the finger technique before inserting the chest tube

    a. Heart
    b. Lung
    c. Esophagus
    d. Aorta
    e. Pulmonary artery
    f. Pulmonary vein
    g. Long thoracic nerve
    h. Mediastinum
    i. Liver
    j. Spleen

11. Leaky underwater-seal apparatus

12. Local cellulitis

13. Local hematoma

14. Mediastinal emphysema

15. Persistent pneumothorax

    a. Large primary leak
    b. Leak at the skin around the chest tube; suction on tube too strong
    c. Leaky underwater-seal apparatus

16. Subcutaneous emphysema (usually at tube site)

17. Recurrence of pneumothorax upon removal of chest tube; seal of thoracostomy wound not immediate

18. Lung fails to expand due to plugged bronchus; bronchoscopy required

III. Pericardiocentesis

A. Monitor the patient's vital signs, CVP, and ECG before, during, and after the procedure.

B. Surgically prepare the xiphoid and subxiphoid areas, if time allows.

C. Locally anesthetize the puncture site, if necessary.

D. Using a #16- to #18-gauge, 6-inch (15 cm) or longer over-the-needle catheter, attach a 35-mL empty syringe with a three-way stopcock.

E. Assess the patient for any mediastinal shift that may have caused the heart to shift significantly.

F. Puncture the skin 1 to 2 cm inferior to the left of the xiphochondral junction, at a 45-degree angle to the skin.

G. Carefully advance the needle cephalad and aim toward the tip of the left scapula.

H. If the needle is advanced too far (into the ventricular muscle) an injury pattern (eg, extreme ST-T wave changes or widened and enlarged QRS complex) appears on the ECG monitor. This pattern indicates that the pericardiocentesis needle should be withdrawn until the previous baseline ECG tracing reappears. Premature ventricular contractions also may occur, secondary to irritation of the ventricular myocardium.

I. When the needle tip enters the blood-filled pericardial sac, withdraw as much nonclotted blood as possible.

J. During the aspiration, the epicardium reapproaches the inner pericardial surface, as does the needle tip. Subsequently, an ECG injury pattern may reappear. This indicates that the pericardiocentesis needle should be withdrawn slightly. Should this injury pattern persist, withdraw the needle completely.

K. After aspiration is completed, remove the syringe, and attach a three-way stopcock, leaving the stopcock closed. Secure the catheter in place.

L. Should the cardiac tamponade symptoms persist, the stopcock may be opened and the pericardial sac reaspirated. The plastic pericardiocentesis needle can be sutured or taped in place and covered with a small dressing to allow for continued decompression en route to surgery or transfer to another care facility.

Complications of Pericardiocentesis

1. Aspiration of ventricle blood instead of pericardial blood
2. Cellulitis
3. Laceration of coronary artery or vein
4. Laceration of ventricular epicardium/myocardium
5. New hemopericardium, secondary to lacerations of the coronary artery or vein, and/or ventricular epicardium/myocardium
6. Local hematoma
7. Pericarditis
8. Ventricular fibrillation
9. Pneumothorax, secondary to lung puncture
10. Puncture of aorta
11. Puncture of inferior vena cava
12. Puncture of esophagus
13. Mediastinitis secondary to puncture of esophagus
14. Puncture of peritoneum
15. Peritonitis, secondary to puncture of peritoneum

Chapter 5:
Abdominal Trauma

Objectives:

Upon completion of this topic, the physician will be able to identify the differences in the patterns of abdominal trauma based on injury mechanism, and to establish management priorities accordingly. Specifically, the physician will be able to:

A. Describe the anatomic regions of the abdomen.

B. Discuss the difference between blunt and penetrating abdominal injury patterns.

C. Identify the signs suggesting retroperitoneal, intraperitoneal, and pelvic injury.

D. Outline the diagnostic and therapeutic procedures specific to abdominal trauma.

E. Discuss diagnostic peritoneal lavage and demonstrate the ability to perform this procedure during the surgical practicum.

Chapter 5:
Abdominal
Trauma

I. Introduction

A. High Index of Suspicion

Unrecognized abdominal injury remains a distressingly frequent cause of preventable death after trauma. Peritoneal signs are often subtle, overshadowed by pain from associated extra-abdominal trauma, or masked by head injury or intoxicants. As many as 20% of patients with acute hemoperitoneum have benign abdominal findings when first examined in the emergency department. Moreover, the peritoneal cavity is a potential reservoir for major occult blood loss. Any patient sustaining significant deceleration injury or a penetrating torso wound must be assumed to have an abdominal visceral injury.

B. Regions of the Abdomen

The abdomen has three distinct anatomic compartments—peritoneal cavity, retroperitoneal space, and pelvis.

The **upper abdomen** is that portion of the peritoneal cavity covered by the bony thorax, and includes the diaphragm, liver, spleen, stomach, and transverse colon. The diaphragm may rise to the fourth intercostal space with full expiration, rendering the viscera at risk after lower chest trauma—particularly penetrating wounds. Fractures of the lower ribs should increase suspicion for hepatosplenic injury.

The **lower abdomen** contains the small bowel and remaining portion of the intra-abdominal colon.

The **retroperitoneal space** contains the aorta, vena cava, pancreas, kidneys, ureters, and portions of the colon and duodenum. Injuries to the retroperitoneal viscera are notoriously difficult to recognize because the area is remote from physical examination and not sampled by peritoneal lavage.

The **pelvis** contains the rectum, bladder, iliac vessels, and in women, the internal genitalia. Early diagnosis of trauma to these structures is similarly compromised because of anatomic location.

II. Assessment

The primary factor in assessing abdominal trauma is not the accurate diagnosis of a specific type of injury, but rather the determination that an abdominal injury exists.

A. History

Details of the incident are particularly helpful in the initial evaluation of blunt multisystem and penetrating trauma. The patient, if conscious, is best prepared to provide most of this information. However, the prehospital care personnel and police may provide critical insight into timing, mechanisms, initial patient presentation, and response to treatment, etc.

B. Physical Examination

The abdominal examination should be conducted in a meticulous, systematic fashion in the standard sequence; ie, inspection, auscultation, percussion, and palpation. These findings, whether positive or negative, should be documented carefully in the medical records.

1. Inspection

The patient must be fully undressed. The anterior and posterior abdomen as well as the lower chest and perineum should be inspected for abrasions, contusions, lacerations, and penetrating wounds. The patient can be **cautiously** log-rolled to facilitate complete examination. (See Chapter 7, Spine and Spinal Cord Trauma, and Skill Station XI, Immobilization Techniques for Neck and Spinal Trauma.)

2. Auscultation

The abdomen should be auscultated for the presence or absence of bowel sounds. Free intraperitoneal blood or enteric contents may produce ileus, resulting in loss of bowel sounds. However, ileus also may occur from extra-abdominal injuries, ie, rib, spine, and pelvic fractures.

3. Percussion

Percussion of the abdomen after injury is done primarily to elicit subtle rebound tenderness. This maneuver generates slight motion of the peritoneum and produces a response similar to asking the patient to cough.

4. Palpation

Palpation of the abdomen results in subjective as well as objective information. Subjective findings include the patient's assessment of pain location as well as magnitude. Early pain is usually visceral in origin, and therefore, poorly localized. Voluntary tensing of the abdominal musculature results from the fear of pain and may not represent significant injury. Involuntary muscle guarding, on the other hand, is a reliable sign of peritoneal irritation. Similarly, unequivocal rebound tenderness indicates established peritonitis.

5. Rectal examination

Digital rectal examination is an important component of the abdominal assessment. Major assessment goals for penetrating wounds are to search for blood that may indicate bowel perforation and to ascertain sphincter tone to assess spinal integrity. After blunt trauma, the rectal wall also should be palpated to detect fractured bony elements and prostate position. A high-riding prostate may indicate posterior urethral disruption.

6. Vaginal examination

Laceration of the vagina may occur from penetrating wounds or bony fragments from pelvic fracture(s). The implications of vaginal bleeding in the pregnant patient are reviewed in Chapter 11, Trauma in Pregnancy.

7. Penile examination

Laceration of the urethra should be suspected if blood is present at the urethral meatus.

A positive physical examination is the most reliable clinical sign of significant intra-abdominal trauma. Conversely, a negative physical examination does not preclude significant intra-abdominal injury. For many patients, abdominal examination may not be diagnostic because of confounding factors or the early absence of clinical signs that may become obvious during subsequent examinations.

C. Intubation

1. Nasogastric tube

Nasogastric intubation is both therapeutic and diagnostic. The primary goal is to remove stomach contents—reducing gastric volume, pressure, and the risk of aspirating gastric contents. The presence of blood in the gastric secretions may suggest upper gastrointestinal tract injury if nasopharyngeal sources are excluded. **Caution:** If severe facial fractures exist, the nasogastric tube should be introduced via the mouth to prevent unintentional intracranial insertion of the tube through a cribriform plate fracture.

2. Bladder catheter

The indwelling urinary catheter serves multiple purposes. The major function is to decompress the bladder and allow for urinary output monitoring as an index of tissue perfusion. Hematuria is an important sign of potential genitourinary trauma, the implications of which are discussed later in this chapter. Consideration also may be given to obtaining a urine drug screen. **Caution:** An examination of the rectum and genitalia should be performed before inserting the urinary catheter, because related findings may contraindicate its placement. A high-riding prostate, blood at the urethral meatus, or scrotal hematoma are contraindications to placing a transurethral bladder catheter until retrograde urethrography confirms an intact urethra.

D. Blood Sampling

Blood should be withdrawn from one of the initial venous access sites and sent to the laboratory for immediate analysis. Blood typing and crossmatching should be performed for the severely injured patient. Laboratory screening for suspected abdominal injury includes a hematocrit, white blood cell count with differential, amylase, urinalysis, pregnancy testing for all females of childbearing age, and alcohol and/or other drug determinations. These baseline tests are important because subsequent changes may be the first sign of occult injury, particularly in the retroperitoneum.

E. Roentgenographic Studies

1. Screening roentgenograms

Roentgenographic studies must be tailored to the patient's overall status as well as injury mechanism. The crosstable lateral cervical spine, anteroposterior chest, and pelvis films take precedence in multisystem blunt trauma. On occasion, abdominal films also may be helpful in identifying abdominal injury. Free air under the diaphragm or extraluminal air in the retroperitoneum signals hollow visceral disruption, and mandates prompt celiotomy. Loss of psoas shadow may suggest retroperitoneal injury. Such roentgenographic studies also should be viewed for bony injuries associated with abdominal injuries. (See Table 1, Associated Injuries.)

Table 1
Associated Injuries

Bony Injuries	Associated Injuries
Lower rib fractures	Liver and/or spleen
Lower thoracic spine injuries	Pancreas, small bowel
Lumbar transverse process fractures	Abdominal viscera, kidneys
Pelvic fractures	Pelvic organ or vessels Retroperitoneal

2. Contrast studies

a. Urethrography

Urethrography should be performed before inserting an indwelling urinary catheter when a urethral tear is suspected. The urethrogram can be performed with a #12-French urinary catheter secured in the meatal fossa by balloon inflation to three milliliters. Undiluted contrast material is instilled with gentle pressure.

b. Cystography

Bladder rupture is established with a gravity flow cystogram. A bulb syringe attached to the indwelling bladder catheter is held 15 cm above the patient, and 250 to 300 mL of water-soluble contrast is allowed to flow into the bladder. Anteroposterior, oblique, and postdrainage views are essential to definitively exclude injury. The order of intravenous pyelogram (IVP) versus cystography is governed by the index of suspicion for upper versus lower tract injury.

c. Excretory urogram

An IVP may be valuable in initial renal evaluation. High-dose intravenous bolus injection should provide evidence of relative kidney function at 5 to 10 minutes. Unilateral nonfunction implies massive parenchymal shattering or vascular pedicle interruption, but may be due to an absent kidney. Nonfunction warrants further surgical evaluation.

In the stable patient, computed tomography (CT) is preferable to the IVP if there is the suspicion of other intra-abdominal and/or retroperitoneal injuries. Intravenous contrast studies should not be performed in the hypotensive, unstable patient.

d. Gastrointestinal

Isolated retroperitoneal gastrointestinal injuries, ie, duodenum, ascending and descending colon, and rectum may not manifest peritoneal signs or abnormalities on diagnostic peritoneal lavage. When these injuries are suspected, specific upper and lower gastrointestinal contrast studies may identify them.

F. Special Diagnostic Studies

If there is early or obvious evidence that the patient will be transferred to another facility, time-consuming tests should **not** be performed. These tests include contrast urologic and gastrointestinal studies, peritoneal lavage, or computed tomography.

Peritoneal lavage or computed tomography should be done for the multiply injured patient if the abdominal examination is:

a. Equivocal (fractured lower ribs, and pelvic and lumbar spine fracture may obscure findings)

b. Unreliable due to head injury, intoxicants, or paraplegia

c. Impractical because of anticipated lengthy roentgenographic studies (angiography) or general anesthesia for extra-abdominal injuries

(See Table 2, Diagnostic Peritoneal Lavage versus Computed Tomography.)

1. Diagnostic peritoneal lavage

Peritoneal lavage is an operative procedure that significantly alters subsequent examinations of the patient and is considered 98% sensitive for intraperitoneal bleeding. Ideally, the procedure should be performed by the surgeon caring for the patient.

The necessity for emergent celiotomy in the patient with multisystem trauma may be difficult to establish and must be sequenced properly among other potential life-saving procedures. For this reason, diagnostic peritoneal lavage (DPL) is a critical step in the evaluation of the severely injured trauma patient.

Since the abdomen, without appearing abnormal, may sequester large amounts of blood, peritoneal lavage should be performed early to evaluate the hypotensive patient. If gross blood is not found, the cause of the patient's hypotension may be an extra-abdominal injury which redirects the focus of the diagnostic and management processes.

The only absolute contraindication to the procedure is an existing indication for celiotomy. Relative contraindications of a DPL include previous abdominal operations, morbid obesity, advanced cirrhosis, and established pre-existing coagulopathy. The use of DPL in advanced pregnancy is controversial. If used, the procedure should be performed superior to the enlarged uterus by the open technique.

If a positive DPL will result in the patient's transfer, the procedure should be done by the referring physician. Any lavage fluid obtained should be sent with the patient. Diagnostic peritoneal lavage has a small but real incidence of technical complications and should be performed only by experienced personnel. The open technique is advocated as a rapid and safe method for performing diagnostic peritoneal lavage. However, the method of employing the Seldinger technique is a suitable alternative to be employed by trained physicians.

2. Computed tomography

Diagnostic peritoneal lavage can be performed rapidly and without delay in the emergency department. By comparison, CT requires transport of the patient to the scan area and time to perform the examination. A complete CT examination, usually using both intravenous and oral contrast material, must include the upper abdomen and pelvis. Therefore, the CT scan should be performed only on stable patients in whom there is no apparent indication for immediate operation. The CT scan provides information relative to specific organ injury and its extent, and also can diagnose retroperitoneal and pelvic organ injuries which are difficult to assess by a physical examination or peritoneal lavage.

Caution: CT may miss some gastrointestinal injuries. In the absence of liver or splenic injuries, the presence of free fluid in the abdominal cavity suggests an injury to the gastrointestinal tract and/or its mesentery, and mandates early surgical intervention.

Table 2
Diagnostic Peritoneal Lavage versus Computed Tomography

	DPL	CT Scan
Time	Faster	
Transport		Required
Sensitive	Greater	
Specific		Greater
Safe	All patients	Stable patients

III. Indications for Celiotomy

1. Hypotension with evidence of abdominal injury

   a. Gunshot wounds
   b. Stab wounds
   c. Blunt trauma with gross blood on DPL

2. Peritonitis—early or subsequent

3. Recurrent hypotension despite adequate resuscitation

4. Extraluminal air

5. Injured diaphragm

6. Intraperitoneal perforation of urinary bladder on cystography

7. CT evidence of injury to the pancreas, gastrointestinal tract, and specific injuries to the liver, spleen, and/or kidney

8. Positive contrast study of upper and lower gastrointestinal tracts

9. Persistent amylase elevation with abdominal findings

IV. Special Problems

A. Blunt Trauma

The abdominal injury pattern of blunt trauma is much different from that of penetrating wounds. Blunt vehicular trauma results from rapid changes in speed in which visceral disruption may occur from a direct blow, shear forces, or closed-loop phenomenon. The liver, spleen, and kidney are the organs predominantly involved following blunt trauma, although the relative incidence of hollow visceral perforation and lumbar spinal injuries increases with incorrect seat belt usage.

Abdominal injury resulting from blunt trauma is difficult to assess and diagnose. The multiplicity of organ systems, alterations in the patient's level of consciousness, and/or variables in prehospital and emergency department care can mask or alter the physical findings of abdominal injuries. Physical findings are often subtle and require a high index of suspicion based on the mechanism of injury. The abdominal examination should be conducted in a meticulous, systematic fashion as previously described. Some injuries are visible on physical examination; others may require more specific studies to be identified.

1. Diaphragm

Blunt tears may occur in any portion of either diaphragm and may involve the pericardium. The most common injury is 5 to 10 cm in length, involving the posterolateral left hemidiaphragm. Abnormalities on the initial chest roentgenogram are usually nonspecific but may be heralded by hemothorax. The position of the nasogastric tube may identify an otherwise occult left-sided tear; a tube above the diaphragm is pathognomonic.

2. Duodenum

Duodenal rupture is classically encountered in the intoxicated, unrestrained driver involved in a frontal-impact motor vehicular accident or by a blow to the abdomen by bicycle handlebars. A bloody nasogastric aspirate or retroperitoneal air should raise one's suspicion. Duodenal "C-loop" diatrizoate meglumine (Gastrografin) studies or double-contrast CT is indicated for the high-risk patient.

3. Pancreas

Pancreatic injury most often results from a direct epigastric blow compressing the organ against the vertebral column. A normal serum amylase level does not exclude major pancreatic trauma; conversely, the amylase level may be elevated from nonpancreatic sources. Even double-contrast CT may not identify significant pancreatic trauma in the immediate postinjury period.

4. Genitourinary

Direct blows to the back or flank resulting in contusions, hematomas, or ecchymosis are markers of potential underlying renal injury. Fractures of posterior lower ribs or spinal transverse processes increase this probability. Similarly, perineal hematomas and anterior pelvic fractures suggest bladder or urethral trauma. Blood at the urethral meatus or the inability to void are overt signs of lower urinary tract injury. Urethral disruptions are divided into those above (posterior) or below (anterior) the urogenital diaphragm. Posterior urethral trauma usually occurs in patients with multisystem injuries and pelvic fracture(s). Anterior urethral injury is due to a straddle impact and may be an isolated injury. Blunt renal artery thrombosis is infrequent and renal pedicle disruption is rare; both lesions may not produce hematuria. In the conscious patient they are associated with severe abdominal pain.

5. Small bowel

Blunt injury to the intestines generally results from sudden deceleration with subsequent tearing near a fixed point of attachment, especially if the patient's seat belt was applied incorrectly. The appearance of transverse, linear ecchymosis on the abdominal wall (seat belt sign) or the presence of an anterior lumbar compression fracture on roentgenogram should alert the physician to the possibility of intestinal injury. Diagnosis may be difficult, especially since minimal bleeding may result from torn intestinal organs. CT is often not diagnostic.

B. Penetrating Trauma

Penetrating injuries may involve indirect effects, such as blast or cavitation, as well as the injury incurred as a result of the anatomic course of the weapon or object inflicting the wound. The injury pattern correlates with the relative size of the abdominal viscera and their proximity to the entrance site. As expected, liver, small bowel, colon, and stomach are commonly involved. Stab injuries traverse adjacent structures, whereas gunshot wounds may have a circuitous trajectory, injuring multiple noncontiguous organs.

Valuable facts in the assessment of penetrating injuries include time of injury, type of weapon, distance from the assailant (particularly for shotgun wounds), number of stab attempts or shots taken, and the amount of blood at the scene. The patient, if conscious, is best prepared to provide most of this information, but police also may glean these data from their preliminary investigation.

Penetrating wounds, particularly gunshot wounds, to the back, flank, or pelvis may produce occult urologic or colon injury. Some perforations of the ureter and bladder may not exhibit hematuria.

1. Lower chest wounds

The lower chest is defined as the area between the fourth intercostal space anteriorly (nipple line), the seventh intercostal space posteriorly (scapular tip), and the costal margins. Because the diaphragm rises to the fourth intercostal space during full expiration, penetrating wounds to this region may involve the underlying abdominal viscera. The safest policy may be celiotomy for lower chest gunshot wounds, while some surgeons may manage stab wounds nonoperatively.

2. Flank and back wounds

Penetrating injuries in the retroperitoneum are particularly difficult to evaluate because of their secluded anatomic location. An overlooked colon perforation can be fatal. The risk of visceral injury following back or flank penetration is significant.

C. Pelvic Fractures and Associated Injuries

Most severe pelvic injuries result from auto-pedestrian, motorcycle, or high-fall incidents. Mortality rates from open pelvic fractures may exceed 50%.

Major hemorrhage from pelvic fractures is an extremely difficult management problem. The large bones of the pelvis have a generous blood supply, and the fractured bone bleeds. The major muscle groups surrounding these bones also are very vascular and may bleed when the pelvis is fractured. Numerous large veins attend the pelvis and are at high risk for disruption. Major arterial injury from pelvic trauma can lead to exsanguinating hemorrhage.

Physical examination should include careful inspection of the perineum for ecchymosis or open wounds, and systematic compression of the bony pelvis. Rectal and genitourinary injuries must be suspected and excluded in all patients with pelvic fractures. Sacral plexus injuries are common. Major hemorrhage usually is associated with posterior pelvic disruption. Single roentgenographic views of the pelvis may underestimate the extent of these injuries, particularly of the posterior elements.

Hypotension in the patient with pelvic fractures represents a difficult problem. The pelvic fracture is rarely an isolated phenomenon. The hypotension may be associated with extrapelvic injury. The patient's hypotension should be the focus of the diagnostic and treatment processes. Causes for blood loss may include:

1. Intra-abdominal from organ or visceral injuries
2. Life-threatening thoracic injuries
3. Retroperitoneal or pelvic vascular injuries
4. Hemorrhage associated with fractured pelvic bones

Initial management priorities in the hypotensive patient with a fractured pelvis include adequate volume replacement, careful hemodynamic monitoring, and a complete patient evaluation to exclude extrapelvic sources of blood loss. Peritoneal lavage should be performed above the umbilicus to avoid the hematoma that frequently extends from the pelvis into the lower anterior abdominal wall. The free flow of **gross blood** indicates an intraperitoneal injury requiring emergency celiotomy. A **positive diagnostic lavage by RBC count** must be interpreted cautiously. Approximately 15% of these patients may not have intraperitoneal injuries, but rather leakage from the retroperitoneal hematoma. If properly performed, **negative peritoneal lavage** reliably excludes serious intraperitoneal bleeding. If the pelvis is unstable, consultation should be obtained for concurrent orthopedic care. Once intraperitoneal bleeding has been controlled, pelvic stabilization, often with an external fixator, can be done without delay.

If significant intraperitoneal bleeding can be excluded by the absence of gross blood on peritoneal lavage, if no distant bleeding source is present (chest, extremities, etc.), and if the patient's hemodynamic stability is not restored by fluid resuscitation, it can be assumed that continuing blood loss is from the retroperitoneal pelvic injury. **In the vast majority of cases, this is due to low-pressure bleeding from either the fracture site, adjacent soft tissue, or venous injuries.** This bleeding is most effectively controlled by stabilizing the pelvis and allowing the closed retroperitoneal space to tamponade. External pelvic fixation is the currently favored method of rapidly stabilizing a mechanically unstable pelvic ring. Until external pelvic fixation can be achieved in the hemodynamically unstable patient, a pneumatic anti-shock garment may be the best alternative, for temporary, emergent splinting of the pelvic ring. Should pelvic stabilization fail to control continuing blood loss, prompt arteriography is indicated. In a small percentage of all patients with pelvic fracture (< 10%), continuing arterial bleeding is identified and may be controlled by embolization of the involved vessel.

In the hemodynamically stable patient, there is less urgency for fixation of the disrupted pelvis. External fixation alone often does not adequately maintain alignment of displaced posterior pelvic ring injuries, and internal fixation is required. Open pelvic fractures require the evaluation described previously, thorough wound debridement, appropriate pelvic stabilization, and a diverting colostomy.

Management of these serious problems, especially in the persistently hypotensive patient, requires a multidisciplinary approach for optimal patient outcome. This often requires transferring the patient to a facility capable of managing the patient's complex problems.

V. Summary

Two major types of abdominal trauma occur: blunt and penetrating. **In either case, early patient evaluation by a surgeon is essential.**

A. Blunt Trauma

Intra-abdominal visceral damage must be strongly suspected following blunt trauma to the abdomen, especially because evidence is frequently subtle and misleading. Diagnosis of such injuries is often difficult, and an aggressive approach is mandatory. Multiple injuries are common, and common signs and symptoms guide the diagnostic process. Assessment of the mechanism of injury may provide some insight. If clinical findings are absent or obscured by other injuries, special techniques must be applied. Peritoneal lavage, properly performed, is a valuable diagnostic tool for these patients. A specific organ injury diagnosis is not necessary—only the finding of an acute abdominal injury.

B. Penetrating Trauma

A surgeon must evaluate all penetrating injuries of the abdomen. Penetrating trauma to the flanks, buttocks, and lower chest may produce intra-abdominal injuries as well and should be regarded with a high degree of suspicion.

C. Management

Management of blunt and penetrating trauma to the abdomen includes:

1. Re-establishing vital functions and optimizing oxygenation and tissue perfusion

2. Delineating the injury mechanism

3. Maintaining a high index of suspicion related to occult vascular and retroperitoneal injuries

4. Repeating a meticulous physical examination, assessing for changes

5. Selecting special diagnostic maneuvers as needed, performed with a minimal loss of time

6. Early recognition for surgical intervention and prompt celiotomy

Bibliography

1. Arajarvi E, Santavirta S, Tolonen J: Abdominal injuries sustained in severe traffic accidents by seat belt wearers. **Journal of Trauma** 1987;27:393-397.

2. Cass AS: Urethral injury in the multiply-injured patient. **Journal of Trauma** 1984;24:901-906.

3. Corriere JN, Sandler CM: Management of the ruptured bladder: seven years of experience with 111 cases. **Journal of Trauma** 1986;26:830-833.

4. Dalal SA, Burgess AR, Siegel JH, et al: Pelvic fracture in multiple trauma: classification by mechanism in key to pattern of organ injury, resuscitative requirements, and outcome. **Journal of Trauma** 1989;29:981-1002.

5. Donohue JH, Federle MP, Griffiths BG, et al: Computed tomography in the diagnosis of blunt intestinal and mesenteric injuries. **Journal of Trauma** 1987;27:11-17.

6. Federle MP, Crass RA, Jeffrey B, et al: Computed tomography in blunt abdominal trauma. **Archives of Surgery** 1982;117:645-650.

7. Flint LM, Brown A, Richardson JD, et al: Definitive control of bleeding from severe pelvic fractures. **Annals of Surgery** 1979;189:709-717.

8. Flint LM, McCoy M, Richardson JD, et al: Duodenal injury-analysis of common misconceptions in diagnosis and treatment. **Annals of Surgery** 1980;191:697-702.

9. Foley WD, Cates JD, Kellman GM, et al: Treatment of blunt hepatic injuries: role of CT. **Radiology** 1987;164:635-638.

10. Gilliland MG, Ward RE, Flynn TC, et al: Peritoneal lavage and angiography in management of patients with pelvic fracture. **American Journal of Surgery** 1982;144:744-747.

11. Griffen WO, Belin RP, Ernst CG, et al: Intravenous pyleography in abdominal trauma. **Journal of Trauma** 1978;18:387-392.

12. Hill AC, Schececter WP, Trunkey DD: Abdominal trauma and indications for exploratory laparotomy. In Mattox, Moore, and Feliciano (eds): **Trauma**. East Norwalk, Connecticut, Appleton and Lange, 1991.

13. Huizinga WKJ, Baker LW, Mtshall ZW: Selective management of abdominal and thoracic stab wounds with established peritoneal penetration: the eviscerated omentum. **American Journal of Surgery** 1987;153:564-568.

14. Kashuk JL, Moore EE, Millikan JS, et al: Major abdominal vascular trauma: a unified approach. **Journal of Trauma** 1982;22:672-679.

15. LeGay DA, Petrie DP, Alexander DI: Flexion-distraction injuries of the lumbar spine and associated abdominal trauma. **Journal of Trauma** 1990;30:436-444.

16. Marx JA, Moore EE, Jorden RC, et al: Limitations of computed tomography in the evaluation of acute abdominal trauma—a prospective randomized comparison with diagnostic peritoneal lavage. **Journal of Trauma** 1985;25:933-937.

17. McAlvanah MJ, Shaftan GW: Selective conservatism in penetrating abdominal wounds: a continuing reappraisal. **Journal of Trauma** 1978;18:206-212.

18. Moreno C, Moore EE, Rosenberger A, et al: Hemorrhage associated with major pelvic fracture-a multispecialty challenge. **Journal of Trauma** 1986;11:987-994.

19. Peitzman AB, Makaroun MS, Slasky BS, et al: Prospective study of computed tomography in initial management of blunt abdominal trauma. **Journal of Trauma** 1986;26:585-592.

20. Robin AP, Andrews JR, Lange DA, et al: Selective management of anterior abdominal stab wounds. **Journal of Trauma** 1989;29:1684-1689.

21. Sirinek KR, Page CP, Root HD, et al: Is exploratory celiotomy necessary for all patients with truncal stab wounds? **Archives of Surgery** 1990;125:844-848.

22. Thal ER: Evolution of peritoneal lavage and local exploration in lower chest and abdominal stab wounds. **Journal of Trauma** 1977;17:642-648.

23. Trafton PG: Pelvic ring injuries. **Surgical Clinics of North America** 1990;70:655-670.

24. Walton CB, Blaisdell FW, Jordan RG, et al: The injury potential and lethality of stab wounds: a Folsom Prison study. **Journal of Trauma** 1989;29:99-101.

25. Whalen G, Argorn IB, Robbs JV: The selective management of penetrating wounds of the back. **Journal of Trauma** 1989;29:508-511.

Skill Station VIII:
Diagnostic Peritoneal Lavage

This surgical procedure, if performed on a live, anesthetized animal, must be conducted in a USDA Registered Animal Laboratory facility. (See *ATLS® Instructor Manual,* Section II, Chapter 9—Policies, Procedures, and Protocols for Surgical Skills Practicum.)

Resources and Equipment

This list is the recommended equipment to conduct this skill session in accordance with the stated objectives for and intent of the procedures outlined. Additional equipment may be used providing it does not detract from the stated objectives and intent of this skill, or from performing the procedure in a safe method as described and recommended by the ACS Committee on Trauma.

1. Live, anesthetized animals

2. Licensed veterinarian (see guidelines referenced above)

3. Animal trough, ropes (sandbags optional)

4. Animal intubation equipment

    a. Endotracheal tubes
    b. Laryngoscope blade and handle
    c. Respirator with 15-mm adapter

5. Electric shears with #40 blade

6. Tables or instrument stands

7. Needles/syringes

    a. 6-mL syringes with #21- or #25-gauge needles
    b. 12-mL syringes

8. Peritoneal dialysis catheter set-ups

9. Surgical instruments

    a. Disposable scalpels with #10 and #11 blades
    b. Tissue forceps
    c. Allis clamps
    d. Hemostats

10. Antiseptic swabs

11. 500- or 1000-mL Ringer's lactate/normal saline with macrodrip and extension tubing

12. Lidocaine with epinephrine

13. Surgical drapes (optional)

14. Surgical garb (gloves, shoe covers, and scrub suits or cover gowns)

Objectives

1. Upon completion of this station, the participant will be able to discuss the indications and contraindications of peritoneal lavage.

2. Upon completion of this station, the participant will be able to describe the procedure for peritoneal lavage.

3. Performance at this station will allow the participant to practice and demonstrate the technique of peritoneal lavage.

4. Upon completion of this station, the participant will be able to discuss complications of this procedure.

The skill procedure for peritoneal lavage is performed via the open-technique method to avoid injury to underlying structures as may occur with the use of the trocar technique. However, the method of employing the Seldinger technique is a suitable alternative to be employed by trained physicians.

Skill Procedure

Diagnostic Peritoneal Lavage

Note: Universal precautions are required whenever caring for the trauma patient.

I. Peritoneal Lavage Technique: Open Technique

A. Decompress the urinary bladder by inserting a urinary catheter.

B. Decompress the stomach by inserting a nasogastric tube.

C. Surgically prepare the abdomen (eg, costal margin to the pubic area and flank to flank, anteriorly).

D. Inject local anesthetic midline and one third the distance from the umbilicus to the symphysis pubis. Use lidocaine with epinephrine to avoid blood contamination from skin and subcutaneous tissue.

E. Vertically incise the skin and subcutaneous tissues to the fascia.

F. Grasp the fascial edges with clamps, elevate, and incise the peritoneum.

G. Insert a peritoneal dialysis catheter into the peritoneal cavity.

H. After inserting the catheter into the peritoneum, advance the catheter into the pelvis.

I. Connect the dialysis catheter to a syringe and aspirate.

J. If gross blood is not obtained, instill 10 mL/kg (body weight) of warmed Ringer's lactate/normal saline (up to 1 liter) into the peritoneum through the intravenous tubing attached to the dialysis catheter.

K. Gentle agitation of the abdomen distributes the fluid throughout the peritoneal cavity and increases mixing with the blood.

L. If the patient's condition is stable, allow the fluid to remain 5 to 10 minutes before allowing it to drain. This is done by putting the Ringer's lactate/normal saline container on the floor and allowing the peritoneal fluid to drain from the abdomen. Make sure the container is vented to promote flow of the fluid from the abdomen.

M. After the fluid has returned, send a sample to the laboratory for erythrocyte and leukocyte counts (unspun). A positive test and the need for surgical intervention are indicated by 100,000 RBCs/mm^3 or more and greater than 500 WBCs/mm^3.

N. A negative lavage, however, does not exclude retroperitoneal injuries, ie, pancreas or duodenum, isolated hollow visceral perforation, or diaphragmatic tears.

Complications of Peritoneal Lavage

1. Hemorrhage, secondary to injection of local anesthetic, incision of the skin, or subcutaneous tissues providing a false-positive study

2. Peritonitis due to intestinal perforation from the catheter

3. Laceration of urinary bladder (if bladder not evacuated prior to procedure)

4. Injury to other abdominal and retroperitoneal structures requiring operative care

5. Wound infection at the lavage site (late complication)

Chapter 6:
Head Trauma

Objectives:

Upon completion of this topic, the physician will be able to demonstrate the techniques of assessment and explain the emergency management of head trauma.

Specifically, the physician will be able to:

A.   Review specific principles of anatomy and physiology related to head injuries.

B.   Identify and discuss the principles of general management of the unconscious patient and delayed complications.

C.   Outline the method of evaluating head injuries using a minineurologic examination.

D.   Identify and discuss management techniques for specific types of head injuries.

E.   Demonstrate the ability to assess various types of head, maxillofacial, and neck injuries, using a head-trauma manikin.

F.   Discuss clinical signs and outline priorities for the initial management of injuries identified during patient assessment.

Chapter 6:
Head Trauma

I. Introduction

Because a head injury occurs every 15 seconds, and a patient dies of a head injury every 12 minutes, a physician dealing with trauma is confronted with a head-injured patient almost every day. Approximately 50% of all trauma deaths are associated with head injury, and more than 60% of vehicular trauma deaths are due to head injury. Because of the immense importance of head injury, the physician who sees patients soon after injury, but is not expert in the comprehensive management of head injuries, must develop a practical knowledge of the initial care of these patients. A neurosurgeon may not be available immediately when a patient with a central nervous system injury is first seen. Therefore, one of the most important responsibilities of physicians initially evaluating such a patient is in the management of ventilation and hypovolemia, thereby obviating potential secondary brain damage. Therefore, a system that incorporates consultation with a neurosurgeon, whose opinion may modify the management of such a patient, is essential. Early transfer of appropriate patients substantially reduces morbidity and mortality.

When conferring with a neurosurgical consultant about a patient with a head injury, the physician should relay the following patient information:

1. Age of patient and mechanism of injury

2. Respiratory and cardiovascular status

3. Results of the neurologic examination, especially the level of consciousness, pupillary reactions, and presence of lateralized extremity weakness

4. Presence and type of noncerebral injuries

5. The results of diagnostic studies, if obtained

Neurosurgical consultation or patient transfer should not be delayed to obtain diagnostic studies, eg, computed tomographic (CT) scan or skull roentgenograms.

II. Anatomy and Physiology

As with all other aspects of medicine, the basis for a rational decision is the integration of the knowledge of anatomy and physiology with the history and physical examination. A short review of these subjects follows.

A. Scalp

The scalp is made up of five layers of tissue covering the bone of the top of the skull (calvarium): (1) skin, (2) subcutaneous tissue, (3) galea aponeurotica, (4) a layer of loose areolar tissue, and (5) periosteum, the "pericranium." The loose areolar tissue, separating the galea from the pericranium, is subject to the commonly encountered subgaleal hematomas, large flaps caused by injury and "scalping" injuries. Because of the scalp's generous blood supply, bleeding from a scalp laceration can result in major blood loss, especially in children.

B. Skull

The skull is composed of the cranial vault (calvarium) and the base. The calvarium is especially thin in the temporal regions. The base of the skull is irregular and rough, allowing injury to occur as the brain moves within the skull during acceleration and deceleration.

C. Meninges

The **dura** is a tough, fibrous membrane that adheres firmly to the internal surface of the skull. Because it is not attached to the underlying arachnoid, a potential space (the **subdural space**) exists into which hemorrhage can occur—usually from veins that traverse the space (bridging veins). In certain places the dura splits into two surfaces forming venous sinuses that provide the major venous drainage from the brain. The midline (superior) sagittal sinus is especially vulnerable to injury.

Meningeal arteries lie between the dura and the internal surface of the skull (**epidural**). The courses of these arteries may be visible on plain skull roentgenograms, if the vessels groove the inner surface of the skull. Laceration of these arteries may result in an epidural hematoma.

Beneath the dura is a second meningeal layer, the thin transparent **arachnoid.** The third layer, the **pia**, is firmly attached to the brain cortex. Between the arachnoid and the pia (**subarachnoid space**), the cerebrospinal fluid (CSF) circulates. Hemorrhage into this space is, by definition, subarachnoid hemorrhage.

D. Brain

The brain consists of the cerebrum, the cerebellum, and the brain stem. The **cerebrum** is composed of right and left hemispheres that are separated by the falx, a dural reflection. The left hemisphere, which usually contains the language centers, is often referred to as the dominant hemisphere. The **frontal lobe** is concerned with emotions and motor function, the **occipital lobe** with vision, and the **parietal lobe** with sensory function. The **temporal lobe** regulates certain memory functions, but can be a relatively silent region on the right side.

The brain can be compared with a funnel. The two cerebral hemispheres comprise the funnel portion. The brain stem, the major neural pathways to and from the hemispheres, comprises the neck of the funnel. The **brain stem** is composed of the midbrain, the pons, and the medulla. The midbrain and upper pons contain the **reticular activating system**, which is responsible for an "awake" state. Vital cardiorespiratory centers reside in the lower brain stem, the **medulla**, which then continues to form the spinal cord. The **cerebellum**, which controls movement, coordination, and balance, surrounds the pons and medulla in the posterior fossa.

E. Cerebrospinal Fluid

Cerebrospinal fluid is produced by the choroid plexus and is discharged into the ventricles of the brain. The fluid leaves the ventricular cavities to circulate through the subarachnoid space.

F. Tentorium

The tentorium divides the head into the supratentorial compartment (comprising the anterior and middle fossae of the skull) and the infratentorial compartment (containing the posterior fossa). The midbrain courses from the cerebrum through the large aperture (incisura) in the tentorium. The third cranial nerve also passes along this opening. Any pathologic process that rapidly increases supratentorial pressure, most commonly hemorrhage or edema, can force the medial aspect of the temporal lobe (the uncus) through this opening. The result (uncal or tentorial herniation) causes compression of the third nerve, producing an ipsilateral and dilated, fixed pupil. Contralateral spastic weakness of the arm and leg, caused by compression of the corticospinal (pyramidal) tract within the cerebral peduncle on the side of herniation, is also an integral component of uncal herniation.

G. Consciousness

Alteration of consciousness is the hallmark of brain injury.

Two types of brain injury—bilateral injury to the cerebral cortices and injury to the reticular activating system of the brain stem—can produce unconsciousness. Increased intracranial pressure and decreased cerebral blood flow, regardless of the cause, can also depress the level of consciousness.

H. Intracranial Pressure

Intracranial pressure can be described as a relationship among volumes of CSF, blood, and brain, and expressed by the equation of the modified Monroe-Kellie hypothesis:

$$\mathbf{K}_{ICP} \sim \mathbf{V}_{CSF} + \mathbf{V}_{Bl} + \mathbf{V}_{Br}$$

Constancy (K) of the intracranial pressure (ICP) relates to the volume (V) of the cerebrospinal fluid (CSF), plus the volume (V) of blood (Bl), plus the volume (V) of the brain (Br).

The volume of CSF is altered by varying rates of absorption depending on the intracranial pressure, since CSF production is constant. Intracranial venous blood volume depends on rates of passive drainage influenced by intracranial pressure and intrathoracic pressure. The arterial blood volume is affected by autoregulation, arterial PCO_2, and may be decreased by autoregulation with hyperventilation. Brain volume is relatively static, except when cerebral edema occurs.

As the volume of mass from an expanding hematoma or cerebral edema increases, CSF or venous blood (or both) are removed from the intracranial compartment at a greater rate than normal. The result of these adjustments is that the intracranial compartment may accommodate an enlarging mass to a volume of 50 to 100 mL, depending on location and rapidity of enlargement. When all normal compensatory measures are exhausted, further small increases in intracranial mass volume cause very large increases in intracranial pressure, resulting in diminution of **cerebral perfusion pressure**. When the mass reaches a critical size, further increases in volume result in a rapid increase in intracranial pressure with brain herniation likely.

Cerebral perfusion pressure is, approximately, the mean systemic arterial pressure minus the intracranial pressure. It is a measure of arterial perfusion of brain tissue, and normally it is greater than 50 mm Hg. Initial elevations of intracranial pressure are often associated with compensatory rises in mean systemic arterial pressure. However, further elevations of intracranial pressure are at the expense of cerebral perfusion pressure (ie, cerebral blood flow), and result in brain ischemia, leading to alterations in the level of consciousness. Brain death occurs when intracranial pressure approaches systemic arterial pressure, thus preventing any blood flow to the brain.

The definitive management of increased ICP is substantially aided by direct measures of arterial, central venous, and intracranial pressures under the direction of a neurosurgeon.

III. Assessment of Head Injuries

A. History

To make the correct management decisions, it is helpful to know what kind of head injury can result from a certain kind of trauma. The cause is usually obvious, but even though a patient may appear to be in good neurologic condition, mechanism-of-injury risk factors should be assessed in deciding how and where to treat the patient (See Chapter 12, Stabilization and Transport). For example, simply knowing that the patient was injured in a fall instead of a vehicular crash quadruples the patient's risk of having an intracranial hematoma.

Prehospital personnel should question observers at the scene about the patient's condition immediately after the incident. Information obtained by ambulance personnel should be documented in writing and provided to the hospital personnel when the patient is delivered to the emergency department.

B. Initial Assessment

The importance of initial assessment is emphasized because it provides the baseline for sequential reassessment, which is the critical basis for many subsequent decisions in patient management.

Because many factors influence the neurologic evaluation, documentation of the cardiorespiratory status must accompany the neurologic examination. **Airway, breathing, and circulatory control and management must take priority.** Care must be exercised in attributing changes in the patient's mental status to head injury if the systolic blood pressure is less than 60 mm Hg or systemic hypoxemia exists. Similarly, a drug screen for alcohol and other nervous system depressants must be obtained, so that toxic factors that may influence head injury assessment are taken into account.

C. Assessment of Vital Signs

Although brain injury may alter the vital signs, it is very difficult to be sure that changes in the vital signs are due to head injury and not to other factors. Some useful clinical rules include:

1. **Never presume that brain injury is the cause of hypotension.** Although bleeding from scalp lacerations can cause hemorrhagic shock (especially in small children), intracranial bleeding will not produce shock from blood loss alone. Hypotension arising from brain injury is a terminal event, resulting from failure of medullary centers.

2. The combination of progressive hypertension associated with bradycardia and diminished respiratory rate (Cushing response) is a specific response to an acute and potentially lethal rise in intracranial pressure. In head injury, the course is usually a lesion demanding immediate operative intervention.

3. Hypertension alone or in combination with hyperthermia may reflect central autonomic dysfunction caused by certain types of brain injury.

D. AVPU + Minineurologic Examination

The AVPU mnemonic is supplemented by a minineurologic examination that is directed toward determining the presence and severity of gross neurologic deficits, especially those that may require urgent operation. The AVPU method, completed in the primary survey, describes the patient's level of consciousness. (See Chapter 1, Initial Assessment and Management and Chart 2, Revised Trauma Score in Chapter 12, Stabilization and Transport.)

The minineurologic examination should be conducted repeatedly for any patient with a head injury. The examination assesses: (1) level of consciousness, (2) pupillary function, and (3) lateralized extremity weakness. **Generally, a patient with abnormalities of all three components will have a mass lesion that may require surgery.**

1. Level of consciousness

a. Glasgow Coma Scale

The Glasgow Coma Scale (GCS) provides a quantitative measure of the patient's level of consciousness. The GCS is the sum of scores for three areas of assessment: (1) eye opening, (2) verbal response, and (3) best motor response. Each is graded separately.

1) Eye-opening response (E score)

Scoring of eye opening is not valid if the eyes are swollen shut. This fact must be documented.

   a) Spontaneous—already open with blinking (normal): **E = four (4) points**

   b) To speech—not necessarily to a request for eye opening: **E = three (3) points**

   c) To pain—stimulus should not be applied to the face: **E = two (2) points**

   d) None: **E = one (1) point**

2) Verbal response (V score)

Scoring of verbal response is invalid if speech is impossible, for example, in the presence of endotracheal intubation. This circumstance must be documented.

a) Oriented—knows name, age, etc: **V = five (5) points**

b) Confused conversation—still answers questions: **V = four (4) points**

c) Inappropriate words—speech is either exclamatory or random, but recognizable words are produced: **V = three (3) points**

d) Incomprehensible sounds—grunts and groans are produced, but no actual words are uttered; do not confuse with partial respiratory obstruction: **V = two (2) points**

e) None: **V = one (1) point**

3) Best motor response (M score)

The **best** response obtained for any extremity is recorded even though worse responses may be present in other extremities. The worst motor activity also is important but is not used for the GCS; worst response should be noted separately. For patients not following verbal command, a painful stimulus is applied to the fingernail or toenail.

a) Obeys—moves limb to command and pain is not required: **M = six (6) points**

b) Localizes—changing the location of the pain stimulus causes purposeful motion toward the stimulus: **M = five (5) points**

c) Withdraws—pulls away from painful stimulus: **M = four (4) points**

d) Abnormal flexion—decorticate posture: **M = three (3) points**

e) Extensor response—decerebrate posture: **M = two (2) points**

f) No movement: **M = one (1) point**

b. Patient categorization

The Glasgow Coma Scale itself can be used to categorize patients:

1) Coma

A patient in **coma is defined as having no eye opening (E = 1), no ability to follow commands (M = 1 to 5), and no word verbalizations (V = 1 to 2).** This means that all patients with a GCS Score of less than eight and most of those with a GCS Score that equals eight are in coma. Patients with a GCS Score more than 8 are not in coma.

2) Head injury severity

On the basis of the GCS, patients are classified as having:

a) Severe head injury if the GCS Score is less than or equal to eight

b)   Moderate head injury if the GCS Score is 9 to 12

c)   Minor head injury if the GCS Score is 13 to 15

2. Assessment of pupillary function

The pupils are evaluated for their equality and response to bright light. A difference in pupil diameters of more than 1 mm is abnormal. Even though eye injury may be present, intracranial injury must be excluded. Light reactivity must be evaluated for the briskness of response; a more sluggish response may indicate an intracranial injury.

3. Lateralized extremity weakness

Spontaneous movements are observed for equality. If spontaneous motion is minimal, the response to a painful stimulus is assessed. A delay in onset of movement, less movement, or need for more stimulus on one side is significant. Often, the motor component of the GCS can be used to score the best and the worst extremity movement. A clearly lateralized weakness suggests an intracranial mass lesion.

4. Purposes of neurologic examination

The purposes of the minineurologic examination are to determine the severity of the brain injury, and detect any neurologic deterioration. The GCS can be used to categorize injuries as mild, moderate, and severe. Irrespective of the GCS, a patient is considered to have a severe head injury if he exhibits **any** of the following:

a.   Unequal pupils

b.   Unequal motor examination

c.   An open head injury with leaking CSF or exposed brain tissue

d.   Neurologic deterioration

e.   Depressed skull fracture

A decrease in the GCS score of two or more points clearly means the patient's condition has deteriorated. A decrease of three or more points is a catastrophic deterioration that demands immediate treatment if the cause is remediable. However, these changes are rather gross and are often preceded by more subtle signs of deterioration. Neurologic deterioration of special concern includes:

f.   Increase in severity of a headache or an extraordinarily severe headache

g.   Increase in the size of one pupil

h.   Development of weakness on one side

It cannot be overemphasized that the initial neurologic examination is only the beginning. The initial findings are only the reference with which to compare results of repeated neurologic examinations to determine whether a patient's condition is deteriorating or improving. **All previous efforts will go to waste if signs of neurologic deterioration are not appreciated.** The brain cannot withstand unrelieved compression for very long before brain damage is irreversible. The neurologic assessment is designed to detect this secondary brain damage so timely treatment can be initiated following neurosurgical consultation.

E. Special Assessment

1. Skull roentgenograms

Skull roentgenograms are of little value in the early management of patients with obvious head injuries, except in cases of penetrating injuries. The unconscious patient should have skull roentgenograms **only** if precise care of the cardiorespiratory system and continuing reassessment can be assured. Physical examination is usually more valuable than skull roentgenograms. (See VII. Scalp Wounds, in this chapter.) Clinical signs of basal fractures are more useful than roentgenograms of the skull base in diagnosing a fracture. Increasingly, skull films are not being obtained on patients with minor head injuries because the information obtained is rarely helpful one way or the other. When in doubt about the patient's condition, the physicians should obtain neurosurgical consultation.

2. Computed tomography

The CT scan has revolutionized diagnosis in patients with head injuries and is the diagnostic procedure of choice for patients who have or are suspected of having a serious head injury. Although not perfect, the CT scan is capable of showing the exact location and size of most mass lesions. Specific diagnosis allows more precise planning of definitive care, including operation. The CT scan has supplanted less specific and more invasive tests, such as cerebral angiography.

Except for patients with minor head injuries, **all head-injured patients will require CT scanning** at some time. The more serious the injury, the earlier and more emergent is the need for the scan. Consequently, injured patients seen first at facilities without CT capability may require transfer to more sophisticated hospitals.

Once initial resuscitation has been undertaken and the need for a CT scan determined, care must be taken to (1) maintain adequate resuscitation during the scan, and (2) assure the best possible quality of the scan. The patient must be attended constantly in the CT suite to monitor vital signs closely and initiate immediate treatment should the patient's status deteriorate.

Patient movement results in artifacts and a poor-quality scan. This artifact may mask significant intracranial lesions requiring urgent surgical intervention. Movement artifact can be eliminated by sedating restless or uncooperative patients. However, extreme caution must be exercised to avoid sedating patients whose restlessness or lack of cooperation is a clinical manifestation of hypoxia. Often endotracheal intubation with controlled ventilation becomes necessary if the scan is considered mandatory, and the patient can be rendered motionless only with paralyzing drugs. **Ideally, the neurosurgeon should examine the patient before the patient is iatrogenically paralyzed or has a CT scan.** However, efficient and correct management of the patient, in certain situations, may dictate otherwise.

3. Other tests

Lumbar puncture, electroencephalogram, and isotope scanning have no role in the acute management of head trauma.

Certain reflexes, eg, oculocephalic and vestibulo-ocular, can reflect the integrity of a portion of the brain-stem neural pathways. Although these may permit more specific diagnosis in some instances, their elicitation can be hazardous, their interpretation difficult, and they add little to the emergency management of the patient. They are best left to the neuro-surgical consultant.

IV. Specific Types of Head Injury

After initial assessment and resuscitation, the emergency management of the patient with a head injury is aimed at (1) establishing a specific anatomic diagnosis of the head injury, (2) assuring the metabolic needs of the brain, and (3) preventing secondary brain damage from treatable causes of elevated intracranial pressure. The need to prevent systemic causes of secondary brain injury, notably hypoxia, ischemia, and hyperthermia, is axiomatic.

Head injuries include (1) skull fractures, (2) diffuse brain injuries, and (3) focal injuries. The pathophysiology, severity, need for urgent treatment, and outcome are different in each group. A review of these head injuries aids in making and simplifying the initial diagnosis.

A. Skull Fractures

Skull fractures are common, but many are not associated with severe brain injury. Likewise, many severe brain injuries occur without skull fracture. Although identifying a skull fracture is important, diagnosing a brain injury does not depend on it. Searching for a skull fracture should never delay patient management. Attention should be directed to the brain injury. The significance of a skull fracture is that it identifies the patient with a higher probability of having or developing an intracranial hematoma. For this reason, all patients with skull fractures should be admitted to the hospital for observation. All patients with skull fractures require neurosurgical consultation.

1. Linear, nondepressed fractures

Linear skull fractures are often seen on the roentgenogram as a lucent line. They may also be stellate. Linear skull fractures require no specific treatment, and management is directed toward the underlying brain injury. Fractures across vascular arterial grooves or suture lines should raise suspicion of the possibility of epidural hemorrhage.

2. Depressed skull fractures

Depressed skull fractures may or may not be neurosurgical emergencies. Management is directed toward the underlying brain injury. To reduce the risk of possible sequelae, such as seizure disorder, any fragment depressed more than the thickness of the skull may require operative elevation of the bony fragment.

3. Open skull fractures

By definition, open skull fractures have a direct communication between a scalp laceration and the cerebral substance, because the dura is torn. This condition can be diagnosed if brain is visible or if CSF is leaking from the wound. Open fractures require early operative intervention, with elevation or removal of the fragments and closure of the dura, to reduce the possibility of infection.

4. Basal skull fractures

These fractures are often not apparent on skull roentgenograms. Indirectly, intracranial air or an opaque sphenoid sinus gives clues.

The diagnosis is based on physical findings such as CSF leaking from the ear (otorrhea) or the nose (rhinorrhea). When CSF is mixed with blood, it may be difficult to detect. An aid is the "ring sign," detected by allowing a drop of the fluid to fall onto a piece of filter paper. If CSF is present, blood remains in the center, and one or more concentric rings of clearer fluid develop.

Ecchymosis in the mastoid region (Battle's sign) also indicates a basal skull fracture, as does blood behind the tympanic membrane (hemotympanum). Cribriform plate fractures are often associated with periorbital ecchymosis (raccoon eyes). These signs may take several hours to appear and may be absent immediately after injury. Whenever a frontal basal skull fracture is present, danger exists of inadvertent intracranial intubation with the insertion of a nasogastric tube. This problem may be prevented by the insertion of the gastric tube through a previously, carefully placed soft, trumpet-style nasal airway, or orally.

B. Diffuse Brain Injuries

Diffuse brain injuries are produced when rapid head motions (acceleration or deceleration) cause widespread interruption of brain function in most areas of the brain. Often as with concussion, the disturbance of neural function is temporary. But with more severe injuries (diffuse axonal injury), microscopic structural damage throughout the brain may cause permanent problems. It is important to try to distinguish these injuries from focal injuries, because diffuse brain injuries do not have mass lesions requiring emergency surgery.

1. Concussion

Concussion is a brain injury accompanied by brief loss of neurologic function. In its milder forms, it may cause only temporary confusion or amnesia. More commonly, concussion causes temporary loss of consciousness. The period of unconsciousness is usually short, but more severe forms exist. Many neurologic abnormalities may be described in the first few minutes after concussion, but these disappear quickly, usually before the patient gets to a medical facility. **Therefore, any neurologic abnormality observed in the patient should not be attributed to a concussion.**

Most patients with a concussion will be awake or awakening when seen in the emergency department, even though some mental confusion may persist. After the confusion clears, the patient may be capable of describing portions of his accident, but may not remember the actual impact. The patient may complain of headache, dizziness, or nausea, but the minineurologic examination will not show localizing signs. These patients should be observed in the hospital and then at home only if their mental state clears completely. Patients sustaining a severe concussion should be admitted for observation, because of the potential for associated serious brain injuries. The decision to admit the patient should be based on the length of unconsciousness and the reliability of the individuals with whom the patient resides. A rule of thumb is that if a patient has been unconscious for five minutes or more, he should be observed in the hospital for 24 hours. The duration of amnesia and/or retrograde amnesia also must be considered. If the patient is under the age of 12 years, it is best to admit for observation. Persistent vomiting and/or convulsions may occur. Any patient whose confusion does not clear completely **must** be admitted.

2. Diffuse axonal injury

Diffuse axonal injury (DAI)—often called brain-stem injury, closed head injury, or diffuse injury is characterized by prolonged coma, often lasting days to weeks. DAI is a frequent injury, occurring in 44% of coma-producing head injuries.

Overall mortality is 33%. In its most severe form, DAI has a 50% mortality, usually from increased intracranial pressure secondary to cerebral edema. DAI results primarily in microscopic damage that is scattered widely throughout the brain, and therefore does not require surgery. Although the length of coma cannot be determined in the emergency department, recognition of DAI is important because it may mimic other injuries that do require emergency surgery. The diagnosis is justified when an emergency CT scan shows no mass lesion in a patient who remains deeply comatose, often with decerebrate or decorticate posturing. Autonomic dysfunction producing high fever, hypertension, and sweating is common. The patient should be transferred to a facility equipped to care for long-term coma patients.

C. Focal Injuries

Focal injuries are those in which macroscopic damage occurs in a relatively local area. They consist of contusions, hemorrhages, and hematomas. These injuries may require emergency surgery because of their mass effects. **Diagnostic efforts during the early postinjury period are primarily aimed at diagnosing focal lesions, because they are treatable and frequently require emergency operative intervention.**

1. Contusion

Cerebral contusions can be single or multiple, small or large. Therefore, the patient may present in several ways. Most commonly, contusions are associated with serious concussions characterized by longer periods of coma and mental confusion or obtundation. Contusions can occur beneath an area of impact (coup contusions) or in areas remote from impact (contrecoup contusions). The tips of the frontal and temporal lobes are especially common sites of contusion. The contusion itself may produce focal neurologic deficit if it occurs near the sensory or motor areas of the brain, but a deficit may not be apparent if the contusion is elsewhere. If the contusion is large or associated with pericontusional edema, the mass effect may cause herniation and brain-stem compression, resulting in secondary or delayed neurologic deterioration. A CT scan of the head determines with certainty the presence, location, and size of contusions.

Patients sustaining cerebral contusion should be admitted to the hospital for observation, because delayed edema or swelling around the contusion may cause neurologic deterioration. Contusions require surgery only if they cause substantial mass effect, but careful observation is necessary to detect patients with delayed bleeding into the contusion. This factor is especially important for patients with measurable blood alcohol levels, because acutely or chronically alcoholic patients have a high incidence of delayed bleeding into their contusions.

2. Intracranial hemorrhages

Intracranial hemorrhages can be classified as meningeal or brain hemorrhages. Due to great variation in location, size, and rapidity of bleeding, there is no typical picture. Computed tomography has made the diagnosis and localization very precise. It must be stressed that epidural hematoma and temporal lobe intracerebral hematoma can mimic each other, because the symptoms and the clinical findings are usually those of tentorial herniation, characteristically seen in epidural hemorrhage.

a. Meningeal hemorrhage
1) Acute epidural hemorrhage

Epidural bleeding almost always occurs from a tear in a dural artery, usually the middle meningeal artery. A small percentage may occur from a tear in the dural sinus. Although epidural hemorrhage is relatively rare (0.5% in unselected head injuries and 0.9% of coma-producing head injuries), it must be considered because it may be rapidly fatal. Such arterial tears are usually associated with linear skull fractures over the parietal or temporal areas that cross the grooves of the middle meningeal artery; however, **this injury is not an absolute requirement for the diagnosis.**

The signs and symptoms of a typical epidural hemorrhage are (1) loss of consciousness (concussion) followed by an intervening lucid interval (the lucid period may not be a return to full consciousness); (2) a secondary depression of consciousness; and (3) the development of hemiparesis on the opposite side. A dilated and fixed pupil on the same side as the impact area is a hallmark of this injury. (Less frequently, the dilated, fixed pupil may be on the side opposite the hematoma or the hemiparesis may be on the same side as the hematoma.) Although the patient is lucid, he may not be entirely symptom free, usually complains of a severe, localized headache, and is sleepy.

This injury requires immediate surgical intervention. If treated early, prognosis is usually excellent, because the underlying brain injury is often not serious. Outcome is directly related to the status of the patient before surgery. For patients not in coma, the mortality from epidural hematoma approximates zero. For those in light coma it is 9%, and for patients in deep coma it is 20%. Secondary brain injury occurs rapidly if the hematoma is not evacuated quickly.

2) Acute subdural hematoma

Subdural hematomas also are life threatening and are much more common than epidural hematomas (30% of severe head injuries). They most commonly occur from rupture of bridging veins between the cerebral cortex and dura, but also can be seen with lacerations of the brain or cortical arteries. A skull fracture may or may not be present. In addition to the problems caused by the mass of subdural blood, underlying primary brain injury is often severe. The prognosis is often dismal, and the mortality remains at 60%. However, recent studies demonstrate improved outcome if the hematoma is evacuated very early.

3) Subarachnoid hemorrhage

This type of hemorrhage results in bloody CSF and meningeal irritation. The patient usually complains of a headache and/or photophobia. No immediate treatment is needed, and the hemorrhage alone is not life threatening. A lumbar puncture is not needed, because the diagnosis can be made with a CT scan.

b. Brain hemorrhages and lacerations
1) Intracerebral hematomas

Hemorrhages within the brain substance can occur in any location. Computed tomography provides a more precise diagnosis. Many small, deep intracerebral hemorrhages are associated with other brain injuries (especially DAI). The neurologic deficits depend on these associated injuries and the region(s) involved, the size of the hemorrhage, and whether bleeding continues. Hemiplegia may occur. Occipital hemorrhages can cause visual defects. Intraventricular and intracerebellar hemorrhages are associated with a high mortality rate.

2) Impalement injuries

All foreign bodies protruding from the skull should be left in place until they can be removed by a neurosurgeon as a formal operation. Roentgenograms of the skull are required to determine the object's angle and depth of penetration.

3) Bullet wounds

The larger the caliber and the higher the velocity of the bullet, the more likely death occurs. Through-and-through and side-to-side injuries, and those lower in the brain, tend to be ominous.

Patients in coma have a very high mortality, especially with an initial GCS Score of less than six. Skull films and a CT scan help plan the surgical approach when operation is deemed necessary. Entrance and exit wounds should be covered with antiseptic-soaked dressings until definitive neurosurgical care is provided. A bullet that does not penetrate the skull may still result in intracranial injury, because of blunt trauma, and such patients require a CT scan.

c. **Time factors**

The earlier the hematoma is recognized and evaluated, the better the prognosis. Epidural hematomas, being arterial in origin, usually develop more rapidly than subdural hematomas of venous origin. Epidural hematomas may require four to six hours to become clinically apparent, whereas subdural hematomas may take 12 to 24 hours to become evident in the absence of other lesions such as intracerebral hematomas or diffuse cerebral edema. However, both types of hematomas may become evident within as little as one hour after injury, especially in children. Therefore, all patients suspected of harboring a developing intracranial hematoma must be observed closely and transferred to the care of a neurosurgeon as rapidly as possible. **Remember**, the decision to **delay transfer** may be as critical a surgical decision as the decision to operate.

V. Emergency Management of Head Injuries

A. Establishing a Specific Diagnosis

The immediate purpose of a specific diagnosis is to determine which patients need an emergency or urgent neurosurgical operation. **This is an issue that demands early participation by the neurosurgical consultant.** Patients requiring emergency surgery are those with massive depressed or open skull fractures and those with large focal mass lesions. The former category is usually obvious, but the latter must be distinguished from diffuse brain injuries where no mass lesion exists.

1. Assessing the need for surgery

Injuries requiring surgery are likely to occur in different circumstances than injuries not requiring surgery. Therefore, a gross estimate of a patient's potential need for surgery can be based on knowledge concerning three factors: (1) whether the patient is comatose; (2) whether the trauma was vehicular or nonvehicular; and (3) whether there is a lateralized motor deficit. (See Table 1, Approximate Percent of Patients Who May Require Surgery.)

Table 1
Approximate Percent of Patients Who May Require Surgery

(Excludes patients with minor injury who are neurologically normal.)

	Not in Coma		Comatose	
	Motor Equal	Unequal	Motor Equal	Unequal
Vehicular	20%	40%	20%	30%
Nonvehicular	40%	70%	60%	80%

2. Diagnostic triage system

Based on the minineurologic examination, a practical and systematic approach can be established for diagnosing head-injured patients. It must be understood that this scheme is only a guideline. (See Figure 1, Head Injury Triage Scheme.) Because of the complexity and multiplicity of brain injuries, this system is not and cannot be either foolproof or all-inclusive. However, it offers one useful approach to determining not only the initial diagnosis, but also the severity of injury, so that emergency treatment decisions can be made.

The first priority is determining the level of consciousness, based on the GCS. If a patient has a score equal to or less than eight, the physician must immediately determine (1) whether the pupils are unequal, or (2) whether there is a lateralized motor deficit. If either of these exist, **a large focal lesion (epidural, subdural, or intracerebral hematoma, or large contusion) must be presumed present.** Preparation must be made for emergency operation to evacuate the lesion. Simultaneously, efforts must be taken to decrease the intracranial pressure. Presumptive evidence of a progressive lesion, capable of producing lethal brain herniation (usually an epidural hematoma), is one of the few neurosurgical emergencies in the injured patient that may require operative intervention within minutes.

A comatose patient with equal pupils and motor responses may still have a surgical mass lesion but is more likely to have diffuse axonal injury, acute brain swelling, or cerebral ischemia. After immediate measures have been taken to reduce intracranial pressure, an emergency CT is needed to exclude a mass lesion.

A patient who is not comatose (ie, GCS >8) still may harbor an injury requiring operation. If pupillary asymmetry or lateralized weakness is present, the patient must be suspected to have a focal lesion that is not (yet) of sufficient size to compress the brain stem and cause coma. A CT scan is urgently required. If the pupils and movements are equal, the presence or absence of an open head injury must be determined by a search for CSF leaking from the nose, ears, or a scalp wound.

If there is no open injury (in the noncomatose patient who has equal pupils and movements), a complete neurologic examination must be performed. If the examination is not normal, a focal lesion must be excluded by CT scan. If the examination is normal, and the patient has been unconscious only briefly and is in the low-risk group for an intracranial lesion (see Table 2, Relative Risk of Intracranial Lesion), discharge from the hospital may be considered after appropriate instructions are given to the patient. If any of these conditions are not met, the patient should be admitted to the hospital for postconcussion observation. **Remember, a normal neurologic examination includes a normal mental status examination.** No patient with signs of head injury should be discharged because he is intact except for being intoxicated. **Do not presume that altered mental status is due to alcohol.** The patient should be observed until his mental status is completely normal, or he should be admitted to the hospital for observation.

Figure 1
Head Injury
Triage Scheme

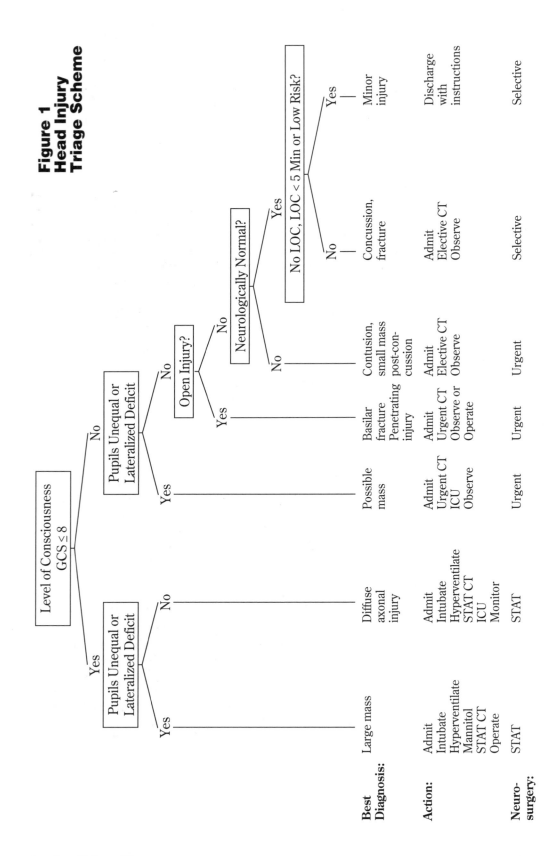

Table 2
Relative Risk of Intracranial Lesion

Low Risk Group	Moderate Risk	High Risk
Asymptomatic	Change of consciousness	Depressed consciousness
Headache	Progressive headache	Focal signs
Dizziness	Alcohol and/or other drug intoxication	Decreasing consciousness
Scalp hematoma	Unreliable history	Penetrating injury
Scalp laceration	Age > 2 years	Depressed fracture
Scalp contusion	Seizure	
Scalp abrasion	Vomiting	
Absence of moderate or high-risk criteria	Amnesia	
	Multiple trauma	
	Serious facial injury	
	Signs of basilar fracture	
	Possible skull penetration	
	Possible depressed fracture	
	Suspected child abuse	

B. Emergency Management

Once a working diagnosis is established, treatment must be commenced; urgency of treatment depends on the nature and severity of injury. Emergency treatment of the seriously injured patient is aimed at protecting the brain from further (secondary) insults by (1) maintaining adequate cerebral metabolism, and (2) preventing and treating intracranial hypertension.

1. Maintenance of cerebral metabolic needs

Cerebral ischemia or hypoxia result in insufficient substrate delivery to the injured brain. These conditions are present in more than 90% of patients who die of head trauma, are associated with poor outcome, and are the most important preventable complications of head injury.

The principal metabolic requirements of the brain are oxygen and glucose, which are normally used at extremely high rates. The injured brain usually has a lowered cerebral metabolism and therefore requires less oxygen and glucose. However, the damaged brain is more susceptible to the lack of these substrates, and thus temporary severe or prolonged moderate deprivation causes worse damage than in the uninjured brain. Therefore, emergency management of head injury includes maintenance of adequate cerebral metabolic fuels.

The physician must assure delivery of adequate levels of glucose and oxygen to the brain. Delivery of these substrates depends on their arterial concentrations and the blood flow to the brain. Blood glucose concentration is not a common problem in trauma, but if it is, correction with supplemental intravenous glucose is needed. However, recent works suggest that hyperglycemia should be avoided.

Oxygen content depends on arterial hemoglobin and oxygen concentrations. Arterial oxygen concentration can be assessed with blood gases and supplemental oxygen delivered to maintain the arterial PO_2 at greater than 80 mm Hg. Blood transfusion may be necessary to provide sufficient hemoglobin to maintain normal oxygen carrying capacity.

Cerebral blood flow is dependent on systemic arterial pressure and arterial PCO_2, especially shortly after head trauma. Normalization of blood pressure and maintenance of $PaCO_2$ at 26 to 28 mm Hg is sufficient to maintain adequate cerebral blood flow under most circumstances. Keep in mind that the $PaCO_2$ cannot be allowed to rise too high as it may aggravate intracranial pressure (see 2.a.).

2. Preventing / treating intracranial hypertension

The purpose of these treatments is to prevent, control, or diminish intracranial hypertension, regardless of its cause. In addition to mass lesions, acute brain swelling (a vascular engorgement phenomena) and brain edema can complicate any primary brain injury by causing or aggravating intracranial hypertension. It is for this reason that, **optimally**, neurosurgical consultation should be obtained when these measures are instituted.

a. Induced hypocapnia

Arterial carbon dioxide concentration profoundly affects cerebral circulation. When abnormally elevated, cerebrovasodilatation occurs, increasing intracranial blood volume and intracranial pressure. (See II. Anatomy and Physiology, H. Intracranial Pressure in this chapter.) Conversely, reduction of $PaCO_2$ reduces intracranial blood volume and, secondarily, intracranial pressure. Additionally, hyperventilation tends to reduce intracerebral acidosis and increase cerebral metabolism, both of which are beneficial. Therefore, hyperventilation is recommended to reduce arterial PCO_2, maintaining it at 26 to 28 mm Hg. This procedure usually requires endotracheal intubation, controlled ventilation, and intermittent iatrogenic paralysis. Intubation should be performed **early** for the comatose patient. Care must be taken to assure that injudicious intubation does not cause further intracranial problems due to increased intracranial pressure elevations from coughing or gagging during intubation. (See Chapter 2, Airway and Ventilatory Management.) Continued intubation may require sedation or iatrogenic paralysis. Hypocapnia can reduce cerebral circulation to the point where cerebral ischemia occurs. Blood gases must be monitored closely.

b. Fluid control

Intravenous fluids should be administered judiciously to prevent overhydration, which augments cerebral edema. Since the nature and volume of fluids administered will depend on the systemic status of the patient, consultations between the trauma surgeon and the neurosurgeon are necessary. Intravenous fluid used for maintenance must not be hyposmolar, as cerebral edema may likewise follow.

c. Diuretics

Diuretics such as mannitol, which cause diuresis by producing intravascular hyperosmolarity, are widely used for severe brain injury. Mannitol undoubtedly can be very effective in shrinking brain volume and lowering intracranial pressure. However, other effects may cause major problems. In the emergency department, this agent should be administered only with the consent of a neurosurgeon or to gain time when neurosurgical capabilities will be delayed and the patient's condition is deteriorating. Mannitol is most commonly and effectively used for a suspected surgical mass lesion when time is needed to prepare for operation (ie, hematoma with deteriorating level of consciousness, hemiparesis, and dilating pupil). For the average patient, 1 g/kg, is administered rapidly and intravenously. Care must be taken to prevent subcutaneous infiltration.

The neurosurgeon also may recommend loop diuretics, such as furosemide, (40 to 80 mg IV for adults). These medications act by medically decompressing the brain and may buy up to several hours of reduced intracranial pressure. A urinary catheter is required.

Because of the rapid production of urine, vascular volume may be significantly affected. Therefore, the patient's blood pressure must be closely monitored, especially if the patient has sustained multiple trauma or is a child. Urine volume may be replaced with isotonic fluids in these patients.

d. Steroids

Steroids are not recommended for the treatment of acute head injury.

VI. Other Manifestations of Head Injury

A. Seizures

Seizures, either full-blown convulsions or focal seizures, can occur with any injury. Seizures are common at the time of injury or shortly thereafter, and do not necessarily portend the development of chronic epilepsy. The neurosurgeon may recommend no treatment. Prolonged or repetitive seizures may be associated with intracranial hemorrhage and should be treated aggressively, because they may cause cerebral hypoxia, brain swelling, and increased intracranial pressure. A common treatment regimen consists of 10 mg of diazepam via an intravenous bolus. Respiratory exchange should be closely monitored. If the patient tolerates diazepam and has another convulsion, the dose may be repeated once **with caution**. Phenytoin, 1 g IV at a rate of 50 mg/minute, should be started as soon as possible, while monitoring the patient's blood pressure and electrocardiogram. If the convulsions persist despite diazepam and phenytoin, the patient should be given phenobarbital or an anesthetic. The injured brain tolerates anesthesia well.

B. Restlessness

Restlessness frequently accompanies brain injury and/or cerebral hypoxia. Its development in a previously quiet patient may be the first clinical expression of an expanding intracranial mass. Restlessness can often be controlled by correcting the cause. Primary attention should be directed to the possibility of cerebral hypoxia and its etiology. Pain from injuries, a distended bladder, painful bandages, tight casts, or systemic hypoxia may also induce restlessness. Only when these etiologic factors have been treated or excluded is the use of drugs justified to control the restlessness.

The relief of severe pain is an important part in the management of the trauma patient. Effective analgesia implies the use of intravenous opiates which may adversely affect the patient. They also may cause respiratory depression and mask neurologic signs. Therefore, for these reasons, opiates and other strong analgesics/sedatives should be withheld, if possible, until neurosurgical consultation has taken place. This presents less of a problem for the neurosurgeon if CT scan is readily available. Chlorpromazine, 10 to 25 mg IV, may be helpful for severe agitation. This agent must be administered carefully to avoid hypotension.

C. Hyperthermia

Hyperthermia is disastrous for the patient with an injured brain. Elevations in body temperature increase the rate of brain metabolism and levels of carbon dioxide. The higher the temperature, the greater the risk to the patient. A head-injured patient with hyperthermia should be placed on a hypothermia blanket, and shivering should be controlled with chlorpromazine.

VII. Scalp Wounds

Despite the dramatic appearance of scalp wounds, they are usually tolerated well and cause few complications. Scalp wounds usually heal well if general principles of good wound management are followed. The location and type of injury to the scalp give the physician a better understanding of the force and direction of the energy transmitted to the brain.

A. Blood Loss

Blood loss from scalp wounds can be extensive, especially in children. If the adult patient is in shock, bleeding from the scalp alone is usually not the cause. The general principles of scalp wound care include locating and stopping the bleeding. In the case of severed large vessels (ie, superficial temporal arteries), the vessels should be clamped with hemostats and ligated. Moderately severe bleeding from a deep scalp laceration can usually be controlled temporarily by applying direct pressure or placing hemostats on the galea and reflecting them backwards. For the unconscious patient, self-retaining retractors can be used.

Most scalp bleeding, with or without direct ligation of bleeding vessels, may be controlled by a snugly applied circumferential head dressing. If necessary, the hair may be clipped to facilitate application.

B. Inspection of the Scalp Wound

One should inspect the wound carefully and search under direct vision for signs of a skull fracture or foreign material. Blind probing with an instrument or the gloved finger should be avoided. Wound inspection also includes looking for CSF leaks, which may indicate not only a skull fracture, but also an arachnoid and dural tear. A neurosurgeon should be consulted before the wound is closed for all cases involving open fractures or depressed fractures of the skull.

C. Repairing the Scalp Wound

The first step in wound care is to irrigate the scalp wound with copious amounts of saline. Debris, including hair, must be removed. **Do not** remove bone fragments, because they may be tamponading intracranial bleeding. The neurosurgeon should remove bone fragments in the operating room. When in doubt, **always consult a neurosurgeon.** If transfer to a definitive-care facility is required, definitive surgical closure of a scalp wound can be delayed. However, temporary repair may be done to prevent further contamination of the wound.

When possible, primary definitive repair should be achieved under sterile technique with meticulous attention to the wound, as **scalp wounds may become infected**. The area immediately around the laceration should be shaved. The galea is closed first, using interrupted sutures. The skin is then sutured and a nonadherent dressing applied. The head wrap, if applied, should be just tight enough to apply mild pressure and prevent subgaleal accumulation of blood.

VIII. Definitive Surgical Management

Within two hours of injury, essential diagnostic studies should be completed. Although meeting this standard is difficult, delay can be extremely costly for the patient. If a neurosurgeon is not available at the facility initially receiving the patient, expeditious transfer of the patient to a hospital with an available neurosurgeon is necessary.

In exceptional circumstances, rapidly expanding intracranial hematomas (usually epidural hematomas) may be imminently life threatening and may not allow time for transfer if neurosurgical care is some distance away. Although this circumstance is rare in urban settings, it may occur occasionally in rural areas. In such circumstances, emergency burr holes can be considered if a surgeon, properly trained in the procedure, is available.

If definitive neurosurgical care is not immediately available, the purpose of an emergency burr hole is to preserve life by evacuating life-threatening intracranial hematomas. The performance of this procedure may be especially important for patients whose neurologic status rapidly deteriorates and for patients who do not respond to nonsurgical measures. However and before proceeding with the procedure, the physician must consider the following problems:

1. Not all severely head-injured patients have hematomas.

2. A burr hole, placed as little as 2 cm away from a hematoma, may not locate it.

3. A burr hole itself may cause brain damage or intracranial hemorrhage.

4. Burr-hole evacuation of a hematoma may not be life saving.

5. A burr hole can consume as much time as getting the patient to a neuro-surgeon.

Performance of emergency burr holes should be done only in exceptional circumstances and only with the advice and consent of a neurosurgeon. The indications for a burr hole performed by a nonneurosurgeon are few, and widespread use as a desperation maneuver is not recommended or supported by the Committee on Trauma. The procedure should be employed only if, in the judgment of a neurosurgeon, the burr hole can be performed in a timely manner, and when definitive neurosurgical care cannot be rendered expeditiously. In almost all instances this means that definitive neurosurgical care is many miles or several hours away.

The neurosurgeon usually recommends the burr hole be placed on the side of the largest pupil in comatose patients with decerebrate or decorticate posturing whose posturing does not respond to endotracheal hyperventilation and dehydrating agents (eg, 1 g/kg mannitol). The Committee on Trauma strongly recommends that those who anticipate the need for this procedure receive proper training in the procedure from a neurosurgeon.

IX. Summary

A. Secure and maintain an open airway.

B. Ventilate the patient to maintain oxygenation and to avoid hypercarbia.

C. Treat shock, if present, and look for cause.

D. Except for shock, restrict fluid intake to maintenance levels.

E. Perform a minineurologic examination.

F. Establish an initial working diagnosis.

G. Prevent secondary brain injury.

H. Search for associated injuries.

I. Obtain roentgenograms or CT scan as needed, but only after the patient is stable.

J. Consult a neurosurgeon and consider early transfer.

K. Should the patient's condition worsen, consider other diagnoses and forms of treatment; consult with a neurosurgeon, and consider transfer.

L. Continually reassess the patient (neurologic examination and GCS Score) to identify changes that necessitate neurosurgical intervention.

Bibliography

1. Anderson DW, McLaurin RL: The national head and spinal cord injury survey. **Journal of Neurosurgery** 1980;53:S1-543.

2. Andrews BT, Pitts LH, Lovely MP, et al: Is computed tomographic scanning necessary in patients with tentorial herniation?: Results of immediate surgical exploration without computed tomography in 100 patients. **Neurosurgery** 1986;19:408-414.

3. Becker DP, Gudeman SK: **Textbook of Head Injury**. Philadelphia, Saunders, 1989.

4. Cooper PR (ed): **Head Injury**, ed 2. Baltimore, Williams and Wilkins, 1987.

5. Gennarelli TA, Spielman GS, Langfitt TW, et al: Influence of the type of intracranial lesion on outcome from severe head injury: a multicenter study using a new classification system. **Journal of Neurosurgery** 1982;56:26-32.

6. Gennarelli TA: Emergency department management of head injuries. **Emergency Medicine Clinics of North America** 1984;2:749-760.

7. Gildenberg PL, Makela M: Effect of early intubation and ventilation on outcome following head injury. In Dacy RG (ed): **Trauma of the Nervous System**. Raven, New York, 1985, pp 79-90.

8. Jennett B, Teasdale G: **Management of Head Injuries**. Philadelphia, Davis, 1981.

9. Masters SJ, McClean PM, Arcarese JS, et al: Skull x-ray examinations after head trauma: Recommendations by a multidisciplinary panel and validation study. **New England Journal of Medicine** 1987;316:84-91.

10. Seelig JM, Becker DP, Miller JD, et al: Traumatic acute subdural hematoma: major mortality reduction in comatose patients treated within four hours. **New England Journal of Medicine** 1981;304:1511-1518.

Chapter 6:
Head Trauma

Skill Station IX:
Head and Neck Trauma
Assessment and Management

Resources and Equipment

This list is the recommended equipment to conduct this skill session in accordance with the stated objectives for and intent of the procedures outlined. Additional equipment may be used providing it does not detract from the stated objectives and intent of this skill, or from performing the procedures in a safe method as described and recommended by the ACS Committee on Trauma.

1. Mr. HURT—Head trauma manikin

2. Ophthalmoscope

3. Otoscope

4. Table and chairs; or gurney, pillows, and sheet

5. Semirigid cervical collar

6. Cervical traction tongs (preferably Gardner-Wells tongs)

7. 2 coconuts

Objectives

1. Performance at this station will allow participants to practice and demonstrate their assessment and diagnostic skills in determining the type and extent of injuries with Mr. HURT (head trauma manikin).

2. Upon completion of this station, the participant will be able to discuss the importance of clinical signs and symptoms found through assessment.

3. Upon completion of this station, the participant will be able to discuss and establish priorities for initial primary management of the patient with head trauma.

4. Participation at this station will allow the student to discuss other diagnostic aids that can be used to determine the area of injury within the brain and the extent of injury.

5. Upon completion of this station, the participant will be able to demonstrate proficiency in the use and application of the cervical traction tongs.

Chapter 6:
Head Trauma

Skill
Station IX

American College of Surgeons

Head and Neck Trauma Assessment and Management

Note: Universal precautions are required whenever caring for the trauma patient.

I. Head Trauma Assessment and Management

A. Primary Survey

1. ABCs

2. Immobilize and stabilize the cervical spine.

3. Perform a brief neurologic examination.

    a. Pupillary response
    b. AVPU

B. Secondary Survey and Management

1. Inspect the head.

    a. Lacerations
    b. Nose and ears for presence of CSF leakage

2. Palpate the head.

    a. Fractures
    b. Lacerations for underlying fractures

3. Inspect all scalp lacerations.

    a. Brain tissue
    b. Depressed skull fractures
    c. Debris
    d. CSF leaks

4. Perform a minineurologic examination and determine the patient's GCS Score.

    a. Eye-opening response
    b. Verbal response
    c. Best limb motor response

5. Palpate the c-spine for fractures and apply a semirigid cervical collar, if needed.

6. Determine the extent of injury.

7. Reassess the patient continuously, observing for signs of deterioration.

    a. Frequency
    b. Parameters to be assessed

C. Head and Neck Injuries

1. Open, depressed skull fracture on the right

This type of injury is indicative of the amount of energy force that has been delivered to the cranium. An open, depressed skull fracture requires early operative intervention, with management directed toward the underlying brain injury.

2. Zygomatic fracture (Le Fort III fracture) on the right

A Le Fort III fracture is a separation of the mid-third of the face at the zygomaticofrontal, zygomaticotemporal, and nasal sutures, and across the orbital floor. It is a compound fracture with major hemorrhage that jeopardizes the integrity of the airway. Airway control and protection of the airway with concomitant immobilization of the cervical spine is imperative. Inability to intubate the patient may be an indication for surgical cricothyroidotomy, depending on the clinical judgment and skill level of the examiner. Nasotracheal intubation is contraindicated.

3. Maxillary fracture (Le Fort I fracture) on the right

Traumatic malocclusion is an important sign indicating a major disruption of the facial bones. Associated bleeding also may compromise the airway. Management includes: (1) securing a patent airway, (2) maintaining c-spine immobilization, and (3) hemorrhage control.

4. Mandibular fracture on the left

This is an important injury to recognize, especially if it occurs in combination with other facial fractures. In the unconscious patient, the tongue falls posteriorly and occludes the airway. Basic airway management procedures, eg, insertion of an oropharyngeal airway, are necessary to prevent airway obstruction.

5. Mandibular/neck laceration on the left

Penetrating injuries of the neck are located in three anatomic areas: (1) Zone 1—structures at the thoracic outlet, (2) Zone 2—between the clavicle and mandible, and (3) Zone 3—between the angle of the mandible and the base of the skull.

This is an important wound to recognize. In this particular manikin, the platysma has been violated. Active bleeding, external or internal, may be present. Control and protection of the airway is necessary in this unconscious patient.

6. Nasal fracture

Bleeding can be significant from nasal fractures and can place the integrity of the airway in jeopardy, especially in the unconscious patient.

7. Multiple fractures, C-6 vertebra

A step-off deformity, although difficult to palpate, is present. Management includes continued immobilization of the c-spine and obtaining a lateral c-spine roentgenogram.

8. **Unequal pupils**

A unilateral, fixed and dilated pupil in an unconscious patient is a sign of grave consequence. Appropriate resuscitation and surgical intervention must be instituted rapidly. The inability of the dilated pupil to react to light denotes one lesion. The third cranial nerve on the side of the dilated pupil may be compressed by increased intracranial pressure due to a mass lesion or epidural bleeding. Rapid neurosurgical intervention is necessary to prevent secondary brain injury. Controlled hyperventilation and fluid resuscitation restriction may be required for this patient. The eyes also are exophthalmic.

9. **Hemotympanum on the right**

This sign denotes a basal skull fracture. Patients with this type of fracture may have significant traumatic CSF leaks. Cribriform plate fractures are often associated with this injury. Insertion of a nasogastric tube and nasotracheal intubation are contraindicated.

II. Application of Cervical Traction Tongs
(Optional Skill Procedure)

Note: Differences of opinion exist among neurosurgeons regarding the indications and techniques for the use of cervical traction in the patient with a **known** cervical spine injury. Therefore, protocols for its use should be established at each local institution in consultation with a neurosurgeon.

This skill procedure is based on the use of Gardner-Wells tongs for the patient with a mid-cervical fracture-dislocation, eg, C-4 on C-5.

A. Identify the site for application of the tongs. The tongs are applied above the ears and below the "equator" (temporal ridges).

B. Surgically prepare the scalp with an antiseptic preparation. It is not necessary to shave the scalp. An aerosol spray that coats and penetrates the hair to the skin is recommended. Then rub in the antiseptic.

C. Locally inject an anesthetic and allow time for it to take effect.

D. If using a spray antiseptic, respray the scalp.

E. Place the tong apparatus with the metal instruction plate facing upward.

F. Advance the spring-loaded points until the 1-mm protrusion indicator within its knob shows that the proper squeeze is being exerted. (As the points are advanced, the skin is stretched increasingly snug, effectively sealing the point of entry and preventing bleeding.)

G. When bone is encountered, the stiff spring yields until the outer end of the spring-loaded point barely protrudes beyond the flat surface of the knurled end. (Indicates 30 pounds of "squeeze" being applied.)

H. Tilt the tong back and forth several times to seat the points. Then check the indicator protrusion and retighten it if necessary.

I. Support the tongs with slight, hand-applied traction, parallel to the bed or patient cart, until the assistant attaches the rope and pulley system.

J. Apply five pounds of weight to the rope, and carefully release hold of the tongs.

K. Additional weight can be applied according to protocol or at the direction of the neurosurgeon.

Contraindications

1. Paget's disease of the skull
2. Neonates or infants
3. Massive open/comminuted skull fracture

Complications

1. Localized sepsis at puncture sites
2. Laceration of a scalp artery

Chapter 7:
Spine and Spinal Cord Trauma

Objectives:

Upon completion of this topic, the physician will be able to identify principles of management, demonstrate the ability to assess spinal trauma, and apply immobilization techniques for patients with vertebral and/or spinal cord injuries.

Specifically, the physician will be able to:

A. Discuss the principles involved in evaluating vertebral and spinal cord trauma.

B. Identify the types of vertebral injuries and outline methods of treatment.

C. Given a simulated patient with suspected cervical vertebral and spinal cord injuries, demonstrate the ability to assess and manage the multiply injured patient.

D. Given a simulated patient with suspected cervical vertebral and spinal cord injuries and appropriate equipment, apply techniques to immobilize the neck and spine safely.

E. Given a series of roentgenograms depicting cervical spine injuries, outline anatomic assessment principles and techniques for detecting abnormalities.

**Chapter 7:
Spine and
Spinal Cord
Trauma**

I. Introduction

The physician must be continually cognizant that injudicious manipulation or movement, and inadequate immobilization can cause additional spinal injury and decrease the patient's overall prognosis.

Vertebral injuries may be present without spinal cord injury. However, the potential for cord injury is always present, and careful patient handling is essential. **A vertebral column injury should be presumed and immobilization of the entire patient should be maintained until screening roentgenograms are obtained and fractures or fracture-dislocations are excluded.** Under many circumstances it is not possible to obtain appropriate roentgenograms of the spine during the initial evaluation of the patient for technical reasons without causing undue delay in the management of serious injuries. Under these circumstances, the physician should maintain continued immobilization of the patient until more specialized help is available. **It is important for the physician to keep in mind that as long as the patient is immobilized, clearance of the spine may be deferred safely, especially in the presence of systemic instability (eg, hypotension, respiratory inadequacy). It is the movement of the nonimmobilized patient with unrecognized, unstable vertebral column injuries that places the spinal cord at risk of damage.**

II. History of Injury

Knowledge of the patient's neurologic condition prior to injury is very important. A description of how the patient sustained the injury is significant in order to understand the mechanism of injury and potential for further injury. Prehospital care personnel can provide valuable information, eg, presence of paralysis immediately postinjury or deterioration of the patient's sensorimotor status. This information is essential to assess and document the site and extent of injury and/or the paralysis present.

Any patient sustaining an injury above the clavicle or a head injury resulting in an unconscious state should be suspected of having an associated cervical spinal column injury. Any injury produced by high-speed vehicles should arouse suspicion of concomitant spine and spinal cord injury.

III. Assessment

A. General

Examination of any suspected case of spinal injury must be carried out with the patient in a neutral position and without any movement of the patient's spine. The neck and trunk must not be flexed, extended, or rotated. The patient should be brought to the emergency department properly immobilized. Although a semirigid cervical collar is useful, securing the head to a spine board and bolster-splinting the neck is more effective. The entire patient should be left immobilized until roentgenograms are taken to exclude vertebral fractures. If the patient must be moved from the spine board, for examination or treatment, a scoop-style stretcher should be used. (See Skill Station XI, Immobilization Techniques for Neck and Spinal Trauma.)

Total spinal immobilization is the goal. Not only the head and neck, but also the chest, pelvis, and lower extremities must be immobilized securely to provide protection to the thoracic and lumbar segments of the spinal column.

A **conscious** patient with paralysis is usually able to identify pain at the site of injury, because loss of sensation is below this level. As the spine is carefully palpated, listen to the patient and watch his face for signs of pain. **Remember**, paralysis and loss of sensation may mask intra-abdominal and lower-extremity injuries.

If the patient is **unconscious**, and the injury is due to a fall or a vehicular collision, the chance of a cervical spine injury is 5% to 10%. Clinical findings that suggest a cervical cord injury in the unconscious patient include:

1. Flaccid areflexia, especially with flaccid rectal sphincter

2. Diaphragmatic breathing

3. Ability to flex, but not extend at the elbow

4. Grimaces to pain above, but not below the clavicle

5. Hypotension with bradycardia, especially without hypovolemia

6. Priapism, an uncommon but characteristic sign

All information obtained from the neurologic examination is carefully documented on the chart for easy identification of any changes. In the paralyzed patient, any movement or sensation at or below the level of the injury is important and may affect the prognosis.

Early consultation with a neurosurgeon and/or orthopedic surgeon is essential. Specific types of neurologic deficit are important only to establish that an injury is present. Once established, consultation and transfer to an institution with neurosurgical and/or orthopedic capabilities are essential.

Spinal immobilization should be continued until removed by the neurosurgical or orthopedic consultant. This usually occurs when no roentgenographic abnormality has been documented, and no symptoms or signs relating to the spine or cord exist.

B. Vertebral Assessment

Vertebral injuries usually are associated with local tenderness, and less often, with palpable deformity. Careful examination of the entire spine from the occiput to sacrum should begin with the patient in a supine position. To visually examine the back, the patient may be log-rolled, **but only to the minimum degree necessary to permit the examination**. This modified log-roll procedure requires the aid of at least four assistants—one to maintain manual, in-line immobilization of the patient's head and neck, one for the torso (including the hips and pelvis), one for the legs, and one to direct the procedure and remove the spine board. (See Skill Station XI, Immobilization Techniques for Neck and Spinal Trauma.)

The physicians should assess for pain, tenderness, and a posterior "step-off" deformity. Pain usually will be localized when an injured spine is palpated, but the pain may radiate to the arms, around the chest and abdomen, or into the lower extremities. Other diagnostic signs and symptoms include prominence of spinous processes, local tenderness, pain with attempted motion, edema, ecchymosis, visible deformity, and muscle spasms. The physicians should also assess for tracheal tenderness or deviation and retropharyngeal hematoma. The position of the head should be noted for muscle spasm and head tilt. These symptoms also help identify and localize the site of injury.

C. Neurologic Assessment of Spinal Cord Injury

The patient is carefully examined for motor strength and weakness, sensory disturbances, reflex changes, and autonomic dysfunction. Autonomic dysfunction is identified by lack of bladder and rectal control and priapism.

Of the many tracts in the spinal cord, only three can be readily assessed clinically. Each is a paired tract that may be injured on one or both sides of the cord. The **corticospinal tract**, in the posterolateral aspect of the cord, controls motor power on the same side of the body and is tested by voluntary muscle contractions or involuntary response to painful stimulus. The **spinothalamic tract**, in the anterolateral aspect of the cord, transmits pain and temperature sensation from the opposite side of the body. It is tested by pinch or pin prick. The **posterior columns** carry proprioceptive impulses from the same side of the body and are tested by position sense of the fingers and toes or tuning fork vibration.

No demonstrable sensory or motor function is exhibited with a **complete spinal cord lesion.** This situation is dismal, because the chance of useful recovery is small. **Incomplete spinal cord lesions** differ considerably, because recovery can occur. Therefore, a careful examination to determine the presence of any sensory or motor function is essential.

Superficial (pin-prick) or deep pain discrimination indicates an incomplete lesion and lateral column preservation. Because the sensation of light touch is conveyed in both the lateral and posterior columns, it may be the one sensory modality preserved when all other sensations are absent. Sparing of sensation in the sacral dermatomes may be the only sign of incomplete injury. To assess sacral sparing, gently lift the leg and assess the anal, perianal, and scrotal areas. The evaluation for sacral sparing should include sensory perception and voluntary contraction of the anus.

D. Neurogenic and Spinal Shock

Neurogenic shock results from impairment of the descending sympathetic pathways in the spinal cord, the results of which are loss of vasomotor tone, and loss of sympathetic innervation to the heart. The former causes vasodilatation of visceral and lower extremity vessels, pooling of blood intravascularly, and consequent hypotension. As a result of loss of cardiac sympathetic tone, the patient may fail to become tachycardic or may be even bradycardic. Therefore, the combination of hypotension and bradycardia due to neurogenic shock is not due to true hypovolemia. The blood pressure is not usually restored by fluid infusion alone, and thus aggressive attempts to treat the hypotension of neurogenic shock by fluid replacement alone may result in fluid overload. The blood pressure often can be restored by the judicious use of vasopressors. This is an exception to the general guideline of not using vasopressors for the treatment of shock. Atropine may be used to counteract the bradycardia. (See Chapter 3, Shock.)

Spinal shock refers to the neurologic condition shortly after spinal cord injury. The "shock" to the injured cord may make it appear completely functionless, even though all areas are not permanently destroyed. This produces flaccidity and loss of reflexes instead of the expected spasticity, hyperactive reflexes, and Babinski signs. Days to weeks later, spinal shock disappears and in areas where no function has returned, spasticity supersedes the flaccid state.

E. Effect on Other Organ Systems

Hypoventilation due to paralysis of the intercostal muscles will result from an injury involving the lower cervical or the upper thoracic spinal cord. If the upper or the middle cervical spinal cord is injured, the diaphragm also will be paralyzed due to involvement of the C-3 through C-5 spinal cord segments, where the motor nerve cells that innervate the diaphragm (via the phrenic nerve) are located. Abdominal breathing and the use of the respiratory accessory muscles will be evident in both instances. The inability to feel pain may mask a potentially serious injury elsewhere in the body, such as the usual signs of an acute abdomen.

F. Roentgenograms

A lateral c-spine roentgenogram should be obtained for every patient sustaining an injury above the clavicle, especially a head injury. In addition, films of the thoracic and lumbar sections of the spine should be obtained for any patient suspected of sustaining a multiple trauma, especially to the trunk. The finding of a c-spine injury mandates radiologic examination of the entire spinal column.

1. Cervical spine

Lateral c-spine roentgenograms should be obtained as soon as life-threatening problems are identified and controlled. **The base of the skull, all seven cervical vertebrae, and the first thoracic vertebrae must be visualized.** The patient's shoulders are pulled down routinely when obtaining the lateral c-spine roentgenogram to prevent missing fractures or fracture-dislocations in the lower c-spine. If all seven cervical vertebrae are not visualized with the lateral roentgenogram, a lateral swimmer's view of the lower cervical and upper thoracic area may be obtained.

After adequate demonstration of all seven cervical and the first thoracic vertebrae, the physician can obtain chest and open-mouth odontoid roentgenograms. Other roentgenograms that can be obtained after the first hour to further evaluate the c-spine include anteroposterior (AP) and oblique cervical views. These or more sophisticated studies should be done for any patient with a normal crosstable lateral roentgenogram who is suspected (either by signs and symptoms or by mechanism of injury) of having cervical injury, because even the best portable films miss 5% to 15% of the injuries. A computed tomographic (CT) scan may be needed to determine the presence of bone fragments within the spinal canal. Alternatively, tomograms may be obtained to confirm a c-spine injury and determine its stability. **Lateral flexion and extension** roentgenograms of the cervical spine may be dangerous and should be done under the direct supervision and control of a knowledgeable physician.

2. Thoracic and lumbar spine

Anteroposterior films of the thoracic and lumbar areas of the spine are standard. Because the crosstable lateral diameter of the body is usually greater than the AP diameter, most portable roentgenographic equipment used in emergency departments provide better bony definition in the AP view. Subsequent films may be obtained in the more elective environment of the radiology department. Oblique thoracic films seldom add further information. Lateral and oblique films of the lumbar spine are obtained if indicated.

IV. Types of Spinal Injuries

A. Fractures and Fracture-Dislocation of the Spine

Roentgenograms of the cervical spine should be examined for:

a. Anteroposterior diameter of the spinal canal

b. Contour and alignment of the vertebral bodies

c. Displacement of bone fragments into the spinal canal

d. Linear or comminuted fractures of the laminae, pedicles, or neural arches

e. Soft-tissue swelling

During the early evaluation of the patient with suspected thoracic and/or lumbar injuries, it usually is sufficient to view only AP films of the vertebral column. These films should be examined for:

f. Bilateral symmetry of the pedicles

g. Height of the intervertebral disc spaces

h. Central alignment of the spinous processes

i. Shape and contour of the vertebral bodies

j. Alignment of the vertebral bodies, should a lateral film be available

1. Cervical spine injuries

Cervical spine injuries result from any one or a combination of these mechanisms of injury: (1) axial loading; (2) flexion; (3) extension; (4) rotation; (5) lateral bending; and (6) distraction. **Cervical spine injuries resulting in unstable fractures, fracture-dislocations, and/or cord injury require transfer to a definitive-care facility.** When in doubt, consult with a neurosurgeon or orthopedic surgeon.

a. C-1 (atlas) fracture

A fracture of C-1 (atlas) usually involves a blowout of the ring (Jefferson fracture). The mechanism of injury of a C-1 fracture is usually an axial load. It appears as a fracture of the lamina on the lateral roentgenogram and is seen best on an open-mouth view of the C-1 and C-2 area. **Remember, one third of these fractures are associated with a C-2 fracture**. They usually are **not** associated with cord injuries. However, they are **unstable** and should be treated initially with the application of a semirigid cervical collar and immobilization of the entire patient on a long spine board.

b. C-1, rotary subluxation

This injury is diagnosed by an odontoid-view roentgenogram. The odontoid will not be equidistant from the two lateral masses of C-1, because of the rotation of the ring of C-1 with reference to the odontoid. This injury is most often seen in children. The patient appears with a torticollis or persistent rotation of the head with reference to the neck. The child should not be forced to overcome the rotation. Rather, he should be immobilized in place and treated. Treatment of subluxation injuries is usually best managed in a definitive-care facility.

c. C-2, odontoid dislocation

Injuries to C-2 may displace the odontoid posteriorly into the spinal canal. Odontoid subluxation occurs because of injury to the transverse ligament that attaches the odontoid to the anterior arch of C-1. Bony injury may not occur, but this diagnosis should be considered whenever the space between the anterior arch of C-1 and the odontoid is greater than 3 mm. Displacement can occur **without** cord injury due to Steel's "Rule of Three": **one third of the spinal canal in the region of the atlas is occupied by the odontoid, one third is occupied by an intervening space, and one third is occupied by the spinal cord**. Room posterior to the odontoid is thus available for displacement. However, this situation is dangerous because excessive head motion can transect the cord. Head and spine immobilization is critical.

d. C-2, odontoid fractures

Three types of fractures may be associated with the odontoid. All can be very difficult to see on routine roentgenograms. If suspected, more views, tomograms, or CT are needed.

1) **Type I** usually occurs above the base of the odontoid and is most often stable.

2) **Type II** occurs at the base of the odontoid and is usually unstable. **Remember**, in children younger than six years, the epiphysis may be present and may appear as a fracture at this level.

3) **Type III** is a fracture of the odontoid that extends into the vertebral body.

Patients with Type I fractures may be treated with a semirigid cervical collar or brace. However, patients with all types should be transported to a definitive-care hospital for further evaluation and possible surgical intervention or halo immobilization.

e. Posterior element fracture of C-2

The "Hangman's Fracture" (name derived from judicial hangings) involves the posterior elements of C-2. The mechanism of this injury is extension and distraction or extension and axial compression. This is an unstable fracture. Patients with a "Hangman's Fracture" should not be placed in cervical traction if the mechanism of injury is secondary to distraction. Rather, such patients should be maintained in external immobilization and transferred to a definitive-care facility.

f. C-3 through C-7, fractures and fracture-dislocations

Various combinations of fractures and/or fracture-dislocations may be seen in C-3 through C-7. The mechanism of injury in **stable** fractures is usually flexion axial loading, extension axial loading, or flexion rotation injuries.

When examining a lateral c-spine film assess the distance between the pharynx and the anterior/inferior border of C-3. The soft-tissue prevertebral thickness at this level should be less than 5 mm between the pharynx and vertebral body. An increase in this area of density is indirect evidence of a vertebral fracture, notoriously associated with a minimally displaced C-2 fracture.

Children normally have prevertebral thickness that is two thirds of the vertebral thickness of C-2. The distance will vary with inspiration and expiration. When assessing for a hematoma at this level in children, **remember that forced expiration or crying increases the distance between the pharynx and the anterior/inferior border of C-3.**

Below the larynx, the tracheal air shadow is further from the anterior vertebral bodies because of the interposition of the esophagus. The best rule for prevertebral hematoma in this area is that the distance to the air shadow should be less than the width of the vertebral body.

Patients with **unstable** vertebral injuries of C-3 through C-7 require transfer to a definitive-care hospital. Typically, these patients include those with one or more of the findings listed herein:

1) A fracture identified by disruption of the anterior and all of the posterior elements

2) A fracture with overriding of a superior vertebra on the adjoining inferior vertebra by more than 3.0 mm

3) A fracture with angulation between two adjoining vertebra greater than 11 degrees

g. Facet dislocations

Facet dislocations also may produce an **unstable** vertebral injury, especially bilateral facet dislocations. Consider a unilateral facet dislocation if the superior vertebra is displaced on the adjoining inferior vertebra by 25%. Consider a bilateral facet dislocation if displacement is greater than 50%. Malalignment of the cervical spinous processes on an AP roentgenogram also is suggestive of unilateral facet dislocation.

2. Cervical spinal cord injuries

A bony fleck off the superior aspect of the vertebral body demonstrates an extension-type injury. It usually is stable and does not involve cord damage. The classic tear-drop sign may be seen with a bone chip off the anterior/inferior aspect of the vertebral body. Cord injuries are often associated with this radiographic tear-drop finding, an ominous sign that may indicate displacement of the disc or posterior fragment of the vertebral body into the spinal canal.

Spinal cord injuries can occur in the c-spine with an otherwise stable compression fracture of the body, because the vertebral body collapses and is displaced posteriorly into the cord. These injuries may range from fracture of the body without displacement and cord damage, to severe vertebral disruption with complete paralysis.

3. Thoracic spine fractures (T-1 through T-10)

Fractures in this region are usually the result of hyperflexion that produces wedge compression of one or more vertebral bodies. The amount of wedging is usually quite small, and the anterior portion of the vertebral body is rarely more than 25% shorter than the posterior body. Because of the rigidity of the rib cage, most of these fractures are stable. Where the kyphosis exceeds 30 degrees, internal stabilization probably will be required to prevent further deformity. The thoracic spinal canal is narrow in relation to the spinal cord, so that thoracic spinal cord injuries commonly are complete. If the deformity is associated with rotation, spinal cord injury is quite common.

4. Thoracolumbar fractures (T-11 through L-1)

Fractures at this level are frequently due to the relative immobility of the thoracic spine compared with the lumbar spine. They most often result from a combination of acute hyperflexion and rotation, and consequently they are commonly unstable. Because the spinal cord terminates at this level, the nerve roots that compose the cauda equina arise at the thoracolumbar junction. An injury at this level will produce bladder and bowel signs from spinal cord injury, and decreased sensation and movement in the lower extremities in various combinations from injury to the cauda equina. Because log-rolling may be destabilizing to this segment of the spine with fractures, this maneuver should be performed only to the minimal degree required under the circumstances to examine the patient's back.

5. Lumbar fractures

Disruption of the posterior ligaments by an acute hyperflexion injury in the lumbar region may produce an unstable vertebral column fracture. The neurologic signs associated with a lumbar fracture may be similar to those of a thoracolumbar fracture. However, lumbar fracture neurologic signs result only from involvement of the cauda equina, which include those nerve roots innervating the bladder.

B. Open Wounds

The most common of open spinal wounds are those caused either by missile injuries or stabbings. A bullet passing through the vertebral canal usually results in complete neurologic deficit. The physician should assess for CSF drainage from the wound. Hemopneumothorax, acute abdomen, or great vessel injury is often associated with an open spinal injury and takes precedence for treatment.

V. Treatment

A. Immobilization

Prehospital care personnel usually immobilize patients before their transport to the emergency department. Any patient with a suspected spine injury must be immobilized above and below the suspected injury site until injury has been excluded by roentgenograms. The proper technique for spinal immobilization is outlined in Skill Station XI. **Remember**, these protective devices must not be removed until absence of c-spine injury is documented. Proper immobilization is achieved with the patient in the neutral position, ie, supine without rotation or bending of the spinal column. It is necessary that proper padding be used to prevent the development of decubiti. Skin injury may occur after two hours of unprotected pressure. The more common sites of injury are the occiput and the sacrum.

Immobilization with a semirigid collar does not necessarily assure stabilization of the c-spine. Immobilization to a spine board with appropriate bolstering devices may be more effective in limiting certain neck motions. **Cervical spine injury requires continuous immobilization of the entire patient with a semirigid cervical collar, backboard, tape, and straps before and during transfer to a definitive-care facility.** Spinal curvature varies with the patient's age and any disease processes. Therefore, padding may be required beneath the shoulders of a pediatric patient and behind the head of an adult patient to avoid hyperextension or flexion of the neck. (See Skill Station XI, Immobilization Techniques for Neck and Spinal Trauma.)

Of special concern is the maintenance of adequate immobilization of the **restless, agitated, or violent patient**. This condition may be due to pain, confusion associated with hypoxia or hypotension, alcohol or drugs, or simply a personality disorder. The physician should search for and correct, if possible, the cause. If necessary, a sedative or tranquilizer, eg, chlorpromazine, may be administered, keeping in mind the need for adequate airway control and ventilation.

B. Intravenous Fluids

Intravenous fluids usually are limited to maintenance levels unless specifically needed for the management of shock. As a result of loss of cardiac sympathetic tone, the patient may fail to become tachycardic or may be even bradycardic. Hypovolemic shock usually can be differentiated from neurogenic shock by tachycardia in the former and bradycardia in the latter. If the blood pressure does not improve after a fluid challenge, the judicious use of vasopressors may be indicated. Overzealous fluid administration may cause pulmonary edema in a patient with a spinal cord injury. A urinary catheter is inserted to monitor urinary output and prevent bladder distention.

C. Medications

Proper limitation of fluid intake usually obviates the need for diuretics. The value of steroids is controversial; however, they are frequently used in the early management of spinal injuries. Steroids may be of value in certain patients with incomplete spinal cord injuries. Their use should be determined in consultation with a neurosurgeon. **A management protocol should be established by prior consultation.**

D. Transfer

Patients with unstable fractures or a documented neurologic deficit should be transferred to a definitive-care facility. For physicians who do not see such injuries routinely, the safest procedure is to transfer the patient after telephone consultation with a specialist. Avoid unnecessary delay. The patient's condition should be stabilized; necessary splints, backboards, and/or semi-rigid cervical collar should be applied; and the patient should be transferred under medical supervision. **Remember, high c-spine injuries can result in partial or total loss of respiratory function.** These patients are best managed by maintaining an adequate airway and ventilation. (See Chapter 2, Airway and Ventilatory Management.)

VI. Summary

A. Attend to life-threatening injuries, avoiding any movement of the spinal column.

B. Establish and maintain proper immobilization of the patient until vertebral fractures or spinal cord injuries have been excluded.

C. Obtain lateral c-spine roentgenograms as soon as life-threatening injuries are controlled.

D. Documentation of the patient's history and physical examination are of paramount importance to establish a baseline for any changes in the patient's neurologic status (ie, ascertaining progress or deterioration of an incomplete lesion).

E. Obtain consultation with a neurosurgeon and/or orthopedic surgeon.

F. Transfer patients with unstable vertebral fractures or spinal cord injury to a definitive-care facility.

Bibliography

1. Bohlman HH: Current concepts review, treatment of fractures and dislocations of the thoracic and lumbar spine. **Journal of Bone and Joint Surgery** 1985;67-A, 1:165-169.

2. Cooper PR (ed): **Management of Posttraumatic Spinal Instability.** Park Ridge, Illinois, American Association of Neurosurgeons, 1990.

3. Geisler FH, Dorsey FC, Coleman WP: Recovery of motor function after spinal-cord injury—a randomized, placebo-controlled trial with GM-1 ganglioside. **The New England Journal of Medicine** 1991;26:1829-1838.

4. Harris P: **Thoracic and Lumbar Spine and Spinal Cord Injuries**. New York, Springer-Verlag, 1987.

5. McCall IW, Park WM, McSweeney T: The radiological demonstration of acute lower cervical injury. **Clinical Radiology** 1973;24:235-240.

6. McGuire RA, Neville S, Green BA, et al: Spine instability and the log-rolling maneuver. **Journal of Trauma** 1987;27:525-531.

7. Moulton RJ, Clifton GL: Injury to the vertebrae and spinal cord. In Mattox KL, Moore EE, Feliciano DV (eds) **Trauma**. Norwalk, Connecticut, Appleton and Lange, 1988, pp 253-269.

8. Podoisky S, et al: Efficacy of cervical spine immobilization methods. **Journal of Trauma** 1983;23:461.

**Chapter 7:
Spine and
Spinal Cord
Trauma**

Skill Station X: Roentgenographic Identification of Spine Injuries

Chapter 7:
Spine and
Spinal Cord
Trauma

Skill
Station X

Equipment and Resources

This list is the recommended equipment to conduct this skill session in accordance with the stated objectives for and intent of the procedures outlined. Additional equipment may be used providing it does not detract from the stated objectives and intent of this skill, or from performing the procedure in a safe method as described and recommended by the ACS Committee on Trauma.

1. Cervical, thoracic, and lumbar spine roentgenograms (available from the ACS, ATLS Division)

2. Identification key to roentgenograms

3. View boxes to display films

Objectives

1. Upon completion of this station, the participant will be able to identify various c-spine injuries by using four specific anatomic guidelines for examining a series of c-spine roentgenograms.

   a. Alignment
   b. Bones
   c. Cartilage
   d. Soft-tissue space

2. Upon completion of this station, the participant will be able to identify various thoracic and lumbar spine injuries by analyzing these areas:

   a. Alignment
   b. Body contour
   c. Disc space
   d. Pedicles
   e. Spinous processes
   f. Canal

3. Given a series of roentgenograms, the participant will be able to:

   a. Diagnose fractures
   b. Delineate associated injuries
   c. Define other areas of possible injury

Chapter 7:
Spine and
Spinal Cord
Trauma

Skill
Station X

Chapter 7:
Spine and
Spinal Cord
Trauma

Skill
Station X

Skill Procedure

Roentgenographic Identification of Spine Injuries

Note: The guidelines outlined herein identify areas of the spine that should be assessed when examining a spine film. Each of these areas should be assessed for potential injury when viewing the roentgenograms associated with this skill station.

I. C-Spine Roentgenograms—Assessing for Injury

A. Identify Presence of All Seven Cervical Vertebrae and Superior Aspect of T-1

B. Anatomic Assessment

1. Alignment—Identify and assess the four lordotic curves.

a. Anterior vertebral bodies
b. Anterior spinal canal
c. Posterior spinal canal
d. Spinous process tips

2. Bone—Assess for:

a. Vertebral body—contour and axial height
b. Lateral bony mass

1) Pedicles
2) Facets
3) Laminae
4) Transverse processes

c. Spinous processes

3. Cartilage—Assess for:

a. Intervertebral discs
b. Posterolateral facet joints

4. Soft-tissue spaces—Assess for:

a. Prevertebral space
b. Prevertebral fat stripe
c. Space between spinous processes

Chapter 7:
Spine and
Spinal Cord
Trauma

Skill
Station X

C. Assessment Guidelines for Detecting Abnormalities

1. Alignment

   a. Vertebral malalignment > 3.0 mm—dislocation

   b. Anteroposterior spinal canal space < 13 mm—spinal cord compression

   c. Angulation of intervertebral space > 11 degrees

2. Bones

   a. Vertebral body

   1) Anterior height < 3 mm posterior height—compression fracture
   2) Oblique lucency—tear-drop fracture

   b. Lack of parallel facets of the lateral mass—possible lateral compression fracture

   c. Lucency through the tip of the spinous process—avulsion fracture

   d. Atlas and axis (C-1 and C-2)

   1) Distance between posterior aspect of C-1 to anterior odontoid process > 3 mm—dislocation
   2) Lucency through the odontoid process of C-2—fracture

3. Soft-tissue space

   a. Widening of the prevertebral space > 5 mm—hemorrhage accompanying spinal injury

   b. Obliteration of prevertebral fat strip—fracture at same level

   c. Widening of space between spinous processes—torn interspinous ligaments and likely spinal canal fracture anteriorly

II. Thoracic and Lumbar Roentgenograms— Assessing for Injury

A. Anteroposterior View

Assess for:

1. Alignment

2. Symmetry of pedicles

3. Contour of bodies

4. Height of disc spaces

5. Central position of spinous processes

Chapter 7:
**Spine and
Spinal Cord
Trauma**

**Skill
Station X**

B. Lateral View

Assess for:

1. Alignment of bodies/angulation of spine

2. Contour of bodies

3. Presence of disc spaces

4. Encroachment of body on canal

III. Review Spine Roentgenograms

**Chapter 7:
Spine and
Spinal Cord
Trauma**

**Skill
Station X**

American College of Surgeons

Skill Station XI: Immobilization Techniques for Neck and Spinal Trauma

Chapter 7:
Spine and
Spinal Cord
Trauma

Skill
Station XI

Equipment and Resources

This list is the recommended equipment to conduct this skill session in accordance with the stated objectives for and intent of the procedures outlined. Additional equipment may be used providing it does not detract from the stated objectives and intent of this skill, or from performing the procedure in a safe method as described and recommended by the ACS Committee on Trauma.

1. Live patient model (participants may serve as patients)

2. Semirigid cervical collar*

3. Long spine board with straps*

4. Rolled towels or similar bolstering devices*

5. Blankets for padding

6. Roller-type dressing/bandage

7. Tape

8. Scoop stretcher (optional)

9. Four assistants (three assistants in addition to the Instructor; participants may serve as assistants)

*Type of equipment used in individual locale.

Objectives

Upon completion of this station the participant will be able to:

1. Discuss and demonstrate the assessment techniques for examining a patient suspected of having neck and/or spinal injuries.

2. Discuss the principles and techniques for immobilizing the patient with neck and/or spinal injuries.

3. Demonstrate the proper method of immobilizing a patient with suspected neck and/or spinal injuries on a long spine board using the modified log-roll technique.

4. Discuss when and demonstrate how to transfer a patient with a possible spine injury from a long spine board to a firm, padded gurney or operating table.

5. Identify when the patient has been properly immobilized in accordance with the techniques and principles outlined during this skill station.

Chapter 7:
Spine and
Spinal Cord
Trauma

Skill
Station XI

Procedures

1. Assessment of neck and spine injuries

2. Patient immobilization and application of a long spine board using the modified log-roll technique

3. Application and use of a scoop stretcher (optional skill)

Note: The procedures outlined in this skill station **must be taught by ATLS physician faculty.** Instructional assistants, eg, paramedic instructor, may assist with the application of these devices. This skill station is conducted in conjunction with Skill Station XII, Extremity Immobilization, Application of the Leg Traction Splint.

Skills Procedures

**Chapter 7:
Spine and
Spinal Cord
Trauma**

**Skill
Station XI**

Assessment and Immobilization of Neck and Spine Injuries

Note: Universal precautions are required whenever caring for the trauma patient.

I. Assessment of Neck and Spine Injuries

A. Assess Respiratory Status

1. Airway patency—establish patent airway as needed while maintaining in-line immobilization of the c-spine

2. Respiratory efforts

B. Assess Patient's Level of Consciousness

C. Obtain Vital Signs

D. Palpate Cervical Spine

Note any abnormality and assess for:

1. Deformity

2. Grating crepitus

3. "Boggy" sensation

4. Increased pain with palpation

E. Assess for:

1. **Pain**

   a. Presence/absence
   b. Level of pain
   c. Location of pain

2. **Paresis**

   a. Presence/absence
   b. Level/location of paresis

3. **Paresthesia**

   a. Presence/absence
   b. Level/location of paresthesia

4. **Paralysis**

   a. Presence/absence
   b. Level/location of paralysis

F. Continually reassess patient's status

Chapter 7:
Spine and
Spinal Cord
Trauma

Skill
Station XI

II. Primary Management: Supine Patient

A. Application of Long Spine Board Using Modified Log-roll Technique

Note: Four individuals are needed to perform this modified log-rolling procedure: (1) one to maintain manual, in-line immobilization of the patient's head and neck; (2) one for the torso (including the pelvis and hips); (3) one for the pelvis and legs; and (4) one to direct the procedure and move the spine board. This procedure maintains the patient's entire body in neutral alignment, minimizing any untoward movement of the spine. This procedure assumes that suspected upper and lower extremity injuries are already immobilized.

1. Prepare the long spine board with straps, placing the board next to the patient's side. The straps are to be positioned for fastening later across the patient's thorax, just above the iliac crests, thighs, and just above the ankles. Straps or tape may be used to secure the patient's head and neck to the long board.

2. Apply gentle, in-line manual immobilization to the patient's head (assistant 1), and apply a semirigid cervical collar (assistant 2).

3. Gently straighten the patient's arms and place them (palm-in) next to the torso.

4. Carefully straighten the patient's legs, placing them in neutral alignment with the patient's spine. Gently, yet firmly, tie the patient's ankles together with roller-type dressing or cravat.

5. Assistant 1 continues to maintain alignment of the patient's head and neck. Assistant 2 reaches across the patient grasping the patient at the shoulder and wrist. Assistant 3 reaches across the patient grasping the patient's hip just distal to the wrist with one hand and with the other hand firmly grasps the roller bandage or cravat that is securing the ankles together.

6. At the direction of assistant 4 (Instructor), the patient is cautiously log-rolled as a unit toward the two assistants at the patient's side, but **only to the minimal degree necessary** to position the board under the patient.

   a. Assistant 1 (at the patient's head) closely observes the log-rolling process and maintains neutral alignment of the patient's head and neck with the torso, avoiding any flexion or hyperextension of the patient's neck.

   b. Assistant 2 controls movement of the patient's torso and maintains neutral alignment of the thoracolumbar spine.

   c. Assistant 3 helps to maintain neutral alignment of the patient's thoracolumbar spine and pelvis with his hand on the patient's hip. Additionally, the legs are maintained in neutral alignment with the torso by firmly grasping the cravat securing the patient's ankles together with the other hand, and elevating them approximately 4 to 6 inches. This latter maneuver helps to maintain neutral alignment of the lumbar spine and avoid pelvic tilt.

**Chapter 7:
Spine and
Spinal Cord
Trauma**

**Skill
Station XI**

7. Assistant 4 (Instructor) places the long spine board beneath the patient.

8. Carefully log-roll the patient back as a unit onto the long board. At the same time, Assistant 4 (Instructor) helps to slide the patient into position in the center of the board. Extreme care is exercised by all assistants during this step to avoid untoward movement and maintain neutral alignment of the patient's spine.

9. The patient is then secured to the long board.

    a. Assistant 1 continues to maintain in-line immobilization of the patient's head and neck.

    b. Assistant 2 securely tightens two straps—one across the patient's upper arms and thorax, and a second just proximal to the iliac crests. The wrists are secured to the patient's sides by this second strap.

    c. Assistant 3 securely tightens two straps—one across the patient's thighs, and one just above the ankles. Blanket rolls, placed on the outer sides of the patient's lower legs, may be required to prevent lateral movement of the lower extremities.

    d. Assistant 4 (Instructor) places padding under the patient's head as necessary to avoid hyperextension and flexion of the neck.

    e. Padding, rolled blankets, or similar bolstering devices are placed on either side of the patient's head and neck. The patient's head is secured firmly to the board by tightening a strap over the lower part of the forehead or using tape. Another strap or piece of tape is placed over the bolstering devices and cervical collar, further securing the patient's head and neck to the long board.

10. Pediatric considerations:

    a. A pediatric-sized, long spine board is preferable when immobilizing the small child. If only an adult-sized board is available, blanket rolls are placed along the entire sides of the child to prevent lateral movement.

    b. The child's head is larger proportionately to his torso than the adult's. Therefore, padding should be placed under the shoulders to elevate the head and maintain neutral alignment of the child's spine. Such padding extends from the child's lumbar spine to the top of the shoulders, and laterally to the edges of the board.

11. Complications

If left immobilized for any length of time on the long spine board, the patient may develop pressure sores at the occiput, scapulae, sacrum, and heels. Therefore, padding should be applied under these areas as soon as possible, and the patient should be removed from the long spine board as soon as his condition permits.

**Chapter 7:
Spine and
Spinal Cord
Trauma**

**Skill
Station XI**

B. Removing a Patient From a Long Spine Board

Movement of a patient with an unstable vertebral spine injury may cause or permanently worsen a spinal cord injury. To reduce the risk of spinal cord damage, mechanical protection is necessary for all patients at risk. Such protection should be maintained until unstable spine injuries have been excluded.

1. As previously described, properly securing the patient to a long spine board is the basic technique for splinting the spine. Generally, this is done in the prehospital setting, so that the patient arrives at the hospital immobilized on a long spine board. The long spine board provides an effective splint and permits safe transfers of the patient with the smallest practical number of assistants. However, the unpadded spine board may soon become uncomfortable for a conscious patient and poses a significant risk for pressure sores on posterior bony prominences—occiput, scapulae, sacrum, and heels. Therefore, as soon as it can be done safely, the patient should be transferred from the spine board to a firm, well-padded gurney or equivalent surface. Before removing the patient from the spine board, c- spine, chest, and pelvis radiographs should be obtained as indicated.

2. A strategy should be developed, dependent upon the patient's needs and the institutional resources, to allow as many appropriate transfers as to be completed while the patient remains on the board. All the necessary assistants must be assembled **before** moving the patient. If a spine injury exists or is strongly suspected, orthopedic and/or neurosurgical consultation should be obtained first.

3. Safe movement of a patient with an unstable or potentially unstable spine requires continuous maintenance of anatomic alignment of the vertebral column. Rotation, flexion, extension, lateral bending, and shearing-type movements in any direction must be avoided. Manual, in-line immobilization best controls the head and neck. No part of the patient's body should be allowed to sag as the patient is lifted off the supporting surface. The transfer options listed herein may be used, depending on available personnel and equipment resources.

   ### a. Modified log-roll technique

   The modified log-roll technique, previously outlined, is reversed to remove the patient from the long spine board. Four assistants are required: (1) one to maintain manual, in-line immobilization of the patient's head and neck; (2) one for the torso (including the pelvis and hips); (3) one for the pelvis and legs; and (4) one to direct the procedure and remove the spine board.

   ### b. Multi-hand or "fireman's" lift

   This procedure may be used instead of log-rolling the patient. Six assistants are needed to maintain the spine in a neutral position while lifting an adult, supine patient off the board. One assistant maintains in-line immobilization of the patient's head and neck. Four assistants—two on each side of the patient's torso, pelvis, and legs—are required to slide their arms under the patient and grasp each other's wrists to provide adequate support to the entire patient when he is lifted. This procedure requires precise coordination by all assistants.

The patient must be lifted in unison as directed by the sixth assistant who removes the spine board as soon as the patient is lifted clear of the board.

c. Scoop stretcher

An alternative to the preceding two techniques is use of the scoop stretcher for patient transfer.

C. Application and Use of the Scoop Stretcher to Transfer a Patient off the Long Spine Board (Optional Skill)

Note: The proper use of this device can provide rapid, safe transfer of the patient from the long spine board onto a firm, padded patient gurney. **Remember**, after the patient is transferred from the back board to the gurney and the scoop stretcher is removed, the patient **must be reimmobilized securely** to the gurney. The scoop stretcher is **not** a device on which the patient is immobilized. Additionally, the scoop stretcher is **not** used to transport the patient, nor should the patient be transferred to the gurney by picking up only the foot and head ends of the scoop stretcher. Without firm support under the stretcher it can sag in the middle, resulting in loss of neutral alignment of the spine.

Five individuals are needed to assist with application of the scoop stretcher, patient transfer, and removal of the device: (1) one at the head of the patient; (2) one at the patient's feet; (3) one on the patient's left side; (4) one on the patient's right side; and (5) one to remove the long board from under the patient.

1. Adjust the scoop stretcher to the length of the patient, and separate it by disconnecting the split frame at both ends.

2. Disconnect the straps and tape used to secure the patient to the long spine board, leaving in place the cervical collar and other bolstering devices used to immobilize the head and neck. Manually immobilize the patient, especially the head and neck. Once assistant 1 manually immobilizes the patient's head and neck it must not be released until the patient has been reimmobilized securely on the gurney.

3. With the straps and tape removed, place the left split frame on top of the long board to the patient's left side and the right frame to the patient's right side. The frames should be placed under any bolstering devices used to immobilize the patient's head and neck.

4. Two assistants carefully slide the split frames beneath the patient, first one side then the other. The assistants should carefully slide their hands under the patient assuring that the patient's clothing or skin will not be caught in the stretcher frame once it is locked into place.

5. With the two frames in place, reconnect the stretcher at both ends, securely locking the components.

6. Reimmobilize the entire patient on the scoop stretcher. Manual immobilization of the patient's head and neck can then be released.

Chapter 7:
Spine and
Spinal Cord
Trauma

Skill
Station XI

7. A minimum of five assistants are required to transfer the patient off the long board — one at the head of the patient, one at the patient's feet, one on either side of the patient, and one to remove the board. With one assistant directing the transfer, carefully lift the scoop stretcher up as a unit approximately four inches. Assistant 5 quickly removes the long board. The patient is then lowered back onto the firm gurney.

8. Reapply manual immobilization, and remove the tape securing the patient's head and neck. Remove the straps securing the patient to the scoop stretcher.

9. Disconnect the locks at either end of the stretcher and gently remove the split frame, one side at a time.

10. **Immobilize** the entire patient, as outlined in II.A., to the gurney.

11. This procedure and device can be used to transfer the patient from one transport device to another or to a previously designated place, eg, x-ray table. **Remember**, the patient must remain securely immobilized until a spine injury is excluded.

III. Continued Management: Reassess the Patient's Status

Chapter 8:
Extremity Trauma

Objectives:

On completion of this topic, the physician will be able to:

A. Identify life- and/or limb-threatening injuries to the extremities, as well as less serious, but potentially disabling injuries.

B. Outline priorities in the assessment of extremity trauma.

C. Outline the proper principles of initial management for extremity injuries.

D. Demonstrate the ability to assess, assign priorities to, and initially manage injuries on a simulated patient, including application of dressings, splints, and traction splints.

Chapter 8:
Extremity
Trauma

American College of Surgeons

I. Introduction

Extremity trauma is rarely life-threatening by itself, but associated injuries can be. Certain injuries and combinations of injuries to the skeleton may be permanently disabling if not properly managed. Appropriate early management of the patient with extremity injuries can reduce the risks of death and disability. Therefore, this chapter focuses on the initial management of extremity injuries, emphasizing related assessment and management procedures that can have a significant impact on the long-term outcome of patients with extremity trauma.

Extremity injuries that pose an immediate threat to life are those with major, uncontrolled hemorrhage. Although this may be external and obvious, life-threatening blood loss also may be internal and thus occult. This is typical of severe pelvic fractures, bilateral femur fractures, and other multiple closed fractures. Severe crush injuries, with large amounts of necrotic tissue, and contaminated open fractures also are potentially fatal, due to renal failure or overwhelming infection (eg, clostridial gangrene). The same is true for traumatic proximal amputations, which may be incomplete or complete. Presence of major fractures increases the risk of multiple organ failure syndrome. This risk can be reduced by a comprehensive plan for early management, including operative fracture stabilization.

Limb-threatening extremity injuries include vascular injuries with distal ischemia, compartment syndromes with localized neuromuscular ischemia, open fractures, crushing-type injuries, and dislocations of major joints.

Extremity injuries usually involve more than one tissue element. Severity is reflected by the extent of damage to each. Therefore, a severe closed fracture may have significant skin and muscle contusion, possible nerve and/or vessel injury, marked comminution and displacement of bone, and is at increased risk of developing a compartment syndrome. In this chapter, fractures are discussed **after** other extremity injuries as a reminder not to allow obvious fractures to distract the physician from a full evaluation of the injured limb.

A. Primary Survey and Resuscitation

1. Airway with cervical spine control

2. Breathing

3. Circulation with hemorrhage control

4. Disability; brief neurologic evaluation

5. Exposure and Environmental control: Completely undress the patient, but prevent hypothermia

During the primary survey, the extremities are assessed only briefly for obvious bleeding that requires immediate control and to assess perfusion. Patients with an apparently isolated extremity injury should be assessed and managed like any other potential multiple trauma patient. However, additional occult injuries may be present, and evaluation and early care of extremity injuries must be an integral part of the overall approach to the patient.

B. Secondary Survey

The secondary survey is the time for detailed evaluation of the extremities, to determine the specifics of any obvious injury, and to identify other injuries that are less apparent or occult. The order of priority is:

1. Assess perfusion.

2. Identify open wounds.

3. Identify closed wounds, including fractures, joint injuries, and contusions (deformity, swelling, tenderness, instability, and crepitus).

4. Assess neuromuscular function (active motion, sensation).

5. Identify abnormal joint mobility.

Once an open wound is inspected, it should be covered promptly with a sterile dressing. If necessary, a splint is then applied to the involved extremity. Although many roentgenograms may be required, these must **not** interfere with other, more urgent aspects of the patient's evaluation and management. Most skeletal radiographs can be deferred until the patient has been treated for life- and limb-threatening injuries or transferred to a more appropriate institution, if required. Ultimately, any extremity with signs or symptoms of injury require adequate roentgenograms but these must not interfere with more urgent priorities.

C. Early Management of Extremity Injuries

1. Immobilize with splints and/or traction. For example, early application of a traction splint to a femoral shaft fracture reduces internal hemorrhage.

2. Restore limb alignment.

3. Perform wound care.

4. Restore perfusion.

II. Extremity Assessment

Except in cases of obvious, exsanguinating hemorrhage, evaluation of extremity injuries is carried out during the secondary survey.

A. History

Information obtained from the patient, relatives, or bystanders at the accident scene should be documented and included as a part of the patient's medical record. Information, pertinent to the patient's extremity trauma, to consider and inquire about includes:

1. Mechanisms of injury

If the patient is injured in a vehicular crash, this information should be determined, if possible: (1) where the patient was in the vehicle (driver, passenger, seat location); (2) where the patient was found (inside the vehicle or ejected), and if ejected, how far; (3) if the vehicle sustained external damage, eg, front, side, or rear impact; (4) if the vehicle sustained internal damage, eg, steering wheel, dashboard, windshield, etc.; and (5) whether a seat belt (lap or shoulder) was worn. Other common mechanisms include vehicle-pedestrian collisions, falls from a height, crushing injuries, and explosions/fires. For each type of injury, efforts should be made to quantify the force of injury in terms of speed, distance, vehicular damage, weight of crushing object, etc, and also the time the injury occurred. (See Resource Document 2, Prehospital Triage Criteria, and Flow Chart 1, Triage Decision Scheme.)

It is essential to estimate the severity of extremity wounds. The injury mechanism provides helpful clues. The most significant issues are the amount of energy absorbed and whether an open wound is present. The actual amount of tissue damage may not be evident until the wound has been explored surgically in the operating room.

2. Environment

Prehospital care personnel should be asked about: (1) patient exposure for any length of time to temperature extremes; (2) patient exposure to toxic fumes or agents; (3) broken glass fragments (which also may injure the examiner); and (4) sources of bacterial contamination (dirt, animal feces, fresh or salt water, etc).

3. Preinjury status and predisposing factors

It is important to determine the patient's baseline condition prior to injury. The patient's overall health, including exercise tolerance and activity level, should be determined. Frequently noted factors that may alter the patient's condition, treatment regimen, and outcome include: (1) ingestion of alcohol and/or other drugs; (2) emotional problems or illnesses; (3) underlying medical illnesses; (4) previous injuries, especially to the same extremity; and (5) allergies.

4. Findings at the incident site

Findings at the incident site that may help the physician identify potential injuries include: (1) the position in which the patient was found; (2) bleeding or pooling of blood at the scene and the estimated amount; (3) bone or fracture ends that may have been exposed; (4) open wounds in proximity to obvious or suspected fractures; (5) obvious deformity or dislocation; and (6) whether or not the patient could move each extremity.

5. Prehospital care

Prehospital observations and care must be reported and documented. Information to obtain, pertinent to extremity injuries, includes: (1) changes in the limb's function, perfusion, or neurologic state; (2) reduction of fractures or dislocations during extrication or splinting at the scene; (3) exposed bone ends that were withdrawn into wounds; (4) dressings and splints applied; (5) extrication procedures; and (6) any delay incurred at the accident site or en route to the hospital.

B. Physical Examination

The patient must be completely undressed for adequate examination. Always compare an injured extremity with the opposite, uninjured one. Assessment of the trauma patient's extremities has three goals: (1) identification of life-threatening injury; (2) identification of limb-threatening injuries; and (3) systematic review to avoid missing any other extremity injury.

1. **Look**

   Visually assess the extremities for: (1) color and perfusion; (2) wounds; (3) deformity (angulation, shortening); and (4) swelling, discoloration, and bruising.

2. **Feel**

   The extremities should be assessed for sensation, tenderness, crepitation (feel carefully but avoid overvigorous manipulation), capillary filling, warmth, and especially pulses.

3. **Movement**

   Active, voluntary motion confirms the function of a muscle-tendon unit. It is rarely normal if the joints involved are injured. However, presence of some active motion does not guarantee a normal joint. **Passive** motion, by the examiner, is most important for identifying motion that should not exist, as in ligament injuries or unstable, occult fractures. If an obvious injury is present, passive motion maneuvers may be unnecessary, painful, and potentially damaging to local soft tissues.

4. **Pelvic stability**

   A pelvic ring injury may produce potentially, life-threatening hemorrhage, and often is associated with other local injuries. Its subtle signs may not be appreciated on a routine pelvic roentgenogram. To identify a mechanically unstable pelvic ring, grasp the iliac crests anteriorly and attempt to rotate them inward toward the midline, and outward away from it. Any motion is abnormal and confirms the presence of a significant pelvic disruption. (See Chapter 5, Abdominal Trauma.)

C. Vascular Injuries

Vascular injuries may result in bleeding or ischemia. Blood loss threatens life. Loss of perfusion distal to an injury threatens survival or function of the injured limb. Brisk bleeding from a wound suggests a major vessel injury. It is notable that complete arterial tears usually bleed less than partial tears, because of the hemostatic contraction and thrombosis of a transected artery. Persistent bleeding is typical of a partial tear. A large hematoma or a neurologic deficit suggests a significant vascular injury.

External bleeding begins at the time and site of injury. The amount of blood shed is not easy to calculate, and the physician may underestimate the degree of prehospital blood loss. Obtaining an accurate history and carefully monitoring the patient's blood volume and response to fluid resuscitation help determine the amount of blood loss. As a rule, hemorrhage from open fractures is far greater than expected.

Closed extremity injuries may produce enough blood loss to cause hypovolemic shock. Patients with multiple closed fractures, particularly those of the femur and pelvis, are at greatest risk. The bleeding may go undetected because it is sequestered in the retroperitoneal space or the injured extremity.

Blood loss from pelvic fractures may be six or more units. Closed femur fractures may account for two or three units of blood loss. However, fractures must **not** be assumed to be the cause of hypovolemic shock in trauma patients until other sources, particularly abdominal and thoracic, are excluded.

Vascular injuries associated with circulatory impairment represent an immediate or potential threat to limb viability. They must be recognized and managed promptly. In a hemodynamically stable patient, pulse discrepancies, coolness, pallor, paresthesia, hypesthesia, and any abnormality of motor function suggest possible impairment of blood flow to the extremity. Such findings may be due to arterial injury or elevated compartmental pressure with impairment of local capillary perfusion. **Examination of distal pulses is crucial for early identification of arterial injuries.** The mere presence of pulses does not exclude vascular injury, especially if the pulse is weak or obtained only by Doppler. Any abnormality of distal pulses strongly suggests a vascular injury and must be explained. **Diminished pulses or pallor of the skin should not be attributed to vasospasm.** It is important to realize that abnormal motor and sensory function may be due to one or more of three potentially coexistent causes—nerve injury, arterial injury, and compartment syndrome.

Vascular injuries are unequivocally indicated by these signs:

1. Brisk, external bleeding
2. Expanding hematoma (rapid, progressive swelling)
3. Abnormal pulses

Additional signs that suggest arterial injury are:

4. Bruit or thrill
5. Pallor
6. Empty veins
7. Decreased capillary refill
8. Relative coolness
9. Wounds close to the course of a major artery
10. Decreased sensation
11. Motor weakness
12. Progressively increasing pain after immobilization of an extremity injury

If any of these abnormalities (particularly any change in pulse) persist after aligning and immobilizing the extremity, a careful investigation for possible vascular injury should be undertaken. With all cases of suspected vascular injury, the physician should (1) check the immobilization device, (2) reassess the fracture alignment, and (3) reassess distal perfusion. If distal perfusion remains abnormal, immediate surgical consultation is mandatory.

If a traction device has been applied to an injured extremity with vascular impairment, its status must be assessed and any necessary adjustments must be made. Vascular impairment can result from failure to align a fracture or dislocation, or from excessive traction. If a circular dressing, splint, or cast has been applied, assess for constriction. Release the device if there is any suspicion of its being too tight.

Blood pressure measurement, with or without Doppler assistance, is useful for evaluation of extremity perfusion. Vascular imaging provides important, additional information in the evaluation of a suspected arterial injury. Imaging studies should be considered whenever the diagnosis is in doubt. The surgeon is responsible for determining what, if any, vascular imaging studies are necessary. This is not to say that arteriography is necessary whenever an arterial injury is present. Roentgenographic studies may interfere with life- or limb-saving therapy. When a limb is ischemic, tissue is dying. Immediate surgical treatment is required. If a fracture or joint injury is involved, both vascular and orthopedic surgeons should be consulted immediately.

An associated injury often guides the surgeon to the site of vascular trauma. If needed, the surgeon can obtain an arteriogram rapidly in the operating room. Roentgenograms and angiograms should **not** be done until the patient's condition is stabilized and the injured extremity is evaluated, dressed, and splinted.

Arteriography is valuable in identifying the site of a vascular injury when more than one is possible and in excluding an occult arterial injury, eg, an incomplete intimal tear that may result in delayed thrombosis with complete arterial occlusion. This is especially likely when a distal pulse remains weak after fracture reduction or after typical injuries, eg, knee dislocations or analogous fractures. If arteriography must be delayed for these patients, careful, frequent clinical monitoring of the injured limb's pulses and neurovascular status is essential. **The goal of managing such patients is to identify and treat vascular injuries before irreversible ischemia develops.**

D. Traumatic Amputation

Amputation is a catastrophic and obvious extremity injury. As a severe open fracture, all but the most distal amputations represent a significant threat to life and to survival of the residual limb. Hemostasis and wound care deserve highest priority in limb management. It is important to recognize that some severe open fractures represent incomplete amputations. An early decision is vital if the patient is to be considered a candidate for replantation or revascularization of the injured limb. However, the potential for replantation should not detract from initial assessment and management efforts. Amputation is the best available treatment for some severe, lower extremity injuries. This possibility should be remembered in communications with the patient and family members.

E. Open Wound

Any skin wound near a fracture or joint must be assumed to communicate with a skeletal injury until proven otherwise. There is no doubt that an open fracture exists when bone ends are seen in the wound or roentgenograms show intra-articular air, etc. Probing the wound is an unreliable method to exclude an open fracture and has an associated significant risk of infection. Serious soft-tissue wounds may not involve bones or joints, but they still pose significant threats to the patient and the limb.

Penetrating injuries may produce lacerations with little tissue necrosis. Examples are knife wounds, low-velocity gunshot wounds, and indirectly produced open fractures (spiral fractures in which a sharp bone spike lacerates the skin from inside-out). These wounds have a significant risk of infection if not managed appropriately.

Small skin wounds may be noted after a direct injury, eg, a leg crushed against a bumper by another speeding car. However, such wounds may have considerable amounts of crushed necrotic muscle. Devascularized bone fragments and neurovascular injuries are often present. Degloving injuries, which occur when skin and subcutaneous tissues separate from the underlying muscle, are common. Progressive swelling poses the risk of compartmental syndrome with further local ischemia. In open wounds, there is little correlation between the severity of injury and the size of any associated skin opening. In addition to crush injuries, which may have no skin opening, high-velocity missile wounds, close-range shotgun wounds, and open fractures due to direct trauma are typical mechanisms for severe soft-tissue wounds.

Severe, open wounds are at greater risk for delayed vascular compromise, compartment syndromes, infection, and disturbances of wound and fracture healing. Their prompt identification and proper surgical management improve outcome.

Open fracture wounds are classified according to severity, as discussed later in this chapter. The risk of tetanus is increased in certain wounds: (1) wounds more than six hours old; (2) contused, abraded, or avulsed wounds; (3) wounds more than one centimeter deep; (4) injuries resulting from high-velocity missiles; (5) injuries due to burns or cold; (6) wounds with significant contamination; and (7) wounds with denervated or ischemic tissue. (See Resource Document 6, Tetanus Immunization.)

F. Compartment Syndrome

Whenever interstitial tissue pressure rises above that of the capillary bed, local ischemia of nerve and muscle occurs. Permanent paralysis and/or necrosis may result. The end-stage is called Volkmann's ischemic contracture.

Elevated tissue pressures typically develop within one or more fascial compartments of the leg or forearm, but can involve any such space (thigh, foot, hand, etc). Prompt recognition of a compartment syndrome is essential so that a fasciotomy can be done to release tight muscle compartments, thereby lowering interstitial pressure and restoring perfusion before necrosis occurs.

Compartment syndromes usually develop over a period of several hours and may not be present when the patient first arrives at the hospital. They may be initiated by crush injuries, closed or open fractures, sustained compression of an extremity in a comatose patient, or after restoration of blood flow to a previously ischemic extremity. The pneumatic antishock garment (PASG) may be associated with compartment syndrome, particularly if applied over an injured leg or legs and left inflated for prolonged periods of time. Prolonged application of the PASG on an **uninjured** extremity also may produce a compartment syndrome.

The signs and symptoms of compartment syndrome are: (1) pain, typically increased by passively stretching involved muscles; (2) decreased sensation of nerves traversing the involved compartment; (3) tense swelling of the involved region; and (4) weakness or paralysis of involved muscles. Diminished distal pulses and capillary filling do not reliably identify compartment syndromes, because they may be intact until late in the evolution of a compartment syndrome, after irreversible changes have occurred. Intracompartmental pressure measurement may help diagnose a suspected compartment syndrome. Tissue pressures greater than 35 to 45 mm Hg suggest impaired capillary blood flow, with the need for fasciotomy. When physical examination cannot exclude a compartment syndrome (swollen limb in an unconscious patient), pressure measurements may permit observation rather than fasciotomy. Experienced surgical judgment is required. Some patients with an intact neuromuscular examination may not require fasciotomy, despite transiently elevated pressures. If neuromuscular compromise and tense swelling are present, fasciotomy is urgent, and pressure measurements only delay necessary treatment.

G. Nerve Injury

Assessment of nerve function usually requires a cooperative patient. For each significant peripheral nerve, distal voluntary motor function and sensation must be systematically confirmed. Muscle testing must include palpation of the contracting muscle, as well as assessment of its strength. (See Tables 1 and 2, Peripheral Nerve Assessment of Lower and Upper Extremities.)

Nerve injuries may be complete, without any motor or sensory function, and with or without any anatomic interruption of the nerve. A significant nerve injury also may be present with only partial loss of function, so that subtle differences deserve further assessment. It is important to remember that impaired sensation and muscle function also may be due to arterial occlusion or compartment syndrome.

H. Joint Injury

Injuries of joints and adjacent structures may be obvious or occult. Even obvious periarticular injuries may be misdiagnosed without careful evaluation, including roentgenograms. Joint injuries include penetrating wounds, dislocations, fracture-dislocations, adjacent fractures, and ligament disruptions that may be complete or partial (sprains). It usually is not possible, without roentgenograms, to differentiate between dislocations and fracture-dislocations, or adjacent fractures.

Local pain and difficulty moving a joint are the most important symptoms of joint injuries. The signs of such an injury are a nearby open wound, deformity, swelling and/or effusion, instability (motion that should not be present), tenderness, impaired motion, and ecchymosis, which usually is delayed. If obvious deformity is present, radiographs are essential before the part is manipulated. Prompt distal nerve and vessel evaluation also is urgent.

In certain injuries, eg, knee dislocations and severely displaced fractures adjacent to the knee, there is a significant risk of an arterial intimal tear with delayed occlusion that may lead to amputation. An arteriogram is often advisable to exclude such occult arterial injuries. The severe deformity of a dislocated joint may result in necrosis of tightly stretched overlying skin, unless reduction is gained promptly. Prolonged delay in reducing a dislocated hip increases the risk of avascular necrosis of the femoral head, with associated permanent disability.

**Table 1
Peripheral Nerve Assessment of Lower Extremities**

Nerve	Motor	Sensation
Femoral	Knee extension	Anterior knee
Obturator	Hip adduction	Medial thigh
Tibial	Toe flexion	Sole of foot
Superficial peroneal	Ankle eversion	Lateral dorsum of foot
Deep peroneal	Ankle/toe dorsiflexion	Dorsal first to second toe web
Superior gluteal	Hip abduction	—
Inferior gluteal	Gluteus maximus contraction with hip extension	—

**Table 2
Peripheral Nerve Assessment of Upper Extremities**

Nerve	Motor	Sensation
Ulnar	Index finger abduction	Little finger
Median—distal	Thenar contraction with opposition	Index finger
Median—anterior interosseous	Index tip flexion	—
Musculocutaneous	Elbow flexion	Lateral forearm
Radial	Thumb extension/abduction	Dorsal web between thumb and index
Axillary	Deltoid contraction with shoulder abduction	Lateral shoulder

All dislocations, even of small joints, are usually painful. They cannot be splinted easily, and pain is difficult to relieve until the dislocation is reduced.

If a joint has no obvious fracture or dislocation, the possibility of an occult ligament injury must be excluded. The physician should assess for abnormal motion—the direction or degree of motion normally prevented by functioning ligaments. For example, in an unstable knee, the leg can be angulated laterally or medially, or there may be excessive anterior or posterior movement of the tibia relative to the femur. Gross instability indicates a major ligament disruption. Pain or lesser degrees of instability also may indicate a significant ligament injury. In children, such instability may be due to an occult growth plate fracture instead of a ligament disruption.

Involvement of a joint by an adjacent wound can be confirmed by attempting to distend the joint with an intra-articular injection of sterile saline solution. Egress of the fluid from the wound confirms communication with the joint.

I. Fractures

Fractures involve not only a broken bone, but the adjacent soft-tissue injury as well. Both injuries must be assessed. Fractures associated with severe soft-tissue injuries (open or closed) have a significant risk of early and delayed complications.

Open fractures are graded according to severity. More severe injuries have absorbed more energy and sustained more soft-tissue damage. (See Table 3, Open Fracture Grading.) **Any** open fracture may have serious consequences because of the high risk of infection if prompt, appropriate surgical treatment is not provided. Therefore, a careful circumferential inspection of the injured limb is essential to avoid overlooking an inconspicuous wound. If a fracture and wound are in proximity, it should be assumed that the fracture is open, even if the bone cannot be seen in the wound. Exploration of open wounds in the emergency department is inappropriate. Such practices often fail to identify an open fracture and increase wound contamination.

Pain, swelling, deformity, tenderness, instability, and crepitus each suggest a fracture. Roentgenograms in at least two planes (anteroposterior and lateral) are required for evaluation of a suspected fractured extremity. However, it is important to realize that definitive evaluation of an extremity fracture must not interfere with higher priority treatment. If the neurovascular status of the limb is satisfactory, and it is splinted so as to prevent further harm, essential extremity radiographs may be postponed until more pressing care is underway.

Fractures are often missed in patients with multiple or severe trauma. Therefore, it is important to be aware of clues to their diagnosis. The most frequent error is to find only one of several injuries.

**Table 3
Open Fracture Grading**

Grade	Injury Description/Characteristics
I.	Small skin laceration by tip of spiral (indirect) fracture
II.	Small to moderate, well-circumscribed wound with little contamination and no significant tissue necrosis or periosteal stripping
IIIA.	Longer laceration, with significant contused or nonviable tissue, but **after debridement**, delayed suture or split-thickness skin graft (STSG) can close the wound
IIIB.	Extensive soft-tissue wound with crush, contamination and/or periosteal stripping; a local or free muscle flap usually is required to close
IIIC.	An open fracture with a vascular injury that requires repair to salvage limb
IV.	Total or subtotal amputation

Modified from Gustilo et al and Tscherne et al. (See Bibliography.)

J. Associated Injury Patterns

Certain musculoskeletal injuries with common mechanisms occur together often enough that the presence of one should lead to a search for the other.

1. The joints above and below a long-bone fracture are **always** suspect.

2. **Hip and pelvis** injuries are frequently associated with femoral shaft fractures, making a pelvis roentgenogram mandatory. Look carefully for a femoral neck fracture, a hip dislocation, an acetabular fracture, or a pelvic ring disruption.

3. **Knee** injuries may be present with either a femur or tibia fracture. They are especially common when both the femur and tibia are involved ("floating knee" injury), which is a reliable indicator of a severely injured patient.

4. **Calcaneal** fractures, usually caused by a fall from a height, may have associated vertebral compression or burst fractures.

5. Shaft fractures of the **radius or ulna** may be associated with injuries of the elbow or wrist joints. A fall onto an outstretched hand may produce injuries at one or more levels in the upper extremity, from the wrist to the shoulder girdle.

K. Occult Skeletal Injuries

Definitive assessment of the multiply injured patient with obvious, life-threatening injuries is a major challenge. Occult fractures and joint injuries may be overlooked easily. Repeated examinations are essential to ensure that all such injuries are identified. The following skeletal regions must be specifically considered.

1. Cervical spine

In cases of head trauma or trauma above the clavicle, cervical spine injuries can be overlooked clinically, especially from C-6 to T-1. They also may be missed roentgenographically or misinterpreted on screening roentgenograms because of the overlying shoulder shadows. Shoulder retraction is necessary and should be routine in obtaining cervical roentgenograms of the trauma patient. If this method fails to demonstrate all seven cervical vertebrae, a swimmer's view should be obtained. An anteroposterior view of the entire cervical spine is essential as well, if injuries are to be excluded reliably. **Remember**, any injury above the clavicles implies a cervical spine injury until it is definitely excluded.

2. Pelvis

Because of its extensive overlying soft-tissue coverage, the pelvis may be seriously injured without obvious external deformity. An anteroposterior screening radiograph and a careful physical examination for tenderness, instability, and leg shortening are essential to avoid overlooking pelvic ring disruptions, acetabular fractures, and dislocations or fractures of the proximal femur.

3. Knee

Significant knee injuries with ligamentous instability but with normal-appearing radiographs are easily overlooked, especially in the unconscious patient. All potential knee injuries must be assessed for instability. This is easiest if the patient is unconscious or anesthetized and is more difficult when pain and tenderness are present. If an adequate stress examination is impossible, it should be assumed that the knee is unstable. Orthopedic consultation is then essential.

4. Shoulder girdle

Fractures and dislocations involving the clavicle, scapula, and proximal humerus may be overlooked easily. They may be associated with thoracic injuries. Careful examination of the patient and inspection of the chest roentgenogram aids in identifying shoulder girdle injuries. (See Chapter 4, Thoracic Trauma, Scapular and Rib Fractures.)

5. Distal injuries

The wrist, hand, ankle, and foot may sustain one or more easily overlooked injuries with significant functional consequences. Tenderness, swelling, and impaired function are clues to occult injuries. Roentgenograms in multiple projections are helpful, but they may appear normal or be hard to interpret when injuries are primarily ligamentous rather than bony, eg, carpal dislocations at the wrist or tarsometatarsal (Lisfranc's) joint injuries in the midfoot.

6. Hand injuries

Space does not permit a complete review of hand injuries in this section. The referenced texts at the conclusion of the chapter should be consulted. Any or several of the complex anatomic structures of the hand may be injured, with little external evidence unless a meticulous examination is carried out. Innocuous wounds may communicate with vital underlying structures. Skin perfusion can be assessed by inspection or pulse oximetry. An injury to the digital nerve that produces distal anesthesia also may involve the adjacent digital artery. Sensation must be assessed systematically in the field of each digital nerve. For initial screening purposes, light touch usually is sufficient. Dislocations and fractures may be obvious, but unless each joint is assessed for tenderness, active and passive motion, and stability, occult injuries may be missed. The function of each tendon must be assessed for each digit. The extrinsic deep flexors act on the distal interphalangeal (IP) joints, and the superficial flexors act on the proximal IP joints. The long extensors primarily extend (dorsiflex) the metacarpophalangeal (MP) joints, while the intrinsic muscles flex the MP joints and extend the IP joints, as well as abducting (dorsal interossei) and adducting (palmar interossei) the MP joints. (See Table 2, Peripheral Nerve Assessment of the Upper Extremity). Adequate, skillfully interpreted, roentgenograms are essential for complete evaluation of an injured hand or wrist.

III. Management

A. Vascular Injuries

Bleeding from an injured extremity usually can be controlled by direct pressure, preferably applied over sterile dressings. Occasionally, direct pressure must be applied to a proximal artery. A tourniquet is used only as a last resort, and with the understanding that it may compromise salvage of the distal extremity. Attempts to explore a wound in the emergency department and clamp vessels are ill-advised. Such measures rarely are successful and often result in injury to adjacent structures.

Distal ischemia may be present when a vascular injury occurs. Perfusion must be restored rapidly by correcting hypovolemia and gross limb deformity. Prompt surgical restoration of blood flow, within four to six hours from injury, is essential to salvage a limb with ischemia. Therefore, surgical consultation is the next step in treatment. **If obvious ischemia is present, an arteriogram may be unnecessary.**

B. Traumatic Amputation

A bulky sterile dressing is applied to the wound, with pressure as needed to control bleeding. Tetanus prophylaxis and antibiotics are given, as for any severe open fracture. Surgical consultation is obtained promptly.

Replantation may be possible. Some patients, particularly those with upper extremity amputations, may be good candidates for replantation. Clean lacerations, rather than crush or avulsion injuries, shorter ischemia times, more distal injuries, and younger, healthier patients have higher replantation success rates.

The techniques and equipment for replantation are highly sophisticated, and usually are found only in specialized replantation centers. Patients with amputation injuries require rapid assessment and consultation with a specialized center. The surgeon at the definitive-care facility who will be treating the patient decides whether or not the patient is a candidate for replantation.

If the patient is a candidate for replantation, the amputated part should be carefully preserved and rapidly transported **with the patient** to the replantation center. Time is of the essence. An amputated part remains viable for only four to six hours at room temperature or up to 18 hours if cooled. The amputated part should be cleansed of any gross dirt or debris, wrapped in a sterile towel moistened with sterile saline, placed in a sterile, sealed plastic bag, and transported in an insulated cooling chest filled with crushed ice and water. **Do not** allow the amputated part to freeze, **do not** place it in dry ice, and make certain that the amputated part accompanies the patient.

If the patient is not a replantation candidate, consider saving some of the amputated parts for grafts to injured areas of the body, including the amputation stump. The treating surgeons make the final decision whether to use such parts.

C. Open Wounds

While minor wounds are routinely treated in the emergency department, major wounds are best treated by a surgeon in the operating room. The same may be true of less extensive wounds in multiply injured patients who require an anesthetic for other injuries. Primary care for such injuries does not require significant efforts at wound toilette in the emergency department. A sterile dressing is applied, and the limb is splinted if necessary. Circumferential dressings must not constrict the limb and interfere with venous drainage. If bone ends are exposed, these may be drawn into the wound to permit correction of gross deformity, and to prevent desiccation. Ensure that the surgical team is informed about all wounds, and the reduction of exposed bone ends. If contamination is significant or a fracture or joint is involved, tetanus prophylaxis and antibiotics are given.

There is no urgency to close open extremity wounds. This may be done after all higher-priority treatment is accomplished. Contaminated wounds need adequate surgical debridement. Delayed closure (five to seven days) reduces the risk of infection.

D. Compartment Syndrome

Once compartmental pressure is high enough to prevent capillary perfusion, irreversible damage occurs to muscles and nerves unless adequate fasciotomy is done within four hours. When symptoms or suspicion of a compartment syndrome are present, all potentially constricting materials, ie, circumferential dressings, casts, etc, must be released. If symptoms do not respond rapidly to external decompression, prompt fasciotomy may be required unless compartment pressure measurements exclude compartment syndrome definitively. Compartmental tissue pressures from 35 to 45 mm Hg may be dangerously elevated. However, other factors are involved, including the duration of ischemia, muscle damage due to blunt trauma, and the difference between mean arterial pressure and intracompartmental pressure. Unless mean arterial pressure is 30 to 40 mm Hg above compartmental tissue pressure, neuromuscular survival is threatened. Immediate surgical consultation is required for a suspected compartment syndrome.

E. Nerve Injury

When a peripheral nerve injury is identified by loss of sensation and motor power, it is important to ensure that the diagnosis is correct and that ischemia (arterial occlusion or compartment syndrome) or central nervous system injuries are not present. Specific emergency treatment for the injured nerve is rarely required, but immediate repair deserves consideration when a clean laceration is the cause of injury. Abundant padding is required when splints are applied to an insensate limb.

F. Joint Injury

Prompt orthopedic consultation should be obtained for all joint injuries. Occasionally the consultant may recommend immediate reduction of a dislocated joint, especially if his examination is delayed. However, reduction of a dislocation should not be attempted without adequate radiographs and preliminary consultation with the orthopedic surgeon. A more or less obvious fracture may be present. All dislocations should be reduced as rapidly as possible. Hip, and occasionally other dislocations, may require a general anesthetic and muscle paralysis for reduction. Since attempts at realignment without reduction may be painful, the limb should be supported in the most comfortable position with pillows, etc.

G. Fractures

1. Open wounds

Any wound associated with a fracture must be managed as if it were an open fracture. Appropriate wound management is essential to minimize the chances of infection which threatens the patient and limb and ultimate functional outcome. Excessive delay risks serious complications. These injuries require consultation and/or transfer to a facility with an orthopedic surgeon.

Primary care involves the removal of only gross contamination from the wound and the prevention of further contamination by applying a sterile dressing. Bulky reinforcement of the dressing is advisable. Open fractures should be aligned with proper splinting techniques. Administer tetanus prophylaxis and appropriate systemic antibiotics without delay.

Tetanus prophylaxis is essential for the multiply injured patient, particularly if open extremity trauma is present. Although most individuals in the industrialized world have had adequate antitetanus immunization, some have not, and immigrants from other areas may be less likely to have completed their immunization series. Therefore, it is essential to determine the patient's immunization status, if possible, and to modify treatment as required by both immunization and the nature of the wound. (See Resource Document 6, Tetanus Immunization.)

Antibiotics, administered intravenously, are recommended for the care of severe extremity wounds associated with open fractures or joint injuries. For all open fractures it is essential to provide adequate coverage for beta-lactamase-producing staphylococci. Antibiotics for Grade III open fractures should include gram-negative coverage as well. If clostridial contamination is likely, high-dose penicillin should be given, in addition to other agents. Intravenous antibiotics should be started early in the management of open fractures, with the choice determined in consultation with the treating surgeon.

Proper surgical care remains the mainstay of wound treatment. It is not replaced by antibiotics.

2. Immobilization

Any fracture or suspected fracture must be immobilized to control pain and prevent further injury. Severely angulated fractures should be aligned first, although alignment should not be forced.

Distal pulses, skin color, temperature, and neurologic status are assessed before and after alignment. Gentle traction, as an adjunct to splinting and to facilitate alignment, is beneficial when immobilizing long-bone fractures. If possible, the splints should extend one joint above and below the fracture site. For dislocations and other joint injuries, immobilize the bone above and below the joint. Roentgenograms, including arteriograms, should **not** be obtained until the extremity is dressed and splinted. (See IV. Immobilization, in this chapter.)

H. Pain Control

Analgesic drugs may prevent prompt identification of serious but occult problems. Always consider the possibility of intracranial lesions, abdominal trauma, and limb ischemia. Limb ischemia is likely to become progressively more painful until ischemic necrosis causes anesthesia. Immobilization of fractures and prompt reduction of dislocations are the safest and most effective means of controlling pain. If they are not successful, intravenous, short-acting narcotics are appropriate to prevent unnecessary suffering. However, the aforementioned conditions must be excluded first, and a determination must be made as to whether the patient may have taken substances that could potentiate the effects of narcotic analgesics. Intramuscular analgesics should **not** be administered to a patient who may be in shock with impaired peripheral perfusion, because the drugs are not absorbed at a predictable time and rate. If a painful procedure must be performed, eg, reduction of a dislocated shoulder, small amounts of carefully monitored sedation (eg, a short-acting benzodiazapine) may be required in addition to an intravenous narcotic.

IV. Principles of Immobilization

Splinting of extremity injuries must be deferred until life-threatening problems are identified and managed. However, all such injuries must be splinted before patient transport. Specific types of splints can be applied for specific fracture needs. The pneumatic antishock garment (PASG) has not proved to be an effective or safe splint for extremity injuries, although it may be helpful temporarily for patients with life-threatening hemorrhage from pelvic injuries. A long spine board provides a "total body splint" for multiple injured patients with possible or definite unstable spine injuries. However, its hard, unpadded surface may cause pressure sores on the patient's occiput, scapulae, sacrum, and heels. Therefore, as soon as possible, the patient should be moved carefully to an equally supportive **padded surface**, using a scoop-style stretcher to facilitate the transfer. The patient should be fully immobilized and an adequate number of personnel should be available during this transfer. (See Chapter 7, Spine and Spinal Cord Trauma and Skill Station XI, Immobilization Techniques for Neck and Spinal Trauma.)

A. Femoral Fractures

Femoral fractures are best provisionally immobilized with traction splints. The traction splint's force is applied distally at the ankle. Proximally, the splint is secured to the thigh and hip area. Traction splints may be used for ipsilateral femoral and tibial fractures. Excess traction may cause skin damage to the foot or ankle, perineal injury, and neurovascular compromise from pressure stretching of anatomic structures. **Hip fractures** can be similarly immobilized with a traction splint, especially if the leg is shortened and malrotated. Alternatively, the injured leg is merely secured to the other leg and/or the stretcher. Hip dislocations may produce a fixed deformity. If gentle realignment of the limb with manual traction is not possible, pillows or other bulky padding and tape may be used to support the limb in the most comfortable position.

B. Knee Injuries

A long-leg splint, a traction-type splint applied with **minimal traction**, or a commercial knee-immobilizer may be used to support the injured knee. Additional stability is provided by splinting to the opposite leg. Padding may be needed to maintain some knee flexion.

C. Tibia Fractures

Tibia fractures are best immobilized with a well-padded board or metal gutter, long-leg splint. A gently inflated pneumatic splint also is good. For proximal fractures, a traction-type splint can be used, but beware of excessive traction. When aligning a tibial fracture in a splint, make sure that rotation is correct.

D. Ankle Fractures

Ankle fractures may be immobilized with a pillow splint or padded-board splint, avoiding pressure over bony prominences. Assess the neurovascular status before and after the splint is applied.

E. Upper Extremity and Hand Injuries

The **hand** can be **temporarily** splinted in an anatomic, functional position, with the wrist slightly dorsiflexed and the fingers gently flexed. This position usually can be achieved by gently immobilizing the hand over a large role of gauze, and using a short arm splint as well.

The **forearm and wrist** are immobilized flat on padded or pillow splints.

The **elbow** is splinted in a flexed position, either by using padded splints or by direct immobilization to the body with a sling and swath device.

The **arm** is immobilized by splinting to the body or simple application of a sling or swath, which can be augmented with splints for unstable fractures.

Shoulder injuries are managed similarly, using bulky padding as necessary.

Circumferential bandages, used to apply molded and padded splints, can have a tourniquet effect. The extremity must be monitored frequently for vascular compromise. All splints must be padded over bony prominences.

All jewelry, including rings, bracelets, etc, must be removed before splinting any extremity injury to prevent pressure on the area and circulatory embarrassment.

V. Summary

The initial assessment and management of extremity trauma are part of the secondary survey in the management of the multiply injured patient. Life-threatening situations must be properly assessed and managed before attention is directed to the injured extremity. The extremity can sustain a variety of injuries, from sprains and fractures to traumatic amputation. It is essential to recognize arterial injuries, compartment syndromes, open fractures, and crush or other severe injuries promptly to assure timely treatment.

A knowledge of the mechanism of injury and history of the injury-producing event enables the physician to diagnose and properly manage the injured extremity. Early alignment of fractures and dislocations and proper splinting techniques can prevent serious complications and late sequelae of extremity trauma. In addition, an awareness of the patient's tetanus immunization status, particularly in cases of open fractures, can prevent serious complications. The astute physician, armed with the proper knowledge and skills, can satisfactorily provide the initial management for most extremity trauma.

In the multiply injured patient with extremity trauma, urgent operative fixation of fractures within the first 24 hours may reduce mortality and morbidity. It is essential to obtain orthopedic consultation early in the patient's management.

Bibliography

1. American Academy of Orthopaedic Surgeons: **Emergency Care and Transportation of the Sick and Injured 4th Edition.** Chicago, 1987.

2. Bone LB, Johnson KD, Weigelt J, et al: Early versus delayed stabilization of femoral fractures: a prospective, randomized study. **Journal of Bone and Joint Surgery** 1989;71A:336-340.

3. Browner BD, Jupiter JB, Levine AM, Trafton PG (eds): **Skeletal Trauma.** Philadelphia, WB Saunders, 1991.

4. Carter PR: Common hand injuries and infections. In: **A Practical Approach to Early Treatment.** Philadelphia, WB Saunders, 1983.

5. Gustilo RB, Anderson JT: Prevention of infection in the treatment of 1025 open fractures of long bones. **Journal of Bone and Joint Surgery** 1976;58A:453.

6. Gustilo RB, Mendoza RM, Williams DN: Problems in the management of type III (severe) open fractures: a new classification of type III open fractures. **Journal of Trauma** 1985;24:742.

7. Heppenstall RB, Sapega AA, Scott R, et al: The compartment syndrome: an experimental and clinical study of muscular energy metabolism using phosphorus nuclear magnetic resonance spectroscopy. **Clinical Orthopedics** 1988;226:138-155.

8. Hoppenfeld S: **Physical Examination of the Spine and Extremities.** New York, Appleton, 1976.

9. Moore EE, Ducker TB, Edlich RF, et al (eds): **Early Care of the Injured Patient 4th Edition.** Philadelphia, Pennsylvania, BC Decker, Inc, 1990, Chapters 19-24.

10. Ododeh M: The role of reperfusion-induced injury in the pathogenesis of the crush syndrome. **New England Journal of Medicine** 1991;324:1417-1421.

11. Rockwood CA, Green DP, Bucholtz R (eds): **Fractures 3rd Edition.** Philadelphia, Pennsylvania, JP Lippincott Co, 1991.

12. Trafton PG: Orthopaedic Emergencies. In Ho MT, Saunders CE (eds): **Current Emergency Diagnosis and Treatment, 3rd Edition.** East Norwalk, Connecticut, Appleton and Lange, 1990.

13. Tscherne H, Gotzen L: **Fractures With Soft Tissue Injuries.** Berlin, Heidelberg, Springer-Verlag, 1984.

Chapter 8:
Extremity
Trauma

Skill Station XII:
Principles and Techniques of
Immobilization for Extremity Trauma

Resources and Equipment

This list is the recommended equipment to conduct this skill session in accordance with the stated objectives for and intent of the procedures outlined. Additional equipment may be used providing it does not detract from the stated objectives and intent of this skill, or from performing the procedure in a safe method as described and recommended by the ACS Committee on Trauma.

1. Live patient model

2. Leg traction splint (type used in individual locale)

3. Blanket

Objectives

Upon completion of this station, the participant will be able to

1. Discuss principles associated with immobilizing extremity injuries.

2. Demonstrate the technique for properly applying a leg traction splint.

3. Identify when the patient's injured extremity has been properly immobilized in accordance with the principles and techniques outlined in this skill station.

**Chapter 8:
Extremity
Trauma**

**Skill
Station XII**

Skill Procedure

Principles and Techniques of Immobilization for Extremity Trauma

Note: Universal precautions are required whenever caring for the trauma patient.

Goal of Splinting: Prevent further injury, and control pain and bleeding.

I. Principles of Extremity Immobilization

A. Assess the ABCs and treat life-threatening situations first.

B. Remove and/or cut open all clothing on the extremity. Remove watches, rings, bracelets, and potentially constricting devices.

C. Assess the neurovascular status of the extremity before applying the splint. Assess for pulses, external hemorrhage, and if possible, motor and sensory function. (See Tables 1 and 2 in this chapter.)

D. Dress any open wounds.

E. Select the appropriate size and type of splint for the injured extremity. The device should extend one joint above and one joint below the injured site.

F. Apply padding over bony prominences that will be covered by the splint.

G. Apply gentle distal and proximal traction to align the extremity before and during application of the splint. Gentle traction should be maintained until the splinting device is secured.

H. Continue to monitor the neurovascular status of the injured extremity.

I. Do not force realignment of deformities near a joint.

J. Obtain orthopedic consultation, especially for fracture-dislocations of the joints.

II. Application of the Leg Traction Splint

A. One person should handle the injured extremity, and another should handle the application of the splint.

B. Measure the **unaffected** leg with the traction splint.

  1. The upper cushioned ring should be placed right under the buttocks and adjacent to the ischial tuberosity.

  2. Two support straps should be above the knee and two below the knee.

C. Cut away clothing (including all foot wear) to expose the injured site. Dress any open wounds.

D.   The first assistant supports the leg, while the second assistant removes the shoe and sock to assess distal circulation and pedal pulses.

E.   The first assistant applies manual traction to the leg, while maintaining support under the fracture site and the calf.

F.   Reassess the distal pulse after applying manual traction.

G.   While the first assistant maintains manual traction on the leg, the second assistant applies the ankle hitch around the patient's ankle and upper foot. The bottom strap should be the same length or preferably shorter than the two upper cross straps.

H.   Gently lift the fractured limb, while maintaining support and traction. Slide the splint under the affected leg, placing the padded upper ring snugly against the ischial tuberosity.

I.   Gently lay the leg on the splint, and extend the leg elevator. Snugly attach the top strap first.

J.   While continuing to support the leg and maintain traction, attach the ankle hitch to the traction hook.

K.   Apply traction gently to the leg by turning the windlass knob until the extremity appears stable, or in the conscious patient, until pain and spasm are relieved.

L.   Reassess the distal, pedal pulses.

M.   Secure the remaining straps, making sure they are not too tight.

N.   Continually reassess the circulation to the affected limb.

Chapter 9:
Injuries Due to Burns and Cold

Objectives:

Upon completion of this topic, the physician will be able to identify methods of assessment and outline measures to stabilize, manage, and transfer patients with burns and cold injuries. Specifically, the physician will be able to:

A. Estimate the burn size and determine the presence of associated injuries.

B. Outline measures of initial stabilization and treatment of patients with burns and patients with cold injury.

C. Identify special problems and methods of treatment of patients with burns and patients with cold injury.

D. Outline criteria for the transfer of burn patients.

**Chapter 9:
Injuries Due to
Burns and Cold**

American College of Surgeons

I. Introduction

Burn and cold injuries constitute a major cause of morbidity and mortality. Attention to basic principles of initial trauma resuscitation and timely application of simple emergency measures should minimize the morbidity and mortality of these injuries.

These principles include a high index of suspicion for the presence of airway compromise in smoke inhalation, the maintenance of hemodynamic stability, and fluid and electrolyte balance. The physician also must have an awareness of measures to be instituted for prevention and treatment of the potential complications of thermal injuries, eg, rhabdomyolysis and cardiac dysrhythmias, as seen in electrical burns. Removal from the injury-provoking environment, cautious temperature control, and observation for definite demarcation of nonviable tissue before major debridement also constitute major principles of thermal injury management.

II. Immediate Life-saving Measures for Burn Injuries

A. Airway

Although the larynx protects the subglottic airway from direct thermal injury, the supraglottic airway is extremely susceptible to obstruction as a result of exposure to heat. Signs of airway obstruction may not be obvious immediately, although if present, they may warn the examiner of potential airway obstruction. When a patient is admitted to the hospital after sustaining a burn injury, the physician should be alert to the possibility of airway involvement, identify signs of distress, and initiate supportive measures. Clinical indications of inhalation injury include:

1. Facial burns

2. Singeing of the eyebrows and nasal vibrissae

3. Carbon deposits and acute inflammatory changes in the oropharynx

4. Carbonaceous sputum

5. History of impaired mentation and/or confinement in a burning environment

6. History of explosion

The presence of any of these findings suggests acute inhalation injury. Such injury requires immediate and definitive care, including airway support, which may involve endotracheal intubation and early transfer to a burn center.

B. Stop the Burning Process

All clothing should be removed to stop the burning process. Synthetic fabrics ignite, burn rapidly at high temperatures, and melt into hot residue that continues to burn the patient. Any clothing with chemical involvement should be removed carefully. Chemical powders (dry) should be brushed from the wound, with the individual caring for the patient avoiding direct contact with the chemical. The involved body surface areas are then rinsed with copious amounts of water.

C. Intravenous Lines

After establishing airway patency and identifying and treating immediately life-threatening injuries, intravenous access must be established. Any patient with burns over more than 20% of the body surface area needs circulatory volume support. Large-caliber (at least #16-gauge catheter) intravenous lines must be established immediately in a peripheral vein. If the extent of burn precludes placement of the catheter through unburned skin, overlying burned skin should not deter placement of the catheter in an accessible vein. The upper extremities are preferable to the lower extremities for venous access because of the high incidence of phlebitis and septic phlebitis in the saphenous veins. Begin infusion with Ringer's lactate solution. Guidelines for establishing the flow rate of Ringer's lactate solution are outlined later in this chapter.

III. Assessing the Burn Patient

A. History

A brief history of the nature of the injury may prove extremely valuable in the management of the burn patient. Associated injuries may be sustained while the victim attempts to escape the fire. Water heater explosions, propane gas explosions, and other explosions may throw the patient some distance and may result in internal injuries or fractures, ie, CNS, myocardial, pulmonary, and abdominal injuries. It is essential that the time of the burn injury be established.

The history, from the patient or relative, should include a brief survey of pre-existing illnesses: (1) diabetes, (2) hypertension, (3) cardiac, pulmonary and/or renal disease, and (4) drug therapy. Allergies and sensitivities also are important. The patient's tetanus immunization status also should be ascertained.

B. Body Surface Area

The "Rule of Nines" is a useful and practical guide to determine the extent of the burn. The adult body configuration is divided into anatomic regions that represent 9%, or multiple of 9%, of the total body surface. Body surface area differs considerably for children. The infant's or young child's head represents a larger proportion of the surface area, and the lower extremities a lesser proportion, than an adult's. The percentage of total body surface of the infant's head is twice that of the normal adult. (See Figure 1, "Rule of Nines".) **Remember, the palm (not including the fingers) of the patient's hand represents approximately 1% of the patient's body surface.** This guideline helps estimate the extent of burns of irregular outline or distribution.

C. Depth of Burn

The depth of burn is important in evaluating the severity of the burn, planning for wound care, and predicting functional and cosmetic results. **First-degree burns** (eg, sunburn) are characterized by erythema, pain, and the absence of blisters. They are not life threatening, and generally do not require intravenous fluid replacement. This type of burn will not be discussed further in this chapter.

Second-degree burns or partial-thickness burns are characterized by a red or mottled appearance with associated swelling and blister formation. The surface may have a weeping, wet appearance and is painfully hypersensitive, even to air current.

Full-thickness or third-degree burns appear dark and leathery. The skin also may appear translucent, mottled, or waxy white. The surface is painless and generally dry. (See Figure 2, Depth of Burn.)

IV. Stabilizing the Burn Patient

A. Airway

Objective signs of airway injury or history of confinement in a burning environment dictates evaluation of the airway and definitive management. Pharyngeal thermal injuries may produce marked upper airway edema, and early maintenance of the airway is important. The clinical manifestations of inhalation injury may be subtle and frequently do not appear in the first 24 hours. If the physician waits for roentgenographic evidence of pulmonary injury or change in blood gas determinations, airway edema may preclude intubation, and a surgical airway may be required.

B. Breathing

The initial treatment of injuries is a graded response based on the patient's signs and symptoms. Major concerns regarding the respiratory status in the patient exposed to smoke and heat are:

1. Direct thermal injury, producing upper airway edema and/or obstruction

2. Inhalation of products of incomplete combustion (carbon particles) and toxic fumes, leading to chemical tracheobronchitis, edema, and pneumonia

Always assume carbon monoxide (CO) exposure in patients burned in enclosed areas. Diagnosis of carbon monoxide poisoning is made primarily from a history of exposure. Cherry-red skin color is rare. Headache, nausea, vomiting, and mental disturbances occur at higher carbon monoxide levels. Because of the increased affinity of carbon monoxide for hemoglobin (240 times that of oxygen), it displaces oxygen from the hemoglobin molecule and shifts the oxyhemoglobin dissociation curve to the left. Carbon monoxide dissociates very slowly, and its half-life is 250 minutes while the patient is breathing room air, compared with 40 minutes while breathing 100% oxygen. Therefore, patients suspected of exposure to carbon monoxide should receive initially, high-flow oxygen via a nonrebreathing mask.

Early management of inhalation injury may require endotracheal intubation and mechanical ventilation. Arterial blood gas determinations should be obtained immediately as a baseline for the evaluation of the pulmonary status. However, measurements of arterial PO_2 do not reliably predict carbon monoxide poisoning, because a carbon monoxide partial pressure of only 1 mm Hg results in carboxyhemoglobin level of 40% or greater. Therefore, baseline carboxyhemoglobin levels should be obtained, and 100% oxygen should be administered.

Figure 1
"Rule of Nines"

The **"Rule of Nines"** is used in the hospital management of severe burns to determine fluid replacement. It also is useful as a practical guide for the evaluation of severe burns. The adult body is generally divided into surface areas of 9% each and/or fractions or multiples of 9%.

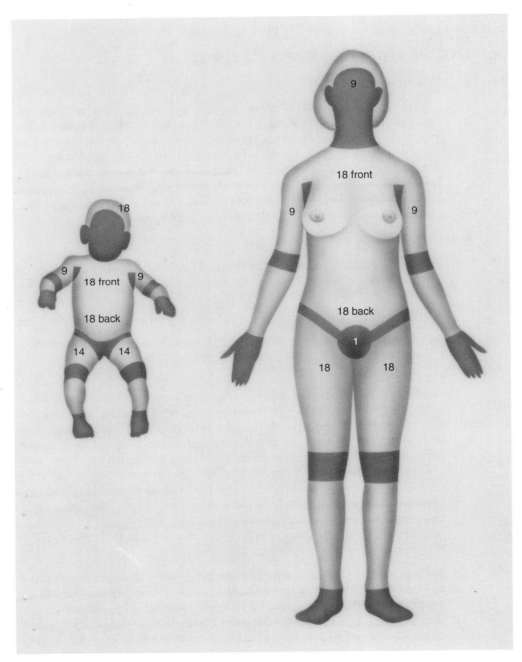

Figure 2
Depth of Burn

	Depth of Burn	Signs and Symptoms
Second-degree or Partial-thickness Burn Injury 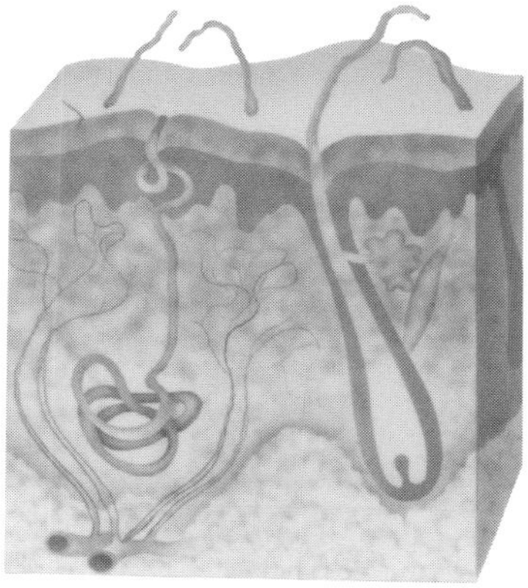	Second-degree burns are deeper than first-degree burns. They commonly result from contact with hot liquids or flash burns from gasoline flames.	Red or mottled appearance Blistered and broken epidermis Considerable swelling Weeping, wet surfaces Painful Sensitive to air
Third-degree or Full-thickness Burn Injury 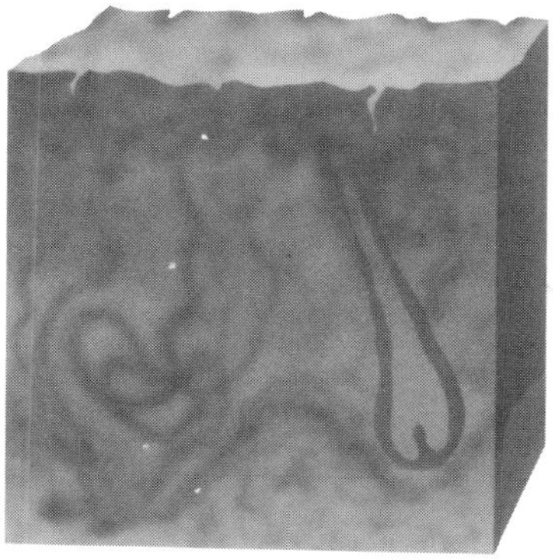	Third-degree burns cause damage to all skin layers, nerve endings and even subcutaneous tissues. They can be caused by fire, prolonged exposure to hot liquids, contact with hot objects, or electricity. Initially, they may resemble second-degree burn injuries.	Pale, white, charred, or leathery appearance Broken skin with fat exposed Dry surface Painless and insensate Edema

C. Circulating Blood Volume

Evaluation of the circulating blood volume is often difficult in the severely burned patient. Blood pressure may be difficult to obtain and may be unreliable. Monitoring hourly urinary outputs reliably assesses circulating blood volume in the absence of osmotic diuresis (eg, glycosuria). Therefore, an indwelling urethral catheter should be inserted. A good rule of thumb is to infuse fluids at a rate sufficient to produce 1.0 mL of urine per kilogram body weight per hour for children who weigh 30 kilograms or less, and 30 to 50 mL of urine per hour in the adult.

The burn patient requires 2 to 4 mL of Ringer's lactate solution per kilogram body weight per percent body surface burn in the first 24 hours to maintain an adequate circulating blood volume and provide adequate renal output. The estimated fluid volume is then proportioned in the following manner: one half of the total estimated fluid is provided in the first eight hours postburn, and the remaining one half is administered in the next 16 hours. To maintain an average urinary output of 1 mL per kilogram per hour in small children who weigh 30 kilograms or less, it may be necessary to calculate and add glucose-containing maintenance fluids to the burn formula.

Any resuscitation formula provides only an estimate of fluid need. Fluid requirement calculations for infusion rates are based on the **time from injury**, not from the time fluid resuscitation is initiated. The amount of fluid given should be adjusted according to the individual patient's response, ie, urinary output, vital signs, and general condition.

D. Physical Examination

The following must be done in order to plan and direct patient management:

1. Estimate extent and depth of burn

2. Assess for associated injuries

3. Weigh the patient

E. Flow Sheet

A flow sheet, outlining the patient's management, should be initiated when the patient is admitted to the emergency department. This flow sheet should accompany the patient when he is transferred to the burn unit.

F. Baseline Determinations for the Major Burn Patient

1. Blood

Obtain samples for CBC, type and crossmatch, carboxyhemoglobin, serum glucose, electrolytes, and pregnancy test in all females of childbearing age. Arterial blood samples also should be obtained for blood gas determinations.

2. Roentgenograms

A chest film should be obtained. An additional film may be required if endotracheal intubation and/or subclavian or internal jugular vein catheterization are accomplished. Other roentgenograms may be indicated for appraisal of associated injuries.

G. Circumferential Extremity Burns—Maintenance of Peripheral Circulation

1. Remove all jewelry.

2. Assess the status of distal circulation, checking for cyanosis, impaired capillary refilling, or progressive neurologic signs (ie, paresthesia and deep tissue pain). Assessment of peripheral pulses in burn patients is best performed with a Doppler Ultrasonic Flow Meter.

3. Circulatory embarrassment in a circumferentially burned limb is best relieved by escharotomy, preferably with surgical consultation. Incision of the eschar to relieve edema pressure can be performed as an emergency procedure without anesthesia, because the incision is limited to insensate full-thickness burn. The incision must extend across the entire length of the eschar in the lateral and/or medial line of the limb including the joints. The incision is limited to nonviable tissue, and to limit blood loss, viable subeschar tissue should **not** be incised. Escharotomy of the fingers is rarely indicated and should be done only in consultation with an experienced burn surgeon.

4. Circumferential burns of the thorax may impair respiratory excursion. Bilateral, escharotomy incisions in the anterior axillary lines should be considered if respiratory excursions are limited.

5. Fasciotomy is seldom required. However, it may be necessary to restore circulation for patients with associated skeletal trauma, crush injury, high-voltage electrical injury, or burns involving tissue beneath the investing fascia.

H. Nasogastric Tube Insertion

Insert a nasogastric tube and attach it to suction if the patient experiences nausea, vomiting, abdominal distention, or if burns involve more than 20% of the total body surface area. Prior to transfer it is essential that a nasogastric tube be inserted and functioning in such patients.

I. Narcotics, Analgesics, and Sedatives

The severely burned patient may be restless and anxious from hypoxemia or hypovolemia rather than pain. Consequently, the patient responds better to oxygen or increased fluid administration, rather than to narcotic analgesics or sedatives that may mask the signs of hypoxemia or hypovolemia. Narcotics, analgesics, and sedatives should be used **sparingly**. If narcotics are necessary, they should be administered in small, frequent doses by the intravenous route only.

J. Wound Care

Partial-thickness (second-degree) burns are painful when air currents pass over the burned surface. Gently covering the burn with clean linen relieves the pain and deflects air currents. Do not break blisters or apply an antiseptic agent. Any applied medication must be removed before appropriate antibacterial topical agents can be applied. Application of cold compresses may cause hypothermia. **Do not apply cold water to a patient with extensive burns.**

K. Antibiotics

Prophylactic antibiotics are **not** indicated in the early postburn period. Antibiotics should be reserved for the treatment of infection.

V. Special Burn Requirements

A. Chemical Burns

Chemical injury can result from exposure to acids, alkalies, or petroleum products. Alkali burns are generally more serious than acid burns, because the alkalies penetrate more deeply. Removal of the chemical and immediate attention to wound care are essential.

Chemical burns are influenced by the duration of contact, concentration of the chemical, and amount of the agent. Immediately flush away the chemical with large amounts of water, using a shower or hose if available, for at least 20 to 30 minutes. Alkali burns require longer irrigation. If dry powder is still present on the skin, brush it away **before** irrigation with water. Neutralizing agents have no advantage over water lavage, because reaction with the neutralizing agent may itself produce heat and cause further tissue damage. Alkali burns to the eye require continuous irrigation during the first eight hours after the burn. A small-caliber cannula can be fixed in the palpebral sulcus for such irrigation.

B. Electrical Burns

Electrical burns result from a source of electrical power making contact with the patient's body. Electrical burns frequently are more serious than they appear on the surface. The body may serve as a volume conductor of electrical energy and the heat generated results in thermal injury of tissue. Different rates of heat loss from superficial and deep tissues account for relatively normal overlying skin coexisting with deep muscle necrosis. Rhabdomyolysis results in myoglobin release, which can cause acute renal failure.

The immediate management of a patient with a significant electrical burn includes attention to the airway and breathing, establishment of an intravenous line, electrocardiographic monitoring, and placement of an indwelling urethral catheter. If the urine is dark, assume that hemochromogens are in the urine. Do not wait for laboratory confirmation before instituting therapy for myoglobinuria. Fluid administration should be increased to ensure a urinary output of at least 100 mL per hour in the adult. If the pigment does not clear with increased fluid administration, 25 grams of mannitol should be administered immediately and 12.5 grams of mannitol should be added to subsequent liters of fluid in order to maintain the diuresis.

Metabolic acidosis should be corrected by maintaining adequate perfusion and adding sodium bicarbonate to alkanize the urine and increase the solubility of myoglobin in the urine.

VI. Criteria for Transfer

A. Types of Burn Injuries

The American Burn Association has identified the following types of burn injuries that usually require referral to a burn center:

1. Partial-thickness and full-thickness burns greater than 10% of the total body surface area (BSA) in patients under 10 years or over 50 years of age

2. Partial-thickness and full-thickness burns greater than 20% BSA in other age groups

3. Partial-thickness and full-thickness burns involving the face, eyes, ears, hands, feet, genitalia, or perineum or those that involve skin overlying major joints

4. Full-thickness burns greater than 5% BSA in any age group

5. Electrical burns, including lightning injury; (significant volumes of tissue beneath the surface may be injured and result in acute renal failure and other complications)

6. Significant chemical burns

7. Inhalation injury

8. Burn injury in patients with pre-existing illness that could complicate management, prolong recovery, or affect mortality

9. Any burn patient in whom concomitant trauma poses an increased risk of morbidity or mortality may be treated initially in a trauma center until stable before transfer to a burn center

10. Children with burns seen in hospitals without qualified personnel or equipment for their care should be transferred to a burn center with these capabilities

11. Burn injury in patients who will require special social and emotional or long-term rehabilitative support, including cases involving suspected child abuse and neglect

B. Transfer Procedure

1. Transfer of any patient must be coordinated with the burn-center physician.

2. All pertinent information regarding tests, temperature, pulse, fluids administered, and urinary output should be recorded on the burn/trauma flow sheet and sent with the patient. Any other information deemed important by the referring or receiving physician also is sent with the patient.

VII. Cold Injury

Severity of cold injury depends on temperature, duration of exposure, and environmental conditions. Lower temperatures, immobilization, prolonged exposure, moisture, the presence of peripheral vascular disease, and open wounds all increase the severity of the injury.

A. Types

Three types of cold injury are seen in the trauma patient:

1. **Frostbite** is due to freezing of tissue from intracellular ice crystal formations and microvascular occlusion. Similar to thermal burns, frostbite is classified into first, second, third, and fourth degree according to depth of involvement.

   a. First degree—Hyperemia, edema without skin necrosis

   b. Second degree—Vesicle formation accompanies the hyperemia and edema with partial thickness necrosis of skin

   c. Third degree—Full-thickness skin necrosis occurs, with necrosis of some underlying subcutaneous tissue

   d. Fourth degree—Full-thickness skin necrosis, including muscle and bone with gangrene

2. **Nonfreezing** injury is due to microvascular endothelial damage, stasis, and vascular occlusion. With ambient temperature above freezing, prolonged exposure leads to "trench foot" over several days while "immersion foot" develops more slowly at higher temperatures. Although the entire foot may appear black, deep tissue destruction may not be present. **Chilblain or pernio**, common among mountain climbers, results from exposure to dry temperatures just above freezing leading to superficial ulceration of the skin of the extremities.

3. **Hypothermia** is a state in which the patient's generalized core temperature drops below 35 degrees centigrade.

Estimation of depth of injury and extent of tissue damage is not usually accurate until demarcation is evident. This often requires several weeks of observation.

B. Management of Frostbite and Nonfreezing Cold Injuries

Treatment should be immediate to decrease duration of tissue freezing. Constricting, damp clothing should be replaced by warm blankets and the patient should be given hot fluids by mouth, if able to drink.

Place the injured part in circulating water at 40 degrees centigrade until the pink color and perfusion return (usually within 20 to 30 minutes). Avoid dry heat.

C. Local Wound Care of Frostbite

The goal of wound care for frostbite is to preserve damaged tissue by preventing infection, avoiding opening noninfected vesicles, and elevating the injured area, which is left open to air. Narcotic analgesics are required.

Tetanus prophylaxis depends on the patient's tetanus immunization status. Antibiotics are administered if infection is obviously present. Only rarely is fluid loss massive enough to require resuscitation with intravenous fluids.

VIII. Hypothermia

Total body hypothermia is defined as a core temperature below 35 degrees centigrade. Clinically, hypothermia may be classified as mild (32 to 35 degrees centigrade), moderate (30 to 32 degrees centigrade), or severe (below 30 degrees centigrade). This drop in core temperature may be rapid, as in immersion in near-freezing water, or slow, as in exposure to more temperate environments. The elderly are particularly susceptible to this condition, because of their impaired ability to increase heat production and decrease heat loss by vasoconstriction. Children also are more susceptible because of relative increased BSA and limited energy sources. Trauma patients also are susceptible to hypothermia. Such hypothermia is preventable with the administration of warmed intravenous fluids and maintenance of a warm environment. Since determination of the core temperature, preferably esophageal, is essential for the diagnosis, special thermometers capable of registering low temperatures are required.

A. Signs of Hypothermia

In addition to a decrease in core temperature, a depressed level of consciousness is the most common feature of hypothermia. The patient is cold to touch and appears gray and cyanotic. Vital signs, including pulse rate, respiratory rate, and blood pressure are all variable, and the absence of respiratory or cardiac activity is not uncommon in patients who eventually recover. Because of severe depression of the respiratory rate and heart rate, signs of respiratory and cardiac activity are easily missed unless careful assessment is conducted.

B. Management of Hypothermia

Immediate attention is devoted to the ABCs, including the initiation of cardiopulmonary resuscitation and the establishment of intravenous access if the patient is in cardiopulmonary arrest.

Prevent heat loss by removing the patient from the cold environment and replacing wet, cold clothing with warm blankets. Administer oxygen via a bag-reservoir device. The patient should be managed in a critical care setting whenever possible. A careful search for associated disorders, such as diabetes, sepsis, and drug or alcohol ingestion, should be conducted. These disorders should be treated promptly. Blood should be drawn for CBC, electrolytes, blood glucose, creatinine, amylase, and blood cultures. Abnormalities should be treated accordingly. For example, hypoglycemia would require intravenous glucose administration.

Determination of death can be very difficult in the hypothermic patient. Patients who appear to have suffered a cardiac arrest or death as a result of hypothermia should not be pronounced dead until they are rewarmed.

The rewarming technique depends on the patient's temperature and his response to simpler measures. For example, treat mild and moderate hypothermia by **passive external rewarming** in a warm room using warm blankets, clothing, and warmed intravenous fluids. Severe hypothermia may require **active core rewarming methods** that may include invasive surgical rewarming techniques, eg, peritoneal lavage, thoracic/pleural lavage, hemodialysis, or cardiopulmonary bypass, all of which are better done in a critical care setting.

The risk of cardiac irritability increases with body temperatures below 30 degrees centigrade, and asystole may occur with body temperatures below 28 degrees centigrade. Cardiac drugs and defibrillation are not usually effective in the presence of acidosis, hypoxia, and hypothermia. Sodium bicarbonate and 100% oxygen should be administered while the patient is warmed to 32 degrees centigrade, and cardiopulmonary resuscitation is continued. Cardiac drugs and defibrillation may then be instituted when the patient is rewarmed, as indicated. Attempts to actively rewarm the patient should not delay transfer to a critical care setting. (See Chapter 3, Shock.)

IX. Summary

A. Burns—Thermal, Chemical, Electrical

Immediate life-saving measures for the burn patient include the **recognition of inhalation** injury and subsequent endotracheal intubation, and the rapid institution of intravenous fluid therapy. **All clothing should be removed rapidly.**

Early stabilization and management of the burn patient include:

1. Identifying the extent and depth of the burn

2. Establishing fluid guidelines according to the patient's weight

3. Initiating a patient-care flow sheet

4. Obtaining baseline laboratory and roentgenographic studies

5. Maintaining peripheral circulation in circumferential burns by performing an escharotomy if necessary

6. Identifying which burn patients require transfer to a burn unit or center

B. Cold Injuries

Diagnose the type of cold injury by obtaining an adequate history and noting the physical findings as well as measuring the core temperature using a low-range thermometer (esophageal temperature probe preferred). The patient should be removed from the cold environment immediately, and vital signs should be monitored and supported continuously. Rewarming techniques should be applied as soon as possible. The patient with hypothermia should not be considered dead until rewarming has occurred.

Early management of cold-injury patients includes:

1. Identifying the type and extent of cold injury

2. Measuring the patient's core temperature

3. Initiating a patient-care flow sheet

4. Initiating rapid rewarming techniques

5. Determining the patient's life or death status after rewarming

Bibliography

1. Amy BW, McManus WF, Goodwin CW Jr, et al: Lightning injury with survival in five patients. **Journal of the American Medical Association** 1985;253:243-245.

2. Cioffi WG, Graves TA, McManus WF, et al: High frequency percussive ventilation in patients with inhalation injury. **Journal of Trauma** 1987;29:350-354.

3. Graves TA, Cioffi WG, McManus WF, et al: Fluid resuscitation of infants and children with massive thermal injury. **Journal of Trauma** 1988;28(12):1656-1659.

4. Halebian P, Robinson N, Barie P, et al: Whole body oxygen utilization during carbon monoxide poisoning and isocapneic nitrogen hypoxia. **Journal of Trauma** 1986;26:110-117.

5. Haponik EF, Munster AM (eds): **Respiratory Injury: Smoke Inhalation and Burns.** New York, New York, McGraw-Hill Inc, 1990.

6. Jurkovich GJ: Hypothermia in the trauma patient. In: Maull KI, Cleveland HC, Strauch GO, et al (eds): **Advances in Trauma.** Chicago, Illinois, Year Book Medical Publishers, Inc, 1989, Volume 4, pp 11-140.

7. Lund T, Goodwin CW, McManus WF, et al: Upper airway sequelae in burn patients requiring endotracheal intubation or tracheostomy. **Annals of Surgery** 1985;201:374-382.

8. McManus WF, Pruitt BA: Thermal injuries. In: Mattox RH, Moore EE, Feliciano CV (eds): **Trauma,** 2nd Edition, East Norwalk, Connecticut, Appleton and Lange, 1991, pp 751-764.

9. Mozingo DW, Smith AA, McManus WF, et al: Chemical burns. **Journal of Trauma** 1988;28:642-647.

10. Pruitt BA Jr: The burn patient: I. Initial care. **Current Problems in Surgery** 1979;16(4):1-55.

11. Pruitt BA Jr: The burn patient: II. Later care and complications of thermal injury. **Current Problems in Surgery** 1979;16(5):1-95.

12. Saffle JR, Crandall A, Warden GD: Cataracts: a long-term complication of electrical injury. **Journal of Trauma** 1985;25:17-121.

13. Sheehy TW, Navari RM: Hypothermia. **Intensive and Critical Care Digest** 1985;4:12-18.

14. Stratta RJ, Saffle JR, Kravitz M, et al: Management of tar and asphalt injuries. **American Journal of Surgery** 1983;146:766-769.

Chapter 9:
Injuries Due to
Burns and Cold

Chapter 10:
Pediatric Trauma

Objectives:

Upon completion of this topic, the participant will be able to:

A. Discuss the unique characteristics of the child as a trauma patient.

   1. Types of injury
   2. Patterns of injury
   3. Anatomic and physiologic differences in children as compared with adults
   4. Long-term effects of injury

B. Discuss the primary management of the following critical injuries in children based on the anatomic and physiologic differences as compared with adults.

   1. Airway management
   2. Shock and maintenance of body heat
   3. Fluid and electrolyte management
   4. Medications and dosages
   5. Cervical spine injuries
   6. Psychologic support

C. Discuss the injury patterns associated with the abused child and the elements that lead to the suspicion of child abuse.

D. Discuss the epidemiology of childhood injury and effective strategies for injury prevention in children.

E. Demonstrate in a simulated situation the following procedures for the pediatric trauma victim.

   1. Endotracheal intubation
   2. Intravenous/intraosseous access
   3. Fluid and drug administration
   4. Management of extremity trauma

**Chapter 10:
Pediatric
Trauma**

American College of Surgeons

I. Introduction

Nearly 22 million children are injured each year in the United States, representing nearly one in every three in the pediatric age group. Injuries surpass all major diseases in children and young adults making it the most serious health care issue for this population cohort. Encounters with motor vehicles, either as an occupant, a pedestrian, or a cyclist, account for the largest fatally injured group followed by drownings, house fires, and homicide. Falls and vehicular crashes account for almost 80% of all pediatric injuries, although distressingly the number of penetrating injuries is on the rise. Multisystem injury is the rule rather than the exception and therefore all organ systems must be assumed to be injured until proved otherwise. **Children with multisystem injuries can deteriorate rapidly and develop serious complications. Therefore, such patients should be transferred early to a facility capable of managing the child with multisystem injuries.**

The order and priorities of assessment and management of the injured child are the same as in the adult. However, the unique anatomic characteristics of the pediatric population require special consideration in the assessment and management of the pediatric trauma victim.

A. Size and Shape

Because of the smaller body mass of children, the energy from the linear forces from fenders, bumpers, and falls results in a greater force applied per unit body area. This more intense energy is further applied to a body with less fat, less elastic connective tissue, and close proximity of multiple organs. The result is the high frequency of multiple organ injuries seen in the pediatric population.

B. Skeleton

The child's skeleton is incompletely calcified, contains multiple active growth centers, and is more pliable. For these reasons, internal organ damage is frequently noted without overlying bony fracture. For example, rib fractures in the child are uncommon, but pulmonary contusion is common. Other soft tissues of the thorax, the heart, and mediastinal structures may sustain significant damage without evidence of bony injury. The identification of rib fractures in a child suggests the transfer of a massive amount of energy and multiple, serious organ injuries should be suspected.

C. Surface Area

The ratio of a child's body surface area to body volume is highest at birth and diminishes as the child matures. As a result, thermal energy loss becomes a significant stress factor in the child. Hypothermia may develop quickly and complicate the management of the hypotensive pediatric patient.

D. Psychologic Status

Psychologic ramifications of caring for an injured child can present significant challenges. In the very young, emotional instability frequently leads to a regressive psychologic behavior when stress, pain, or other perceived threats intervene in the child's environment. The child's ability to interact with unfamiliar individuals in strange and difficult situations is limited, making history-taking and cooperative manipulation, especially if it is painful, extremely difficult. The physician who understands these characteristics and is willing to cajole and soothe an injured child is more likely to establish a good rapport. This facilitates comprehensive assessment of the child's psychologic as well as physical injuries.

E. Long-term Effects

A major consideration in dealing with injured children is the effect that injury may have on subsequent growth and development. Unlike the adult, the child must not only recover from the effects of the traumatic event, but also must continue the normal process of growth and maturation. The physiologic and psychologic effects of injury on this process should not be underestimated, particularly in those cases involving long-term function, growth deformity, or abnormal subsequent development. Children sustaining even a minor injury may have prolonged disability in either cerebral function, psychologic adjustment, or organ system disability. Recent evidence suggests that as many as 60% of children who sustain severe multisystem trauma have residual personality changes at one year following hospital discharge, and 50% show cognitive and physical handicaps. Social, affective, and learning disabilities are present in one half of seriously injured children. In addition, childhood injuries have a significant impact on the family structure, with personality and emotional disturbances in two thirds of uninjured siblings. Frequently, a child's injuries impose a strain on the family's marital relationship, including the financial and sometimes employment hardships. Inadequate or inappropriate care in the immediate posttraumatic period may affect not only the child's survival, but perhaps just as importantly, the quality of the child's life for years to come.

F. Equipment

Immediately available equipment of the appropriate size is essential for successful initial management of the injured child. (See Table 5 at the end of this chapter.) The recently available Broselow Pediatric Resuscitation Measuring Tape is an ideal adjunct for rapid determination of weight based on length for appropriate drug doses and equipment size. (See Skill Station IV, Vascular Access and Monitoring.)

II. Airway Management

The primary goal of initial assessment and triage of the injured child is to restore, or maintain, adequate tissue oxygenation. Oxygen delivery is as essential to the injured child as to the adult. The standard principles of airway control, breathing, and circulation are applied to the injured child as they are to the adult. The child's airway is the first priority of assessment.

A. Anatomy

The smaller the child, the greater is the disproportion between the size of the cranium and the midface. This produces a greater propensity for the posterior pharyngeal area to buckle as the relatively larger occiput forces passive flexion of the cervical spine. The child's airway is thus protected by a slightly superior and anterior position of the midface, known as the "sniffing position." Careful attention to maintaining this position while providing maximum protection to the cervical spine is especially important in the obtunded child. Soft tissues in the infant's oropharynx (ie, tongue, tonsils) are relatively large compared with the oral cavity, which may make visualization of the larynx difficult.

A child's larynx has a slightly more antero-caudal angle and is frequently more difficult to visualize for direct cannulation in the slightly head-flexed position assumed by the supine child. The infant's trachea is approximately five centimeters in length and grows to seven centimeters by about 18 months. Failure to appreciate this short length may result in intubation of the right mainstem bronchus, inadequate ventilation, and mechanical injury to the delicate bronchial tree.

B. Management

In a spontaneously breathing child, the airway should be secured by the chin lift or jaw thrust maneuver. After the mouth and oropharynx have been cleared of secretions or debris, supplemental oxygen should be administered. If the patient is unconscious, mechanical methods of maintaining the airway may be necessary.

Before attempts are made to mechanically establish an airway, the child should be oxygenated.

1. Oral airway

The practice of inserting the airway backwards and rotating it 180 degrees is not recommended for the pediatric patient. Trauma with resultant hemorrhage into soft-tissue structures of the oropharynx may occur. The oral airway should be gently inserted directly into the oropharynx. The use of a tongue blade to depress the tongue may be helpful. As in the adult, the oral airway should not be used in the conscious child.

2. Orotracheal intubation

Endotracheal intubation is the most reliable means of ventilating the child with airway compromise. Uncuffed tubes of appropriate size should be used to avoid subglottic edema, ulceration, and disruption of the infant's fragile airway. The smallest area of the child's airway is at the cricoid, which forms a natural seal with the endotracheal tube. Therefore, cuffed endotracheal tubes are not needed. A simple technique to gauge the size of the endotracheal tube is to approximate the diameter of the external nares or the child's fifth (small) finger with the tube diameter.

Orotracheal intubation under direct vision with adequate immobilization and protection of the cervical spine is the preferred method of obtaining initial airway control. Nasotracheal intubation should not be performed in children. Nasotracheal intubation requires blind passage around a relatively acute angle in the nasopharynx toward an anterior and cranially located glottis, making intubation by this route difficult. Inadvertent penetration of the cranial vault or damage to nasopharyngeal soft tissues also makes the nasotracheal route for airway control ill-advised.

Once past the glottic opening, the endotracheal tube should be positioned 2.0 to 3.0 cm below the level of the vocal cords and carefully secured in place. Auscultation of both hemithoraces **in the axillae** should be performed to ensure that right mainstem bronchial intubation has not occurred, and that both sides of the chest are being adequately ventilated. Any movement of the head may result in displacement of the endotracheal tube. Breath sounds should be evaluated periodically to ensure that the tube remains in the appropriate position and to identify the possibility of evolving ventilatory dysfunction.

3. Cricothyroidotomy

Surgical cricothyroidotomy is rarely indicated for the infant or small child, and if absolutely necessary, it should be performed by a surgeon. When airway access and control cannot be accomplished by bag-valve-mask or orotracheal intubation, needle cricothyroidotomy is the preferred method. Needle jet insufflation via the cricothyroid membrane is an appropriate, temporizing technique for oxygenation, but it does not provide adequate ventilation and hypercarbia may occur.

4. Ventilation

Children should be ventilated at a rate of approximately 20 breaths per minute, while infants require 40 breaths per minute. Tidal volumes of 7 to 10 mL per kilogram are appropriate for both infants and children. Although most bag-valve-mask devices for use with pediatric patients are designed to limit the amount of pressure that can be exerted manually on the child's airway, the physician should remember the fragile nature of the immature tracheobronchial tree and alveolae to minimize the potential for iatrogenic bronchoalveolar injury.

The most common acid-base abnormality that develops during pediatric resuscitation is acidosis secondary to **hypoventilation**. If adequate ventilation and perfusion have been re-established, the injured child should be able to maintain a relatively normal pH. **Remember**, in the absence of adequate ventilation and perfusion, sodium bicarbonate does **not** correct the evolving acidosis and may lead to further hypercapnea.

5. Tube thoracostomy

Injuries that disrupt pleural to pleural apposition, eg, hemothorax, pneumothorax, or hemopneumothorax, occur with equal frequency in children as adults with the same physiologic consequences. These injuries are managed with pleural decompression. Chest tubes are obviously of smaller size (see table at the end of this chapter) and are placed into the thoracic cavity by tunneling the tube over the rib above the thoracostomy site.

III. Shock

Every injured child with evidence of hypotension or inadequate organ system perfusion must be evaluated by a surgeon as soon as possible.

A. Recognition

Injury in childhood frequently results in significant blood loss. The increased physiologic reserve of the child allows the maintenance of nearly normal vital signs even in the presence of severe shock. This early state of "compensated" shock may be misleading and may mask a major reduction in circulating blood volume. Tachycardia and poor skin perfusion are the keys to recognizing this problem and to instituting appropriate crystalloid resuscitation.

The primary response to hypovolemia in the child is tachycardia. However, caution must be exercised when monitoring only the child's heart rate because tachycardia also may be caused by pain, fear, and psychologic stress. Blood pressure and indices of adequate organ perfusion, eg, urinary output, should be monitored closely.

Hypotension in the child represents a state of uncompensated shock and indicates severe blood loss and inadequate resuscitation. Changes in vital organ function are outlined in Table 1, Systemic Responses to Blood Loss in the Pediatric Patient. Although signs of severe hypovolemic shock may be unmistakable, signs of early hypovolemic shock may be extremely subtle. Careful, repeated evaluation is imperative.

The association of tachycardia, cool extremities, and a systolic blood pressure of less than 70 mm Hg are clear indicators of evolving shock. Early compensated shock may present with normal vital signs. As a rule, a child's blood pressure should be 80 mm Hg plus twice the age in years, and the diastolic pressure should be two thirds of the systolic blood pressure. (See Table 2, Vital Signs.)

Table 1
Systemic Responses to Blood Loss in the Pediatric Patient

	< 25% Blood Volume Loss	25% - 45% Blood Volume Loss	> 45% Blood Volume Loss
Cardiac	Weak, thready pulse; increased heart rate	Increased heart rate	Hypotension, tachycardia to bradycardia
CNS	Lethargic, irritable, confused	Change in level of consciousness, dulled response to pain	Comatose
Skin	Cool, clammy	Cyanotic, decreased capillary refill, cold extremities	Pale, cold
Kidneys	Decreased urinary output; increased specific gravity	Minimal urine output	No urinary output

Table 2
Vital Signs

	Pulse Rate (Beats/min)	Blood Pressure (mm Hg)	Respiratory Rate (Breaths/min)
Infant	160	80	40
Preschool	120	90	30
Adolescent	100	100	20

B. Fluid Resuscitation

Approximately a 25% diminution in blood volume is required to produce minimal clinical manifestations of shock. When shock is suspected, a fluid bolus, using warmed fluids whenever possible, of 20 mL/kg of crystalloid solution is an appropriate initial bolus. This represents 25% of the normal blood volume of a child (20 mL/kg divided by 80 mL/kg = 25%).

The injured child should be monitored carefully with respect to the adequacy of organ perfusion and response to the initial fluid challenge. Return of hemodynamic stability is indicated by:

1. Slowing of the heart rate (< 130 beats/minute)
2. Increased pulse pressure (> 20 mm Hg)
3. Decrease in skin mottling
4. Increased warmth of extremities
5. Clearing of sensorium
6. Urinary output of 1 mL/kg/hour
7. Increased systolic blood pressure (> 80 mm Hg)

Failure to improve hemodynamic abnormalities following the first bolus of resuscitation fluid mandates prompt involvement of a surgeon, raises the suspicion for continuing hemorrhage, and prompts the need for the administration of a second 20-mL/kg bolus of crystalloid fluid. Serious consideration should be given to the prompt infusion of 10 mL/kg of type-specific blood or O-negative packed red blood cells (P-RBCs) in this situation.

The resuscitation flow diagram is a useful aid in the initial management of the injured child. (See Table 3, Resuscitation Flow Diagram for the Stable and Unstable Pediatric Patient.)

C. Blood Replacement

The child in severe hypovolemic shock who does not respond to an initial crystalloid bolus must have restoration of the circulating red blood cell mass to ensure adequate tissue oxygen delivery. Rapid transfusion of warmed, red blood cells should be considered as soon as adequate venous access has been established in the hypovolemic child. Children who have received the initial two boluses of 20 mL/kg of Ringer's lactate and have not responded clearly require immediate blood transfusion as well as ongoing crystalloid infusion. Further, children who respond initially, but whose conditions later deteriorate also are candidates for prompt infusion of red blood cells. Until type-specific blood is available, warmed type O, Rh-negative packed red blood cells (10 mL/kg) is appropriate. **Remember, evaluation by a surgeon is essential.**

D. Venous Access

Severe hypovolemic shock usually occurs as the result of disruption of intrathoracic or intra-abdominal organ systems. Venous access should preferably be established by a percutaneous route. The common femoral veins should be avoided in infants and children whenever possible because of the high incidence of venous thrombosis and the possibility of ischemic limb loss. If percutaneous access is unsuccessful after two attempts, consideration should be given to intraosseous infusion in children younger than six years of age or direct venous cutdown in children six years of age or older. Venous cutdown may be considered at these sites:

1. Greater saphenous at the ankle
2. Median cephalic vein at the elbow
3. Main cephalic vein higher in the upper arm
4. External jugular, which also may be cannulated percutaneously

Table 3
Resuscitation Flow Diagram for the Stable and Unstable Pediatric Patient

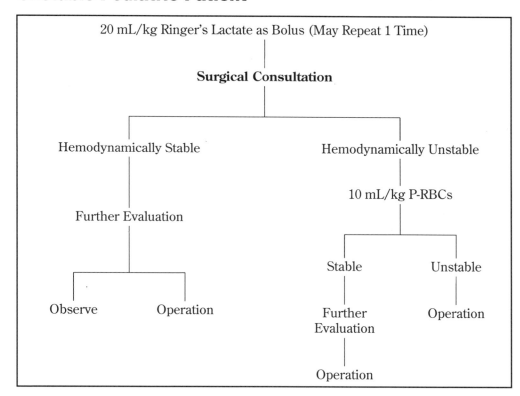

Intravenous access in the hypovolemic child younger than six years of age is a perplexing and challenging problem, even in the most experienced hands. **Intraosseous infusion**, cannulating the marrow cavity of a long bone in an **uninjured** extremity, is an emergent-access procedure for the critically ill or injured child. The intraosseous route is safe, efficacious, and requires less time than venous cutdown. However, intraosseous infusion should be discontinued when suitable peripheral venous access has been established.

Indications for intraosseous infusion are limited to children six years of age or younger, for whom venous access is impossible due to circulatory collapse or for whom percutaneous peripheral venous cannulation has failed on two attempts. Complications of this procedure include cellulitis and rarely, osteomyelitis. The preferred site for intraosseous cannulation is the proximal tibia, below the level of the tibial tuberosity. If the tibia is fractured, the needle may be inserted into the distal femur. Intraosseous cannulation should not be performed distal to a fracture site. (See Figure 1, Site for Intraosseous Infusion.)

Using a #16- or #18-gauge, one-half inch long, bone marrow aspiration/transfusion needle, entry is directed distally in the tibia and superiorly in the femur, with the bevel directed up to avoid the joint space and the physis. Aspiration of bone marrow contents identifies adequate needle position. Needle position also can be verified by the lack of resistance to infusion without soft-tissue extravasation. Crystalloids, blood products, and drugs may be administered via the intraosseous route. Circulation time from the marrow cavity to the heart is generally less than 20 seconds. Effective volume resuscitation can be accomplished by this method.

Figure 1
Site for Intraosseous Infusion

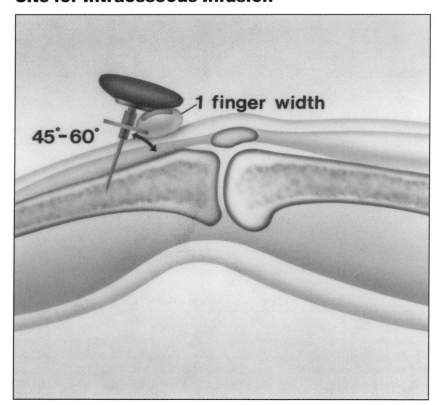

E. Thermoregulation

The high ratio of body surface area to body mass in children increases the facility with which heat exchange occurs with the environment, and directly affects the child's ability to regulate core temperature. Thin skin and the lack of substantial subcutaneous tissue contribute to increased evaporative heat loss and caloric expenditure. Hypothermia may render the injured child refractory to treatment, prolong coagulation times, and adversely affect central nervous system function. While the child is exposed during the initial survey and resuscitation phase, overhead heat lamps or heaters or thermal blankets may be necessary to maintain body temperature. Warming the room as well as intravenous fluids and blood products is necessary to preserve body heat.

IV. Chest Trauma

Blunt thoracic trauma is common in children and often requires immediate intervention to establish adequate ventilation. The child's chest wall is very compliant, allowing for the transfer of energy to the intrathoracic soft tissues, frequently without any evidence of injury to the external chest wall itself. The specific abnormalities caused by thoracic trauma in the child are identical to those encountered in the adult, and usually can be treated without thoracotomy. The management approach is the same.

Mobility of mediastinal structures makes the child more sensitive to tension pneumothorax and flail segments. The pliable chest wall increases the frequency of pulmonary contusions and direct intrapulmonary hemorrhage, usually without overlying rib fractures. **However, the identification of rib fractures in young children implies massive energy transfer, severe associated organ system injury, and a poorer prognosis. Therefore, children sustaining multiple rib fractures should be transported to a facility capable of providing optimal management.**

Children sustain bronchial injuries and diaphragmatic ruptures more frequently than adults due to blunt crushing forces. Injury to the great vessels is infrequent compared with that in the adult. Significant injuries rarely occur alone and are frequently a component of major multisystem injury.

Penetrating thoracic injury is rare in the preadolescent child; however, it represents an increasing cause of injury after 10 years of age. Penetrating trauma to the chest is managed in the same manner as in the adult.

V. Abdominal Trauma

Most pediatric abdominal injuries occur as the result of blunt trauma, primarily in the situations involving motor vehicles and falls.

Penetrating abdominal injuries, which increase during adolescence (both intentional and unintentional), dictate prompt involvement by the surgeon. As in the adult, the hypotensive child who has sustained penetrating abdominal trauma should be assumed to have major intra-abdominal injury and requires operative resuscitation.

A. Assessment

The conscious infant and young child are generally frightened by the events preceding admission to the emergency department, and this may influence the examination of the abdomen. While talking **quietly** and calmly to the child, ask questions about the presence of abdominal pain, and gently assess the tone of the abdominal musculature. Deep painful palpation of the abdomen should be avoided at the onset of the examination to prevent voluntary guarding that may confuse the abdominal findings. Almost all infants and young children who are stressed and crying will swallow a large amount of air. Decompression of the stomach by inserting a gastric tube, as in the adult, should be a part of the resuscitation phase. Orogastric intubation is preferred in infants. Tenseness of the abdominal wall will often decrease as gastric distention is relieved. The abdomen then can be carefully and more reliably evaluated. Abdominal examination in the unconscious patient will not vary greatly with age. Decompression of the urinary bladder will facilitate abdominal evaluation.

B. Peritoneal Lavage

Although the interpretation of the results of peritoneal lavage is the same for the pediatric and the adult patient, the procedure is performed less often in children. Peritoneal lavage is a useful technique in the evaluation of the hemodynamically unstable child.

As in the adult, use a buffered Ringer's lactate solution in volumes of 10 mL/kg up to 1000 mL, with the solution running over a 10-minute period. The fluid should be warmed. It is important to remember that the child's abdominal wall is relatively thinner than in the adult. Sudden penetration of the abdominal cavity can produce iatrogenic injury to the abdominal contents, even using the open technique. Peritoneal lavage has utility in diagnosing injuries to intra-abdominal viscera only. Retroperitoneal organs cannot be evaluated reliably by this technique.

Because nonoperative management requires surgical supervision, diagnostic peritoneal lavage in a child should be performed only by the surgeon who will care for the patient.

C. Computed Tomography

Many surgeons use computed tomographic (CT) scanning in place of peritoneal lavage, and some use both. CT scans may be useful in the assessment of abdominal injuries in the hemodynamically stable child. If CT scanning is used to evaluate the abdomen of children sustaining blunt trauma, it must be immediately available, performed early, and **not delay further treatment**. The identification of intra-abdominal injuries by CT scan in otherwise stable pediatric patients may allow nonoperative management by surgeons when a positive lavage would have mandated celiotomy.

D. Nonoperative Management

Selective nonoperative management of children with blunt abdominal injuries is performed in many trauma centers. These children **must** be managed in a facility offering pediatric intensive care capabilities, and under the supervision of a qualified surgeon. Intensive care must include continuous nursing staff coverage, continuous monitoring of vital signs, and **immediate** availability of surgical personnel and operating room resources.

Nonoperative management of confirmed abdominal, visceral injuries requires the direction of a surgeon. The decision to manage the patient nonoperatively, to continue to manage the patient nonoperatively, or to operate is a surgical decision. Therefore, a surgeon's involvement in the early management of the pediatric patient is absolutely necessary.

VI. Head Trauma

Information provided in Chapter 6, Head Trauma, also applies to pediatric patients. This section emphasizes additional points peculiar to children.

Most head injuries in the pediatric population are the result of motor vehicle crashes, bicycle accidents, and falls. Data from the National Pediatric Trauma Registry indicate that an understanding of the interaction between the central nervous system and extracranial injuries is imperative. Determinants of survival in this population are related more to associated injuries (lack of attention to the ABCs) than the head injury itself. As in the adult, hypotension is rarely, if ever, caused by head injury alone, and other explanations for this finding should be investigated aggressively.

A. Assessment

Children and adults may differ in their response to head trauma, which may influence the evaluation of the injured child. The principal differences include:

1. Although children generally recover from head injuries better than adults, children younger than three years old have worse outcomes from severe head trauma than older children. Children are particularly susceptible to the effects of the secondary brain injury that may be produced by hypoxia, hypotension with reduced cerebral perfusion, seizures, or hyperthermia. **Adequate restoration of an appropriate circulating blood volume is mandatory and hypoxia must be avoided.**

2. Although an infrequent occurrence, infants may become hypotensive from blood loss into either the subgaleal or epidural space. Treatment is directed toward appropriate volume restoration as it is with blood loss from other body regions.

3. The young child with an open fontanelle and mobile cranial suture lines is more tolerant of an expanding intracranial mass lesion. Signs of an expanding mass may be hidden until rapid decompensation occurs. Therefore, an infant who is not in coma, but who has a a bulging fontanelle or suture diastases **should be treated as having a more severe injury.** Early neurosurgical consultation is essential.

4. Vomiting is common after head injury in children and does not necessarily imply increased intracranial pressure. However, persistent vomiting or vomiting that becomes more frequent is of concern and demands CT of the head. Gastric decompression is essential, because of the risk of aspiration.

5. Seizures occurring shortly after head injury are more common in children and are usually self-limiting. Recurrent seizure activity requires investigation by CT scanning.

6. Children tend to have fewer focal mass lesions than adults, but elevated intracranial pressure due to cerebral edema is more common. In children, a lucid interval may be prolonged, and the onset of neurologic deterioration may be delayed for this reason. Although rapid restoration of appropriate circulating blood volume is necessary, overhydration, especially with hypotonic fluids, should be avoided. Emergency CT is vital to identify those children who require emergency surgery.

7. The Glasgow Coma Scale (GCS) is useful when applied to the pediatric age group. However, the verbal score must be modified for children younger than four years of age. (See Table 4, Pediatric Verbal Score.)

Table 4
Pediatric Verbal Score

Verbal Response	V-Score
Appropriate words or social smile, fixes and follows	5
Cries, but consolable	4
Persistently irritable	3
Restless, agitated	2
None	1

8. Because of the frequency for developing increased intracranial pressure in children, intracranial pressure monitoring should be considered **early** in the course of resuscitation for children with:

    a. A GCS Score of eight or less, or motor scores of one or two

    b. Multiple injuries who require major volume resuscitation, immediate life-saving thoracic or abdominal surgery, or for whom stabilization and assessment will be prolonged

9. Medication dosages must be adjusted as dictated by the child's size, and in consultation with a neurosurgeon. Frequently used drugs in children with head injuries include:

    a. Phenobarbital—2 to 3 mg/kg

    b. Diazepam—0.25 mg/kg, slow IV bolus

    c. Phenytoin—15 to 20 mg/kg, administered at 0.5 to 1.5 mL/kg/minute as a loading dose, then 4 to 7 mg/kg/day for maintenance

    d. Mannitol—0.5 to 1.0 g/kg

B. Management

Successful management of diffuse axonal injury in children involves:

1. Rapid, early assessment and management of the airway, respiration, and circulatory system

2. Appropriate neurosurgical involvement from the beginning of treatment

3. Appropriate sequential assessment and management of the brain injury with attention directed toward the prevention of secondary brain injury, ie, hypoxia and underperfusion. Early endotracheal intubation with adequate oxygenation and ventilation are indicated to avoid progressive central nervous system damage. Attempts to orally intubate the trachea in the uncooperative, head-injured child may be difficult and actually increase intracranial pressure. Based on the intubation skills of the physician, iatrogenic paralysis to facilitate intubation potentially risks the life of the patient. Therefore, this modality should be employed only by the physician who has considered the risks and benefits of intubating the child and who is confident of his intubation abilities.

4. Continuous reassessment of all parameters

VII. Spinal Cord Injury

Information provided in Chapter 7, Spine and Spinal Cord Trauma, also applies to pediatric patients. This chapter emphasizes the peculiarities of pediatric spinal injury.

Spinal cord injury in children is fortunately rare. Only 5% of all spinal cord injuries occur in the pediatric age group. For children younger than 10 years of age, motor vehicle crashes most commonly produce these injuries. For children aged 10 to 14 years, motor vehicles and sporting activities account for an equal number of spinal injuries.

A. Anatomic Differences

1. Interspinous ligaments and joint capsules are more flexible.

2. The uncinate articulations are poorly developed and incomplete.

3. Vertebral bodies are wedged anteriorly and tend to slide forward with flexion.

4. The facet joints are flat.

5. The child has a relatively large head compared with the adult, and more angular momentum can be generated during flexion or extension, resulting in greater energy transfer.

B. Roentgenographic Considerations

Pseudosubluxation—About 40% of children younger than seven years of age show anterior displacement of C-2 on C-3. About 20% of children up to 16 years of age exhibit this phenomenon. Although this radiographic finding is seen less commonly at C-3 to C-4, more than 3 mm of movement can be seen when these joints are studied by flexion and extension maneuvers.

Increased distance between the dens and the anterior arch of C-1 occurs in about 20% of young children. Gaps exceeding the upper limit of normal for the adult population are frequently seen.

Skeletal growth centers can resemble fractures. Basilar odontoid synchrondrosis appears as a radiolucent area at the base of the dens, especially in children younger than five years of age. Apical odontoid epiphyses appear as separations on the odontoid roentgenogram and are usually seen between the ages of five and eleven years. The growth center of the spinous process may resemble fractures of the tip of the spinous process.

Children may sustain spinal cord injury without radiographic abnormality more commonly than adults. A normal spine series can be found in up to two thirds of children suffering spinal cord injury. Therefore, if spinal cord injury is suspected, based on history or results of the neurologic examination, normal spine roentgenograms do not exclude significant spinal cord injury. **When in doubt about the integrity of the cervical spine, assume that an unstable injury exists, maintain immobilization of the child's head and neck, and obtain appropriate consultation.**

VIII. Extremity Trauma

The initial priorities in the management of skeletal trauma in the child are similar to those for the adult, with the additional concerns about potential injury to the growth plate.

A. History

History is of vital importance. In the younger child, roentgenographic diagnosis of fractures and dislocations is difficult because of the lack of mineralization around the epiphysis and the presence of a physis (growth plate). Information about the magnitude mechanism and time of the injury facilitates better correlation of the physical findings and roentgenograms. Radiographic evidence of fractures of differing ages should alert the physician to possible child abuse.

B. Blood Loss

Blood loss associated with long bone and pelvic fractures is proportionately greater in the child than in the adult. Even a small child can lose up to one unit of blood into the muscle mass or the thigh, and hemodynamic instability may develop as the result of a fractured femur.

C. Physeal (Growth Plate) Fractures

Bones lengthen as new bone is laid down by the physis near the articular surfaces. Injuries to, or adjacent to, this area before the physis has closed can potentially retard the normal growth or alter the development of the bone in an abnormal way. Crush injuries, which are often difficult to recognize radiographically, have the worst prognosis.

D. Fractures Unique to the Immature Skeleton

The immature, pliable nature of bones in children may lead to a so-called "greenstick" fracture. Such fractures are incomplete, with angulation maintained by cortical splinters on the concave surface. The torus or "buckle" fracture, seen in small children, involves angulation due to cortical impaction with a radiolucent fracture line. Supracondylar fractures at the elbow or knee have a high propensity for vascular injury as well as injury to the growth plate.

E. Principles of Immobilization

Simple splinting of fractured extremities in children is usually sufficient until definitive orthopedic evaluation can be performed. Injured extremities with evidence of vascular compromise require emergent evaluation to prevent the adverse sequelae of ischemia. A single attempt at reduction of the fracture to restore blood flow is appropriate followed by simple splinting or traction splinting of the femur.

IX. The Battered, Abused Child

The battered, abused child syndrome refers to any child who sustains a nonaccidental injury as the result of acts by parents, guardians, or acquaintances. Children who die within the first year of life from injury usually do so as the result of child abuse. Therefore, a history and careful evaluation of the child suspected of being abused is critically important to prevent eventual death, especially in children who are younger than one year of age. A physician should suspect abuse if:

1. A discrepancy exists between the history and the degree of physical injury.

2. A prolonged interval has passed between the time of the injury and the seeking of medical advice.

3. The history includes repeated trauma, treated in different emergency departments.

4. Parents respond inappropriately or do not comply with medical advice, eg, leaving a child in the emergency facility.

5. The history of injury changes or differs between parents or guardians.

These findings, on careful physical examination, should suggest child abuse and indicate more intensive investigation:

1. Multiple subdural hematomas, especially without a fresh skull fracture

2. Retinal hemorrhage

3. Perioral injuries

4. Ruptured internal viscera without antecedent major blunt trauma

5. Trauma to the genital or perianal areas

6. Evidence of frequent injuries typified by old scars or healed fractures on roentgenogram

7. Fractures of long bones in children younger than three years of age

8. Bizarre injuries such as bites, cigarette burns, or rope marks

9. Sharply demarcated second- and third-degree burns in unusual areas

In every state, physicians are bound by law to report incidences of child abuse to governmental authorities, even cases where abuse is only suspected. Abused children are at increased risk for fatal injuries, and no one is served by failing to report. The system protects physicians from legal liability for identifying confirmed or even suspicious cases of abuse. Although the reporting procedures may vary from state to state, it is most commonly handled through local social service agencies or the state's Health and Human Services Department.

X. Epidemiology of Injury in Children and Strategies for Injury Control

Considering the devastating impact that childhood injuries may have on the child, and his/her family, the physicians involved in the care of children have an obligation to be engaged in efforts directed toward injury prevention. Blunt injuries predominate in the pediatric population, but penetrating injuries appear to be on the increase, particularly in adolescents and teenagers. If physicians can convince the lay public that "accidents" are not random events beyond the control of society, then much can be done to prevent injuries. Programs for injury prevention should begin in the home. Parents should be counseled on appropriate supervision during play time activities, poison prevention, fall precautions, and should be encouraged to take classes in cardiopulmonary resuscitation. Bicycle safety programs should be introduced into the school curricula of all elementary schools. The use of the bicycle helmets has been shown to effectively reduce the number and seriousness of head injuries, and these programs should be introduced and encouraged for all cyclists. Given the fact that even minor head injuries may have profound influences on the physical, cognitive, emotional, and social aspects of development, all efforts in the area of head injury prevention are certainly justifiable.

Identification of children at risk for injury is somewhat more problematic. Epidemiologists have identified preliminary risk factors that are worthy of consideration, and involve environmental and social characteristics that can be recognized. Signs of stress and discord within family units have been statistically associated with increased risk of injury. Other related factors to the potential for injury, though perhaps not causally, include a chronic medical condition, weight in the lowest 25th percentile, birth order third or later, and maternal education level greater than high school.

The issues concerning whether children who sustain one injury are at higher risk for subsequent injuries and the concept of the "accident-prone" child are controversial. However, studies have produced evidence that suggests that a significantly greater proportion of school-aged children who sustained more than one injury did so at a rate greater than could have been accounted for by chance alone. A group of recurrently injured children, composing only one percent of the injured pediatric population, sustained nearly one fifth (20%) of all the injuries identified. Further, injuries occurred more frequently in school systems with "open" classrooms, junior high schools, extended hours, magnet curricula, and those with active athletic programs. The association of these factors with childhood trauma is an important marker for the development of injury awareness programs in the community. Children at potentially greater risk for injury might be identified.

The problem of social violence is increasing throughout the United States and the pediatric age group is not immune. The association of pediatric injury with the increasing use of drugs and other substances of abuse is suggestive, but it lacks confirmatory evidence. No doubt, the availability and access to hand guns and other weapons contribute to the problem. While preventive measures in scenarios involving violence may be difficult to identify prospectively, school-sponsored drug and alcohol awareness programs, gun control, gun safety, and even programs designed to teach appropriate measures for dealing with anger and conflict would be beneficial. Physicians should be able to identify parents who lack sufficient parenting skills or reside in pathologic environmental situations. Referrals to appropriate social agencies who could render assistance would be prudent in these situations. It may be unfortunate that often the families in need of such services are identified after the fact, but an opportunity does exist for the physician to intervene when circumstances suggest correctable social, psychologic, or environmental predisposing factors.

Legislative activity to mandate safety (seat belt laws, child restraint legislation, requirements for helmets for cyclists, gun control, etc) is laudable. However, successful preventive programs must begin at the "grass roots" level. Physicians are in a unique position not only to identify the problem, but also to serve as role models and community leaders in this area. Despite the fact that all the answers to the problems of injury prevention do not exist, the medical community cannot afford to waste any opportunities considering the enormity of the impact of injuries in children.

XI. Summary

The recognition and management of pediatric injuries require the same astute skills as for adults. However, the unwary physician can make serious errors unless he is fully cognizant of the unique features of the pediatric trauma patient. These unique characteristics include airway anatomy and management, fluid requirements, diagnosis of extremity fractures, and the recognition of the battered, abused child.

Early involvement of the surgeon or the pediatric surgeon is imperative in the management of the injured child. Nonoperative management of abdominal visceral injuries should be performed only by surgeons in facilities equipped to handle any contingencies in an expeditious manner. All physicians should be engaged in efforts to expand injury awareness and prevention in their communities.

Bibliography

1. Becker D, et al: The outcome from severe head injury with early diagnosis and intensive management. **Journal of Neurosurgery** 1977;47:491.

2. Boyce WT, Sobolewiski S: Recurrent injuries in schoolchildren. **American Journal of Diseases of Children** 1989;143:338-342.

3. Bruce D: Outcome following severe head injuries in children. **Journal of Neurosurgery** 1978;48:697.

4. Chesire DJE: The paediatric syndrome of traumatic myelopathy without demonstrable vertebral injury. **Paraplegia** 1977;15:74-85.

5. Eichelberger MR, Mangubat EA, Sacco WS, et al: Comparative outcomes of children and adults suffering blunt trauma. **Journal of Trauma** 1988;28:430-434.

6. Harris BH, Schwaitzberg SD, Seman TM, et al: The hidden morbidity of pediatric trauma. **Journal of Pediatric Surgery** 1989;24:103-106.

7. Kraus JF, Fife D, Cox P, et al: Incidence, severity and external causes of pediatric brain injury. **American Journal of Diseases of Children** 1986;140:687-693.

8. Luna GK, Dellinger EP: Nonoperative observation therapy for splenic injuries: a safe therapeutic option. **American Journal of Surgery** 1987;153:462-468.

9. O'Neill JA, Meacham WF, Griffen PO, et al: Patterns of injury in the battered children syndrome. **Journal of Trauma** 1973;13:332.

10. Orgood GJ, Prakash A, Warsenberger J, et al: Pediatric gunshot wounds. **Journal of Trauma** 1987;27:1272-1278.

11. Pang D, Wilberger JE: Spinal cord injury without radiographic abnormalities in children. **Journal of Neurosurgery** 1982;57:114-129.

12. Powell RW, Green JB, Oschner MG, et al: Peritoneal lavage in pediatric patients sustaining blunt abdominal trauma: a reappraisal. **Journal of Trauma** 1987;27:6-10.

13. Ramenofsky ML, Luterman A, et al: Maximum survival in pediatric trauma: the ideal system. **Journal of Trauma** 1984;24(9):818.

14. Rivara FP, Calonge N, Thompson RS: Population based study on unintentional injury incidence and impact during childhood. **American Journal of Public Health** 1989;79:990-998.

15. Salter EJ, Bassett SS: Adolescents with closed head injuries: a report of initial cognitive defects. **American Journal of Diseases of Children** 1988;142:1048-1051.

16. Spivak H, Prothrow-Stith D, Hansman AJ: Dying is no accident: adolescents, violence, and intentional injury. **Pediatric Clinics of North America** 1988;35:1339-1347.

17. Tepas JJ, Ramenofsky ML, et al: The pediatric trauma score as a prediction of injury severity: an objective assessment. **Journal of Trauma** 1987;28:425-429.

18. Thompson RS, Rivara FP, Thompson DC: A case controlled study of the effectiveness of bicycle safety helmets. **New England Journal of Medicine** 1989;320:1361-1367.

19. Waller AE, Baker SP, Szocka A: Childhood injury deaths: a national analysis and geographic variations. **American Journal of Public Health** 1989;79:310-315.

Table 5
Pediatric Equipment

Age / Weight (kg)	Airway/Breathing							Circulation		Supplemental Equipment				
	O₂ Mask	Oral Airways	Bag-Valve Mask	Laryngo-scope Blades	ET Tubes	Stylet	Suction	BP Cuff	IV Catheter	NG Tubes	Chest Tubes	Urinary Catheter	C-collar
Premie 3 kg	Premie Newborn	Infant	Infant	0 – Straight	2.5-3.0 Uncuffed	6 Fr	6-8 Fr	Premie Newborn	22 Gauge	12 Fr	10-14 Fr	5 Fr Feeding	—
Newborn 0-6 mos 3.5 kg	NB	Infant Small	Infant	1 – Straight	3.0-3.5 Uncuffed	6 Fr	8 Fr	Newborn Infant	22 Gauge	12 Fr	12-18 Fr	5-8 Fr Feeding	—
6-12 mos 7 kg	PED	Small	PED	1 – Straight	3.5-4.5 Uncuffed	6 Fr	8-10 Fr	Infant Child	22 Gauge	12 Fr	14-20 Fr	8 Fr	Small
1-3 yrs. 10-12 kg	PED	Small	PED	1 – Straight	4.0-4.5 Uncuffed	6 Fr	10 Fr	Child	20-22 Gauge	12 Fr	14-24 Fr	10 Fr	Small
4-7 yrs. 16-18 kg	PED	Medium	PED	2 – Straight or Curved	5.0-5.5 Uncuffed	14 Fr	14 Fr	Child	20 Gauge	12 Fr	20-32 Fr	10-12 Fr	Small
8-10 yrs. 24-30 kg	Adult	Medium Large	PED Adult	2-3 – Straight or Curved	5.5-6.5 Cuffed	14 Fr	14 Fr	Child Adult	18-20 Gauge	12 Fr	28-38 Fr	12 Fr	Medium

Chapter 10:
Pediatric
Trauma

Chapter 11:
Trauma in Pregnancy

Objectives:

Upon completion of this topic, the participant will be able to:

A. Discuss anatomic and physiologic alterations of pregnancy that affect initial management of the injured pregnant patient.

B. Discuss mechanisms of injury unique to the pregnant patient and fetus.

C. Outline the priorities and method of evaluating the injured pregnant patient.

D. Outline indications for surgical intervention unique to the injured pregnant patient.

E. Recognize the possibility of isoimmunization and its early treatment in Rh-negative mothers following trauma.

F. Recognize indications for obstetric intervention and consultation in the injured pregnant patient.

Chapter 11:
Trauma in
Pregnancy

I. Introduction

Pregnancy causes major physiologic changes and altered anatomic relationships involving nearly every organ system of the body. These changes of structure and function may influence the evaluation of the traumatized pregnant patient by altering the signs and symptoms of injury, as well as the results of diagnostic laboratory tests. Pregnancy may also affect the patterns of injury or severity of injury. **Treatment priorities for an injured pregnant patient remain the same as for the nonpregnant patient.** However, resuscitation and stabilization should be modified to accommodate the unique anatomic and physiologic changes of pregnancy. The physician attending a pregnant trauma victim must remember that he does, in fact, have two patients. A thorough understanding of this special relationship between a pregnant patient and her fetus is essential if the best interests of both are to be served. The best treatment for the fetus is the provision of optimum treatment for the mother. Monitoring and evaluation techniques should allow not only assessment of the mother but also of the fetus. The use of roentgenograms, if indicated during critical management, should not be withheld because of the pregnancy. **A qualified surgeon and obstetrician should be consulted early in the evaluation of the pregnant trauma patient.**

II. Anatomic and Physiologic Alterations of Pregnancy

A. Anatomic

The uterus remains an intrapelvic organ until the 12th week of gestation, when it begins to rise out of the pelvis and encroach on the peritoneal cavity. By 20 weeks, the uterus is at the umbilicus. At 36 weeks, it reaches its maximal supraumbilical extent—the costal margin. During the last two to eight weeks of gestation, the fetus slowly descends as the fetal head engages the pelvis. As the uterus enlarges, it reduces the confines of the intraperitoneal space, restricting the intestines to the upper abdomen. Likewise, the intrauterine environment gradually changes from very protective to very vulnerable.

During the first trimester, the uterus is a thick-walled structure of limited size, confined within the safety of the bony pelvis. During the second trimester, the uterus leaves its protected intrapelvic location, but the small fetus remains mobile and cushioned by a relatively generous amount of amniotic fluid. The amniotic fluid itself could be a source of amniotic fluid embolism and disseminated intravascular coagulation following trauma. By the third trimester, the uterus is large and thin walled. The head is usually fixed in the pelvis with the remainder of the fetus exposed above the pelvic brim. The placenta reaches its maximum size by 36 to 38 weeks and is devoid of elastic tissue. This lack of placental elastic tissue predisposes to shear forces between the placenta and uterine wall leading to such complications as abruptio placentae. The placental vasculature is maximally dilated throughout gestation, yet it is exquisitely sensitive to catecholamine stimulation. Direct trauma to the placenta or uterus may reverse the normal protective hemostasis of pregnancy by releasing high concentrations of placental thromboplastin or plasminogen activator from the myometrium. All of these changes make the uterus and its contents more susceptible to injury, including penetration, rupture, abruptio placentae, and premature rupture of membranes.

B. Hemodynamic

1. Cardiac output

After the 10th week of pregnancy, cardiac output is increased by 1.0 to 1.5 liters per minute. This increased output is greatly influenced by the maternal position as term nears. Vena cava compression in the supine position may decrease cardiac output by 30% to 40%. As maternal blood volume decreases due to trauma, placental blood flow is preferentially reduced.

2. Heart rate

Heart rate increases throughout pregnancy. During the third trimester, it reaches a rate of 15 to 20 beats per minute more than in the nonpregnant state. This change in heart rate must be considered in interpreting the tachycardic response to hypovolemia.

3. Blood pressure

Pregnancy results in a 5- to 15-mm Hg fall in systolic and diastolic pressures during the second trimester. Blood pressure returns to near-normal levels at term. Some women may exhibit profound hypotension (supine hypotensive syndrome) when placed in the supine position. This condition is relieved by turning the patient to the left lateral decubitus position.

4. Venous pressure

The resting central venous pressure (CVP) is variable with pregnancy, but the response to volume is the same as in the nonpregnant state. Venous hypertension in the lower extremities is normal during the third trimester.

5. Electrocardiographic changes

The axis may shift leftward by approximately 15 degrees. Flattened or inverted T waves in leads III, AVF, and the precordial leads may be normal. Ectopic beats are increased during pregnancy.

C. Blood Volume and Composition

1. Volume

At 34 weeks' gestation, plasma volume increases by 40% to 50%. A smaller increase in red blood cell (RBC) volume occurs, resulting in a decreased hematocrit (physiologic anemia of pregnancy). In late pregnancy, a hematocrit of 31% to 35% is normal. Blood volume overall increases by 48%. With hemorrhage, otherwise healthy pregnant women may lose 30% to 35% of their blood volume before exhibiting symptoms.

2. Composition

The white blood cell (WBC) count increases during pregnancy to a high of 20,000/mm^3. Levels of serum fibrinogen and many clotting factors are elevated. Prothrombin and partial thromboplastin times may be shortened but bleeding and clotting times are unchanged. The serum albumin level falls to 2.2 to 2.8 g/dL during pregnancy, causing a drop in serum protein levels by approximately 1.0 g/dL. Serum osmolarity remains at about 280 mOsm/L throughout pregnancy.

D. Respiratory

Minute ventilation increases primarily as a result of an increase in tidal volume. This is attributed to an increased level of progesterone—a known respiratory stimulant. Hypocapnea ($PaCO_2$ of 30 mm Hg) is therefore common in late pregnancy. Although the forced vital capacity (FVC) fluctuates slightly during pregnancy, it is largely maintained throughout pregnancy due to equal and opposite changes in inspiratory capacity (which increases) and residual volume (which decreases). Anatomic alterations in the thoracic cavity appear to account for the decreased residual volume that is associated with diaphragmatic elevation with increased lung markings and prominence of the pulmonary vessels seen on chest roentgenogram.

The FEV_1/FVC does not change significantly during pregnancy, suggesting no obstruction to air flow.

Oxygen consumption is usually increased during pregnancy so that maintenance of adequate arterial oxygenation is particularly important in the resuscitation of the injured pregnant patient.

E. Gastrointestinal

Gastric emptying is greatly prolonged during pregnancy, and the physician should assume that the stomach is full. Therefore, early nasogastric tube decompression is particularly important in order to avoid aspiration of gastric contents. The intestines are relocated to the upper part of the abdomen and may be shielded by the uterus. Position of the patient's spleen and liver are essentially unchanged by pregnancy.

F. Urinary

The glomerular filtration rate and the renal plasma blood flow increase during pregnancy. Levels of creatinine and serum urea nitrogen (BUN) fall to approximately one half of normal prepregnancy levels. Glycosuria is common during pregnancy. Excretory urography reveals a physiologic dilatation of the renal calyces, pelves, and ureters outside of the pelvis.

G. Endocrine

The pituitary gland gets 30% to 50% heavier during pregnancy. Shock may cause necrosis of the anterior pituitary, resulting in pituitary insufficiency.

H. Musculoskeletal

The symphysis pubis widens by the seventh month (4 to 8 mm). The sacroiliac-joint spaces also increase. These factors must be considered in interpreting roentgenograms of the pelvis.

I. Neurologic

Eclampsia is a complication of late pregnancy that may mimic head injury. Eclampsia should be considered if seizures occur with or without hypertension, especially if hyperreflexia is present.

III. Mechanisms of Injury

Mechanisms of injury are similar to those in the nonpregnant patient. However, certain differences must be recognized in the pregnant patient.

A. Penetrating Injury

As the gravid uterus increases in size, the remainder of the viscera is relatively protected from penetrating injury, while the likelihood of uterine injury increases. The dense uterine musculature can absorb a great amount of energy from penetrating missiles and decreases the missile velocity and transfer of energy to other viscera. Also, the amniotic fluid and conceptus contribute to slowing of the penetrating missile. The resulting low incidence of associated maternal visceral injuries accounts for the generally excellent maternal outcome in penetrating wounds of the gravid uterus.

B. Blunt Injury

The amniotic fluid acts as a buffer to direct fetal injury from blunt trauma. Direct injuries may occur when the abdominal wall strikes an object such as the dashboard or steering wheel or is struck by a blunt instrument. Indirect injury of the fetus may occur from rapid compression, deceleration, contra-coup effect, or a shearing force.

Seat belts decrease maternal injury and death by preventing ejection. However, the type of restraint system affects the frequency of uterine rupture and fetal death. The use of a lap belt alone allows forward flexion and uterine compression with possible uterine rupture. Also a lap belt worn too high could produce uterine rupture because of direct force transmission to the uterus on impact. The use of shoulder restraints improves fetal outcome presumably because of the greater surface area over which the decelerative force is dissipated as well as the prevention of forward flexion of the mother. Therefore, determination of the type of restraint device worn by the pregnant patient is important in the overall assessment.

IV. Severity of Injuries

Severity of maternal injuries determines not only maternal but also fetal outcome. Therefore, the method of treatment also is dependent on the severity of maternal injuries. All pregnant patients with major injuries require admission to a facility with surgical obstetrical capabilities since there is a 24% maternal mortality rate and 61% fetal mortality rate in this group of patients. Eighty percent of females admitted to the hospital in hemorrhagic shock have an unsuccessful fetal outcome. Even the pregnant patient with minor injuries should be carefully observed since occasionally even minor injuries are associated with such complications as feto-maternal hemorrhage (the presence of fetal RBCs in the maternal circulation). Fetal injuries usually tend to occur in late pregnancy, the most common being skull fractures and intracranial hemorrhage, although any injury could occur.

V. Diagnosis and Management

A. Initial Assessment

1. Patient position

Uterine compression of the vena cava reduces venous return to the heart, thereby decreasing cardiac output and aggravating the shock state. Elevated caval pressures below the point of compression can lead to extension of placental separation. Therefore, **unless a spinal injury is suspected**, the pregnant patient should be transported and evaluated on her left side. If the patient is in a supine position, the right hip should be elevated and the uterus should be displaced manually to the left side to relieve pressure on the inferior vena cava.

2. Primary survey

Follow the ABCs and administer supplemental oxygen. If ventilatory support is required, consideration should be given to hyperventilating the patient. **Because of the increased intravascular volume and the rapid contraction of the uteroplacental circulation shunting blood away from the fetus, the pregnant patient can lose up to 35% of her blood volume before tachycardia, hypotension, and other signs of hypovolemia occur. Thus, the fetus may be "in shock" and deprived of vital perfusion, while the mother's condition and vital signs appear stable.** Crystalloid fluid resuscitation and early type-specific blood administration are indicated to support the physiologic hypervolemia of pregnancy. Avoid administering vasopressors to restore maternal blood pressure, because these agents further reduce uterine blood flow, resulting in fetal hypoxia.

B. Secondary Assessment

The secondary survey should follow the same pattern as in the nonpregnant patient. Indications for diagnostic peritoneal lavage are the same and this may be conducted safely if the incision is made in the midline well above the fundus of the uterus. The examination of the patient should include an assessment of uterine irritability, fundal height and tenderness, fetal heart tones, and fetal movement. Use a Doppler ultrasound stethoscope or fetoscope to auscultate fetal heart tones. Pay careful attention to the presence of uterine contractions suggesting early labor; or tetanic contractions accompanied by vaginal bleeding, suggesting premature separation of the normally implanted placenta. The evaluation of the perineum should include a formal pelvic examination. The presence of amniotic fluid in the vagina, evidenced by a pH of 7 to 7.5, suggests ruptured chorio-amniotic membranes. Cervical effacement and dilatation, fetal presentation, and the relationship of the fetal presenting part to the ischial spines should be noted. Because vaginal bleeding in the third trimester may indicate disruption of the placenta and impending death of the fetus, an obstetrician ideally should carry out the vaginal examination or be called immediately if blood is coming from the cervical os. The decision regarding an emergency cesarean section should be made in conjunction with an obstetrician.

Admission to the hospital is mandatory in the presence of vaginal bleeding, uterine irritability, abdominal tenderness, pain or cramps, evidence of hypovolemia, changes in or absence of fetal heart tones, or leakage of amniotic fluid. Care should be provided at a facility with appropriate fetal and maternal monitoring and treatment capabilities. **The fetus may be placed in jeopardy even with apparent, minor maternal injury.**

C. Monitoring

1. Patient

If possible, the patient should be monitored on her left side after physical examination. Monitoring of the CVP response to fluid challenge is extremely valuable in maintaining the relative hypervolemia required in pregnancy.

A correlation between maternal serum bicarbonate level and fetal outcome has been suggested. Therefore, it may be useful to monitor the material serum bicarbonate level in addition to other hemodynamic parameters. It should be noted that serum bicarbonate level may be depressed in these patients when large volumes of normal saline are infused. The requirement for saline infusion itself may be a reflection of severity of injury and blood loss opposed to the bicarbonate itself.

2. Fetus

Fetal distress can occur at any time and without warning. Although fetal heart rate can be determined with any stethoscope, the fetal heart rate and rhythm is best monitored continuously using the ultrasonic Doppler cardioscope. The fetus should be monitored continually to ensure early recognition of fetal distress. Inadequate accelerations of fetal heart rate in response to fetal movement, and/or late or persistent decelerations of fetal heart rate in response to uterine contractions indicate fetal hypoxia.

Indicated radiographic studies should be performed, because the benefits certainly outweigh potential risk to the fetus. However, unnecessary duplication of films should be avoided.

D. Definitive Care

In addition to the spectrum of injury found in a nonpregnant patient, trauma during pregnancy may cause uterine rupture. The uterus is protected by the bony pelvis in the first trimester, but it becomes increasingly susceptible to injury as gestation progresses. Traumatic rupture may present a varied clinical picture. Massive hemorrhage and shock may be present or only minimal signs and symptoms may be present.

Roentgenographic evidence of rupture includes extended fetal extremities, abnormal fetal position, or free intraperitoneal air. Suspicion of uterine rupture mandates surgical exploration.

Placental separation from the uterine wall (abruptio placentae) is the leading cause of fetal death after blunt trauma. Abruption can occur following relatively minor injuries especially late in pregnancy. With separation involving 25% of the placental surface, external vaginal bleeding and premature labor may begin. Larger areas of placental detachment are associated with increasing fetal distress and demise. Other than external bleeding, signs and symptoms may include abdominal pain, uterine tenderness, uterine rigidity, expanding fundal height, and maternal shock. Uterine ultrasonography will frequently demonstrate the lesion.

With extensive placental separation or with amniotic fluid embolization, widespread intravascular clotting may develop causing depletion of fibrinogen, other clotting factors, and platelets. This consumptive coagulopathy may emerge rapidly. In the presence of life-threatening amniotic fluid embolism and/or disseminated intravascular coagulation, uterine evacuation should be accomplished on an urgent basis.

Consequences of fetomaternal hemorrhage include not only fetal anemia and death, but also isoimmunization if the mother is Rh-negative. Since as little as 0.01 mL of Rh-positive blood will sensitize 70% of Rh-negative patients, the presence of fetomaternal hemorrhage in an Rh-negative mother should warrant Rh immunoglobulin therapy. This should be undertaken early in consultation with and under the direction of an obstetrician. Although a positive Kleihauer-Betke test (a maternal blood smear allowing detection of fetal RBCs in the maternal circulation) indicates fetomaternal hemorrhage, a negative test does not exclude minor degrees of fetomaternal hemorrhage that are capable of sensitizing the Rh-negative mother. Where this test is readily available, increasing ratios of fetal to maternal RBCs demonstrated in sequential maternal blood smears may be used as an index of increasing fetomaternal hemorrhage. All pregnant Rh-negative trauma patients should be considered for Rh immunoglobulin therapy unless the injury is so minor or remote from the uterus as to make fetomaternal hemorrhage unlikely. In situations where there is doubt as to the severity of the injury or the presence of fetomaternal hemorrhage, then the traumatized pregnant Rh-negative patient should receive Rh immunoglobulin therapy. Three hundred micrograms of Rh immunoglobulin therapy is required for every 30 mL of fetomaternal hemorrhage. In 90% of cases the volume of fetomaternal hemorrhage is less than 30 mL. Immunoglobulin therapy should be instituted within 72 hours of injury.

The large, engorged pelvic vessels that surround the gravid uterus can contribute to massive retroperitoneal bleeding after blunt trauma with associated pelvic fractures.

Initial management is directed at resuscitation of the pregnant patient and stabilization of her condition because the fetus' life at this point is totally dependent on the integrity of the mother's. Fetal monitoring should be maintained after satisfactory resuscitation and stabilization of the mother's condition.

Obstetric consultation is necessary for the care of the fetus.

VI. Summary

Important and predictable anatomic and physiologic changes occur during pregnancy that may influence the evaluation and treatment of the injured pregnant patient. Vigorous fluid and blood replacement should be given to correct and prevent maternal as well as fetal hypovolemic shock. A search should be made for conditions unique to the injured pregnant patient, such as blunt or penetrating uterine trauma, abruptio placentae, amniotic fluid embolism, isoimmunization, and premature rupture of membranes. Attention also must be directed toward the second patient of this unique duo—the fetus—after its environment has been stabilized. A qualified surgeon and obstetrician should be consulted early in the evaluation of the pregnant trauma patient.

Bibliography

1. Berry MJ, McMurray RG, Katz VL: Pulmonary and ventilatory responses to pregnancy, immersion, and exercise. **Journal of Applied Physiology** 1989;66(2):857-862.

2. Buchsbaum HG, Staples PP Jr: Self-inflicted gunshot wound to the pregnant uterus: report of two cases. **Obstetrics and Gynecology** 1985;65(3):32S-35S.

3. Esposito TJ, Gens DR, Smith LG, et al: Trauma during pregnancy—a review of 79 cases. **Archives of Surgery** 1991;126:1073-1078.

4. Higgins SD, Garite TJ: Late abruptio placenta in trauma patients: implications for monitoring. **Obstetrics and Gynecology** 1984;63(3):10S-12S.

5. Kissinger DP, Rozycki GS, Morris JA, et al: Trauma in pregnancy—predicting pregnancy outcome. **Archives of Surgery** 1991;126:1079-1086.

6. Maull KI, Pedigo RE: Injury to the female reproductive system. In: Moore EE, Feliciano DV, Mattox KL (eds): **Trauma.** East Norwalk Connecticut, Appleton and Lange, 1991, pp 587-595.

7. Mollison PL: Clinical aspects of Rh immunization. **American Journal of Clinical Pathology** 1973; 60:287.

8. Pearlman MD, Tintinalli JE, Lorenz RP: Blunt trauma during pregnancy. **New England Journal of Medicine** 1991;323:1606-1613.

9. Rose PG, Strohm PL, Zuspan FP: Fetomaternal hemorrhage following trauma. **American Journal of Obstetrics Gynecology** 1985;153:844-847.

10. Rothenberger D, Quattlebaum FW, Perry JF, et al: Blunt maternal trauma: a review of 103 cases. **Journal of Trauma** 1978;18(3):173-179.

11. Schoenfeld A, Ziv E, Stein L, et al: Seat belts in pregnancy and the obstetrician. **Obstetrical and Gynecological Survey** 1987;42(5):275-282.

12. Stuart GCE, Harding PGR, Davies EM: Blunt abdominal trauma in pregnancy. **Canadian Medical Association Journal** 1980;122:901-905.

13. Towery RA, English P, Wisner DW: Kleihauer-Betke test, uterine ultrasound, and external fetal monitoring in pregnant women after blunt injury. **Journal of Trauma** 1992 (in press).

Chapter 12: Stabilization and Transport

Objectives:

Upon completion of this topic, the physician will be able to define and outline general principles for the **optimal** stabilization and **most appropriate** transportation of trauma patients.

Specifically, the physician will be able to:

A. Identify those injured patients who may require transfer from a primary care institution to a facility capable of providing the necessary level of trauma care.

B. Outline procedures to **optimally** stabilize and prepare the trauma patient for safe transport to a higher-level trauma care facility via the appropriate mode of transportation.

**Chapter 12:
Stabilization
and Transport**

I. Introduction

This course is designed to train the students to be more proficient in their ability to assess, stabilize, and prepare the patient for definitive care. If definitive care cannot be rendered at the local hospital, the patient requires transfer to a hospital better suited to his needs. Ideally, this facility should be an **appropriately** designated trauma center, the level of which depends on the patient's needs. The decision to transfer the patient to another facility depends on the victim's injuries and the local resources. Decisions as to which patients should be transferred, and when, are matters of medical judgment. Recent evidence supports the view that trauma outcome is enhanced if critically injured patients are cared for in facilities prepared for and dedicated to the needs of the acutely injured. **No longer should the trauma patient be transferred to the closest hospital, but rather to the closest appropriate hospital, preferably a designated trauma center.**

The major principle of trauma management is to **do no further harm**. Indeed, care of the trauma patient should consistently improve with each step, from the scene of the incident to the facility that can provide the patient with the necessary, proper treatment. All those who care for trauma patients must ensure that the level of care never declines from one step to another.

II. Determining the Need for Patient Transfer

The vast majority of patients receive their total care in the local hospital, and movement beyond that point is not necessary. **It is essential that physicians assess their own capabilities and limitations, and those of their institution. This allows for early recognition of patients who may be safely cared for in the local hospital, and those who require transfer to an institution that can provide optimal care.** Once the need for transfer is recognized, arrangements should be expedited and not delayed for diagnostic procedures (eg, peritoneal lavage, computed tomographic scan) that do not change the immediate plan of care.

Patient outcome is directly related to time from injury to properly delivered definitive care. In those institutions in which there is no full-time, in-house emergency department coverage, the timeliness of transfer is partly dependent on the response of the physician to the emergency department. Consequently, it is recommended that appropriate communication with the prehospital system be developed such that those patients can be identified who require the presence of a physician in the emergency department at the time of arrival. Subsequently, the attending physician should be committed to respond to the emergency department prior to the arrival of these critically injured patients. Identification of those patients requiring prompt attention can be based on physiologic measurements, specific identifiable injuries, and mechanism of injury.

The timing of interhospital transfer varies based on the distance of transfer, the available skill levels for transfer, circumstances of the local institution, and intervention that is necessary before the patient can be transferred safely. Life-threatening injuries that can be stabilized, operatively or nonoperatively, at the primary care facility **must** be treated prior to transport. This treatment may require operative intervention to ensure that the patient is in the best possible condition for transfer. **Intervention prior to transfer is a surgical decision.**

To help the physician determine **which** patients might need care at a higher-level facility, the ACS Committee on Trauma recommends using certain physiologic indices, injury mechanisms and patterns, and historical information. These factors also help the physician decide which **stable** patients might benefit from transfer.

Certain clinical measurements of physiologic status are useful in determining the need for transfer to an institution that provides a higher level of care. Patients who exhibit evidence of shock, significant physiologic deterioration, or progressive deterioration in neurologic status require the highest level of care and should benefit from timely transfer.

Patients with certain specific injuries, combinations of injuries (particularly those involving the brain), or who have historical findings indicating high-energy transfer may be at risk for death and are candidates for early transfer to a trauma center. Criteria suggesting the necessity for early transfer are outlined in Table 1, Interhospital Triage Criteria.

Alcohol and/or other drug abuse are common to all forms of trauma and are particularly important to identify. Physicians should recognize that alcohol and drugs can alter pain perception and mask significant physical findings. Alterations in the patient's responsiveness may be related to alcohol and drugs, but absence of cerebral injury should never be assumed in the presence of alcohol or drugs. If the examining physician is unsure, transfer to a higher-level facility may be appropriate. Death of another individual involved in the incident suggests the possibility of severe, occult injury in survivors. **A thorough and careful evaluation of the patient, even in the absence of obvious signs of severe injury, is mandatory.**

III. Transfer Responsibilities

A. Referring Physician

The referring physician is responsible for the initiation of transfer of the patient to the receiving institution **and** for the selection of an appropriate mode of transportation and level of care required for optimal management of the patient en route. The referring physician should consult with the receiving physician and should be thoroughly familiar with the transporting agencies, their capabilities, and with the arrangements for patient management during transport.

The referring physician is responsible for stabilizing the patient's condition, within the capabilities of the initial institution, **before** the patient is actually transferred to another facility. Initiation of the transfer process should begin while resuscitative efforts are in progress.

Transfer agreements must be established to provide for the consistency and efficient movement of patients between institutions. These agreements allow for feedback to the referring hospital and enhance the efficiency and quality of the patient's management during transfer. (See Resource Document 9, Transfer Agreement.)

B. Receiving Physician

The receiving physician must be consulted with regards to the transfer of a trauma patient to his institution. The receiving physician must assure that his institution is qualified, able and willing to accept the patient, and is in agreement with the intent to transfer. The receiving physician may assist the referring physician in arrangements for the appropriate mode and level of care during transport.

The quality of care rendered en route also is of vital importance to the patient's outcome. Only by direct communication between the referring and receiving physicians can the details of patient transfer be clearly delineated. If adequately trained ambulance personnel are not available, a nurse or physician should accompany the patient. All monitoring and management rendered en route should be documented.

IV. Modes of Transportation

The principle of "Do No Further Harm" is the most important principle when choosing the mode of patient transportation. Ground and air transportation modalities can be safe and effective in fulfilling this principle.

Keys to successful patient transport are the availability of appropriately trained personnel and proper equipment to manage problems specific to the patient's condition, whether transportation is by ground or air. The choice of transport mode is based on the availability of these personnel, and which mode provides the safest and most rapid method of transportation. Weather considerations are crucial in this decision-making process.

V. Transfer Protocols

Where protocols for patient transfer do not exist, the following guidelines are suggested.

A. Referring Physician

The local physician wishing to transfer the patient should speak directly to the physician accepting the patient at the receiving hospital and provide this information:

1. Identification of the patient

2. A brief history of the incident, including pertinent prehospital data

3. Initial patient findings in the emergency department, and the patient's response to the therapy administered

B. Information to Transferring Personnel

Information regarding the patient's condition and needs during transfer should be communicated to the transporting personnel. This information should include, but not be limited to:

Table 1
Interhospital Triage Criteria

Central Nervous System
Head Injury — Penetrating injury or depressed skull fracture
— Open injury with or without CSF leak
— GCS score < 14 or GCS deterioration
— Lateralizing signs
Spinal cord injury

Chest
Widened mediastinum
Major chest wall injury
Cardiac injury
Patients who may require protracted ventilation

Pelvis
Unstable pelvic-ring disruption
Pelvic-ring disruption with shock and evidence of continuing hemorrhage
Open pelvic injury

Multisystem Injury
Severe face injury with head injury
Chest injury with head injury
Abdominal or pelvic injury with head injury
Major burns or burns with associated injuries, (see Transfer Criteria in
Chapter 9, Injury Due to Burn and Cold)
Multiple fractures

Evidence of High-energy Impact
Auto crash or pedestrian injury—velocity ≥ 25 mph
Rearward displacement of front axle or front of car (20 inches or 50 cm)
Ejection of patient or rollover
Death of occupant in same car

Comorbid Factors
Age < 5 years or > 55 years
Known cardiorespiratory or metabolic diseases

Secondary Deterioration (Late Sequelae)
Mechanical ventilation required
Sepsis
Single or multiple organ system failure (deterioration in central nervous,
cardiac, pulmonary, hepatic, renal, or coagulation systems)
Major tissue necrosis

(Adapted with permission, ACS Committee on Trauma: *Resources for Optimal Care of the Injured Patient.*
Chapter 14, 1993.)

    1. Airway maintenance

    2. Fluid volume replacement

    3. Special procedures that may be necessary

    4. Revised Trauma Score, resuscitation procedures, and any changes that may occur en route

C. Documentation

A written record of the problem, treatment given, and patient status at the time of transfer, as well as certain physical items, must accompany the patient. These should include:

    1. Initial diagnostic impression

    2. Patient's name, address, hospital number, age; and name, address, and phone number of next of kin

    3. History of injury or illness

    4. Condition at the time of admission to the hospital

    5. Vital signs prehospital, during stay in emergency department, and at time of transfer

    6. Treatment rendered, including medications given and route of administration

    7. Laboratory and roentgenographic findings, appropriate laboratory specimens (eg, lavage), and all roentgenograms

    8. Fluids given by type and volume

    9. Name, address, and phone number of the referring physician

    10. Name of physician at the receiving institution who has been contacted about the patient

D. Prior to Transfer

The patient should be resuscitated and attempts made to stabilize his or her condition as completely as possible based on this suggested outline.

    1. Respiratory

        a. Insert an airway or endotracheal tube, if needed.

        b. Determine rate and method of administration of oxygen.

        c. Provide suction.

        d. Provide mechanical ventilation when needed.

        e. Insert a chest tube if needed.

        f. Insert a nasogastric tube to prevent aspiration.

    2. Cardiovascular

        a. Control external bleeding.

        b. Establish two large-caliber IVs and begin crystalloid solution infusion.

    c. Restore blood volume losses with crystalloid or blood, and continue replacement during transfer.

    d. Insert an indwelling catheter to monitor urinary output.

    e. Monitor the patient's cardiac rhythm and rate.

3. Central nervous system

    a. Maintain controlled hyperventilation for head-injured patients after neurosurgical consultation.

    b. Administer mannitol or diuretics, if needed, after neurosurgical consultation.

    c. Immobilize head, neck, thoracic, and/or lumbar spine injuries.

4. Diagnostic studies

    a. Roentgenograms of cervical spine, chest, pelvis, and if indicated, extremities

    b. Hemoglobin, hematocrit, type and crossmatch, arterial blood gas determinations, and pregnancy test on all females of childbearing age

    c. Blood alcohol and/or other drugs as indicated

    d. Electrocardiogram

    e. Urinalysis (include drug screen as indicated)

5. Wounds

    a. Clean and dress

    b. Tetanus toxoid

    c. Tetanus Immune Globulin, if indicated

    d. Antibiotics, when indicated

6. Fractures: Appropriate splinting and traction

E. Management During Transport

1. Continued support of cardiorespiratory system

2. Continued blood volume replacement

3. Monitoring of vital signs

4. Use of appropriate medications as ordered by a physician or as provided by written protocol

5. Maintenance of communication with a physician or institution during the transfer

6. Maintenance of accurate records during transfer

VI. Transfer Data

The information accompanying the patient should include both demographic and historical information pertinent to the patient's injury. Uniform transmission of information is enhanced by the use of an established transfer form. Examples of appropriate data to include on a transfer form are outlined on Chart 1, Transfer Form, at the conclusion of this chapter. Other data that should accompany the patient are outlined on Chart 2, Revised Trauma Score (this chapter), and the Pediatric Trauma Score (Resource Document 7). In addition to the information already outlined, space should be provided for recording data in an organized, sequential fashion—vital signs, CNS function, and urinary output—during the initial resuscitation and transport period. (See Resource Document 8, Trauma Flow Sheet.)

VII. Summary

A. The major principle of trauma management is to do no further harm.

B. The treating physician should know his own capabilities and his institution's capabilities, and the indications for transfer.

C. The referring physician and receiving physician should communicate directly.

D. Transfer personnel should be adequately skilled to administer the required patient care en route.

Bibliography

1. American College of Surgeons Committee on Trauma: **Resources for Optimal Care of the Injured Patient.** 1987 and 1990.

2. American College of Surgeons Committee on Trauma: Field categorization of trauma patients. **Resources for Optimal Care of the Injured Patient** 1990, pp 15-18.

3. American College of Surgeons Committee on Trauma: Optimal care in the rural setting. Ibid, pp 19-20.

4. American College of Surgeons Committee on Trauma: Interhospital transfer of patients. Ibid, pp 61-65.

5. Champion HR, Sacco WJ, Copes WS, et al: A revision of the Trauma Score. **Journal of Trauma** 1989;29(5):623-629.

Chart 1
Sample Transfer Form
(Suggested Information to Send With The Patient)

A. Patient's Name:

    Address:
    Address:
    Age: Sex: Weight:

    Next of Kin:
    Address:
    Address:
    Phone Number:

B. Time

    Of Injury:
    Admitted to ED:
    Admitted to OR:
    Transfer:

C. History of Current Injury:

    Mechanism of Injury:

    AMPLE History:

D. Condition on Admission:

    Pulse: Respiratory Rate:
    Blood Pressure: Rhythm:
    Temperature:

E. Initial Diagnostic Impressions:

F. Diagnostic Studies:

    1. Laboratory Data—Attach all
        results to form

    2. Basic Radiographic Studies—
        Send films with patient

    3. Electrocardiogram

    4. Send appropriate specimens,
        eg, peritoneal lavage fluid

G. Treatment Rendered:

    1. Medications: Amount and Time

    2. IV Fluids: Type and Amount

    3. Other:

H. Status of Patient When Transferred:

I. Management During Transport:

J. Referring Physician:
    Referring Hospital:
    Phone Number:

K. Receiving Physician:
    Receiving Hospital:

Chart 2
Revised Trauma Score

(Adherence to these guidelines is thought to enhance interhospital transfer.)

	Variables	Score	Start of Transport	End of Transport
A. Respiratory Rate, Breaths/minute	10 - 24	4		
	25 - 35	3		
	≥ 36	2		
	1 - 9	1		
	0	0	_____	_____
B. Systolic Blood Pressure, mm Hg	> 89	4		
	70 - 89	3		
	50 - 69	2		
	1 - 49	1		
	0	0	_____	_____
C. Glasgow Coma Scale Score Conversion C = D + E + F	13 - 15	4		
	9 - 12	3		
	6 - 8	2		
	4 - 5	1		
	< 4	0	_____	_____

	Variables	Score	Start of Transport	End of Transport
D. Eye Opening	Spontaneous	4		
	To voice	3		
	To pain	2		
	None	1	_____	_____
E. Verbal Response	Oriented	5		
	Confused	4		
	Inappropriate words	3		
	Incomprehensible words	2		
	None	1	_____	_____
F. Motor Response	Obeys command	6		
	Localizes pain	5		
	Withdraw (pain)	4		
	Flexion (pain)	3		
	Extension (pain)	2		
	None	1	_____	_____
Glasgow Coma Score (Total D + E + F)			_____	_____
REVISED TRAUMA SCORE = A + B + C			_____	_____

(Charts 1 and 2 adapted with permission, ACS Committee on Trauma: *Resources for Optimal Care of the Injured Patient.* Chapter 14, 1993.)

**Chapter 12:
Stabilization
and Transport**

ATLS Resource Documents

These resource documents provide additional information to enhance the physician's knowledge of trauma-related issues.

Contents

1. Trauma Prevention 307
   Figure 1, Trimodal Death Distribution 308
   Figure 2, Haddon Matrix 311
   Figure 3, Ten Basic Strategies for Injury Control 311
   Figure 4, Motorcycle Fatalities 313

2. Prehospital Triage Criteria 317
   Flow Chart 1, Triage Decision Scheme 318

3. Kinematics of Trauma 319
   Figure 1, Cavitation 320
   Figure 2, Frontal Impact, Unrestrained Driver 322
   Figure 3, Rear Impact, Improper/Proper Headrest Use 323
   Figure 4, Proper versus Improper Lap Belt Application 325
   Figure 5, Adult Pedestrian Injury Triad 326
   Figure 6, Cavitation Results 329
   Figure 7, Ballistics Tumble and Yaw 329
   Table 1, Missile Kinetic Energy 331

4. Protection of Personnel From Communicable Diseases 333

5. Roentgenographic Studies 335
   Table 1, Spine Roentgenographic Suggestions 338
   Table 2, Chest Roentgenographic Suggestions 342
   Table 3, Pelvic Roentgenographic Suggestions 343
   Table 4, Abdominal Roentgenographic Suggestions 347
   Table 5, Extremity Roentgenographic Suggestions 350

6. Tetanus Immunization 353
   Table 1, Nontetanus- and Tetanus-Prone Wounds 356
   Table 2, Tetanus Prophylaxis 357

7. Pediatric Trauma Score 359
   Table 1, Pediatric Trauma Score 360

8. Trauma Flow Sheet 361

9. Transfer Agreement 365

Contents continued

10. **Transfer Record** 367

11. **Organ and Tissue Donation**...369

12. **Preparations for Disaster**..371

13. **Ocular Trauma** (Optional Lecture) 373

14. **ATLS and the Law** (Optional Lecture) 381

Resource Document 1: Trauma Prevention

I. Introduction

Reduction of trauma morbidity and mortality remains a perplexing problem in today's society. The ATLS Course for Physicians focuses on reducing morbidity and mortality by presenting well-established treatment methods and approaching trauma care in a systematic manner. The physician participant in this course receives a concise method for establishing assessment and management priorities in the care of the trauma patient. Adhering to these principles of trauma care can result in a reduction of trauma morbidity and mortality.

Trauma morbidity and mortality also can be reduced through prevention. This document focuses on: (1) the basic strategies and concepts of trauma prevention; (2) the active role that physicians can take in preventing trauma through the implementation of these strategies, and (3) suggestions for establishing trauma prevention programs in their local communities. The leadership role of the physician can be extended to and involve other trauma care providers (eg, nurses and prehospital care personnel) in similar leadership roles. By identifying specific trauma-related problems in a community and instituting the appropriate prevention effort, a reduction in injuries should follow.

II. Reducing Trauma Morbidity and Mortality

Trauma is the leading cause of death in the first four decades of life. Trauma deaths occur in a trimodal distribution. (See Figure 1, Trimodal Death Distribution.) The **third peak** (late deaths) represents trauma deaths that occur days or weeks after an injury, primarily from multisystem organ failure and sepsis. Organized trauma care systems, improvements in patient care, and research reduce deaths occurring during this period of time. The **second peak** represents early deaths within the first few hours of injury. The primary focus of the ATLS Course is on the first hour of trauma management, when rapid assessment and resuscitation can be initiated to reduce this second peak of trauma deaths. Reduction of death in this category also occurs when regionalized trauma care systems are implemented.

The **first and largest peak** represents more than half of all trauma deaths. These deaths occur at the scene as a result of major injuries to the brain, spinal cord, heart, or great vessels. Research breakthroughs, advancements in patient care, and improved systems of trauma care do **not** impact on these immediate deaths.

Because these deaths are usually related to injury severity, effective prevention programs can reduce fatalities.

Physicians who manage trauma patients even infrequently need to become involved in trauma prevention. There is reluctance to accept this challenge, primarily because of the belief that such efforts prove futile. However, it is becoming increasingly apparent that physicians can be and should be an essential component of any comprehensive trauma prevention strategy.

Figure 1
Trimodal Death Distribution

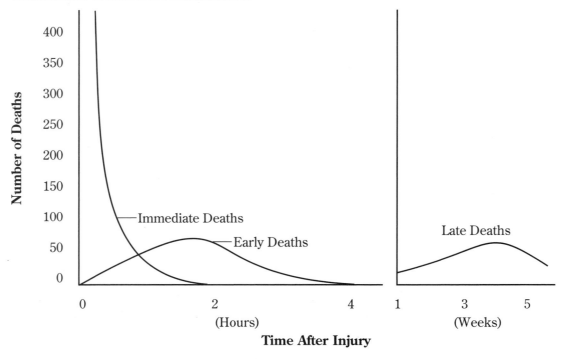

Trimodal distribution of trauma deaths is observed when the death rate for a large enough sample of such deaths is plotted as a function of time after injury. The graph is based on a sample of 862 trauma deaths recorded over a two-year period by the author's group at San Francisco General Hospital.

Used with permission, ACS Pre and Postoperative Care Committee: *Care of the Surgical Patient*, Vol I, Section IV, Chapter 6. New York, NY, Scientific American, Inc, 1988-91, pp 3-4.

III. Reducing the Financial Burden of Trauma Care

The costs associated with trauma care are staggering. According to the Centers for Disease Control, injuries account for one of the most expensive health problems—more than 180 billion dollars annually, directly and indirectly. However, injury research receives less than two cents of every federal dollar expended for research on health problems. As the competition increases for the limited health care dollar, physicians must increasingly justify the expenses related to trauma care. The implementation of effective trauma prevention programs can reduce these costs significantly by reducing the actual number of trauma incidents.

IV. Basic Concepts of Trauma Prevention

Prevention may be defined as primary, secondary, or tertiary. **Primary prevention** refers to the elimination of the trauma incident altogether. For example, an increased risk of pedestrian versus motor vehicular injury was recognized at one specific location in North Carolina. Overhead lighting and a sidewalk were installed along this section of the highway, reducing the number of pedestrian injuries. **Secondary prevention** refers to reducing the severity of injuries during the trauma incident. Safety restraints and motorcycle helmet usage are examples of effective secondary prevention efforts. **Tertiary prevention** includes all efforts following the trauma incident that optimize outcome, thereby preventing complications, long-term disability, or death. Regionalized trauma care systems, indeed ATLS itself, are examples of effective tertiary prevention programs.

The first step in developing trauma prevention strategies is to recognize that the term "accident" is often inappropriate and misleading. This term suggests that injury-producing events are capricious and beyond control. Traumatic events do **not** occur randomly. By and large, they occur in predictable, high-risk groups. Injury-producing events, especially among the high-risk groups, can be analyzed and specific etiologic factors can be defined. These etiologic factors can be modified, and the number and severity of injury-producing events can be reduced. For example, male teenagers account for a disproportionate percentage of automobile crashes in relation to their distribution in the population. Boys between the ages of one and five years, are at an increased risk for pool drowning. The elderly are at an increased risk for self-inflicted injuries.

Prevention strategies are more successful when they focus on these specific high-risk groups rather than on the entire population. However, individuals in these high-risk groups often are resistant to the necessary behavioral changes that would reduce their potential for injury. Strategies that rely on changing an individual's behavior are less likely to succeed than those providing automatic protection. For example, although it is worthwhile to educate male teenagers on the dangers of drunk and reckless driving, it is more important to mandate the use of devices such as seat belts, air bags, shatter-proof glass windows, and collapsible steering wheels. It is estimated that if all cars were equipped with air bags, thousands of lives and approximately eight billion dollars could be saved annually. Teaching young children to swim is an important step in safeguarding them from drowning. However, it is less effective than requiring them to wear life jackets while boating or supporting legislation that demands outdoor pools be fenced or covered when not in use.

An effective approach in developing injury-reducing strategies is to identify as many potential intervention options as possible, and then to select those with the greatest potential for success at the lowest cost. To facilitate this process, Haddon introduced the concept of a matrix to analyze vehicular crashes. (See Figure 2, Haddon Matrix.) Subsequently, this matrix has been used to evaluate other injury-producing events. Additionally, Haddon developed a list of 10 basic strategies for trauma prevention. (See Figure 3, Ten Basic Strategies for Injury Control.) This matrix and strategies can be used to develop intervention strategies for a wide variety of injury-producing events.

Since communities differ in the types of traumatic injuries encountered most frequently, it is important to understand the general principles related to injury control. Society is exposed to increased risks as people fly, jog, cycle, and drive more miles each year. There also is an ever-expanding list of products (eg, all-terrain vehicles, mopeds, ultralight aircraft, high-powered jet skis, snowmobiles, and hang gliders) that encourage risk-taking behavior. Innovative injury-reducing strategies must be identified and implemented if the number and severity of injuries are to be reduced.

V. Automatic Protection and Elimination of Environmental Hazards

After identification, trauma intervention strategies should be ranked in terms of potential effectiveness and cost. Injury-reducing strategies that promote automatic protection through product design or through elimination of environmental hazards are the most cost effective and rank the highest in priority for implementation. Examples of environmental modifications include placement of barriers on the center dividers of freeways, placement of stop signs and lights at busy and hazardous intersections, and removal of roadside obstacles on highways. Product design has the potential for saving millions of dollars. The introduction of air bags in all cars, the modification of cigarettes to reduce the potential for ignition, and greater side reinforcement for automobiles would save countless lives and millions of dollars.

Another cost-effective approach to trauma prevention is the passage of laws that mandate modification of high-risk behavior, such as requiring motorcyclists to wear protective helmets. However, the least effective strategy in trauma prevention appears to be educational programs designed to modify risk-taking behavior. For example, drivers' education programs, often lauded for their attempts to impart the importance of responsible driving, actually have resulted in a higher number of deaths among young drivers in many communities. This occurs because such programs increase the total number of 16-year-old drivers, who, for a given number of miles, are in the highest-risk group for crash exposure. This example underscores the necessity for considering outcome analysis in establishing or maintaining any proposed trauma prevention program.

The development of successful trauma prevention strategies requires astute observation and careful, critical analysis. Although physicians usually do not consider themselves a part of life-saving product design or responsible for the elimination of environmental hazards, they can serve an essential role in both areas. Physicians usually are among the first to directly observe the consequences of unsafe products and environmental hazards. It is critical that they discipline themselves to analyze the factors that lead to the injuries they treat. Mechanisms for reporting observations to appropriate authorities should be established to facilitate the identification of both local and national safety hazards. Trauma registries that record the circumstances involved in serious injuries enable physicians to identify causes of injuries that would remain unidentified under systems with less-organized data control. For example, a midwestern surgeon, who identified a subtle pattern in child injuries related to a specific type of garage door spring, notified the public and the manufacturer of the product's defect. His observation and responsible action consequently reduced the chances of other children being injured by this poorly engineered device.

Figure 2
Haddon Matrix

	Factors			
Phases {	Human	Vehicles and Equipment	Physical Environment	Socio-economic Environment
Precrash				
Crash				
Postcrash				
Losses	Damage to People	Damage to Vehicles and Equipment	Damage to Physical Environment	Damage to Society

Haddon Matrix. Reprinted with permission: "Approaches to the Prevention of Injuries," by W. Haddon, Jr., as read before the American Medical Association Conference on Prevention of Disabling Injuries, Miami, 1983.

Figure 3
Ten Basic Strategies for Injury Control

Strategy 1	Prevent the creation of the hazard in the first place.
Strategy 2	Reduce the amount of the hazard brought into being.
Strategy 3	Prevent the release of the hazard into the environment.
Strategy 4	Modify the rate or spatial distribution of the release of the hazard.
Strategy 5	Separate the hazard in time or space from that which is to be protected.
Strategy 6	Separate the hazard and its potential victim by a physical barrier.
Strategy 7	Modify the basic nature of the potential vehicle for energy transfer.
Strategy 8	Increase the resistance of that which is protected to the adverse consequences of an interaction with the hazard.
Strategy 9	Detect and evaluate damage that is occurring and counteract its continuation and extension.
Strategy 10	Restore maximum functional potential to that which has been damaged.

Reprinted with permission: "On the Escape of Titers: An Ecologic Note," by W. Haddon, Jr., American Journal of Public Health 1970;60:2229-2334.

VI. Legislation

Another effective strategy in reducing trauma death and disability is through legislative efforts. A classic example of the success of this approach can be seen by plotting motorcycle fatalities per number of motorcycles between 1959 and 1980. (See Figure 4, Motorcycle Fatalities per 10,000 Motorcycles.) The Highway Safety Act of 1966 withheld highway construction funds from states that lacked mandatory helmet laws. By 1975, 47 states required motorcyclists to wear helmets, which drastically reduced motorcycle fatalities. However, in 1976, a new Highway Safety Act restricted the federal government's ability to withhold funds, and by 1983, 28 states had weakened or repealed their helmet laws. This resulted in a dramatic increase in motorcycle fatalities.

Some existing legislation needs strengthening, and physicians should be active in helping to accomplish this goal. For example, current legislative efforts to reduce the incidence of drinking and driving have encountered limited success in many communities. Drinking and driving laws tend to be loosely enforced, and judges are lenient in punishing offenders. Evidence suggests that these laws would be more effective if potential offenders perceived a high probability of detection and rapid enforcement of strict penalties, eg, jail sentences and loss of drivers' licenses.

The single, greatest obstacle in passing trauma prevention legislation is the public's fear of infringement on their individual rights. When public opinion tends to favor the individual's right to seek pleasure while engaging in a high-risk activity, eg, riding a motorcycle without a helmet, preventative legislation often encounters public resistance. Physicians are perceived by members of the community as being knowledgeable leaders in promoting community health. Therefore, physicians can make important contributions to injury-prevention programs by voicing their support for appropriate legislation and strategies that prevent injury and death, and by demonstrating how reducing costs associated with trauma ultimately benefits the community. Physicians should take an active role in formulating legislation and lobby aggressively those legislators whose votes guarantee its passage. An example is the Tennessee pediatricians' success in promoting the passage of the first statewide infant "buckle up" law.

VII. Education

Physicians are most familiar with educational approaches to trauma prevention. Using education to promote trauma prevention assumes that the targeted audience is motivated and ready to change their risk-taking behaviors. Although this assumption is seldom true, education has enjoyed some success. For example, educational campaigns to reduce cigarette smoking in the general population have resulted in an actual decrease in the number of new and habitual smokers.

Educational programs also may encounter the challenge of the audience's rather complex, repetitive patterns of undesired behaviors. Even when positive behavioral changes occur, transient lapses can be equally detrimental. Parents may be strongly motivated to provide pool safety for their children, yet a momentary attention lapse may lead to a drowning. Smokers who faithfully avoid smoking in bed may doze off on their couches and set themselves ablaze in their living rooms. For these reasons, it is advisable to provide additional automatic-prevention strategies to back up educational programs, eg, fences around pools and pool covers, self-

Figure 4
Motorcycle Fatalities per 10,000 Motorcycles: 1959-1979

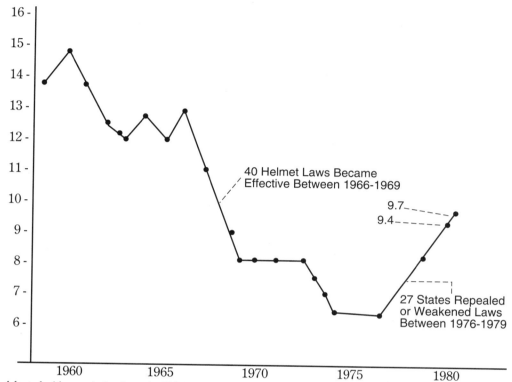

40 Helmet Laws Became
Effective Between 1966-1969

9.7
9.4

27 States Repealed
or Weakened Laws
Between 1976-1979

Adapted with permission from the U.S. DOT, National Highway Safety Administration: The effects of helmet
law repeal on motorcycle fatalities. DOT HS 1986; 807:065.

extinguishing cigarettes, and smoke detectors. In addition, evidence suggests that
citizens are more likely to cooperate with educational programs directed at trauma
prevention if the financial burden of automatic-prevention strategies is reduced,
eg, free smoke detectors and coupons for bicycle helmets.

The Orange County Trauma Society has found that peer education programs are
effective in making teenagers more aware of the risks of drinking and driving and
in identifying acceptable alternatives to such behavior. Mothers Against Drunk
Drivers (MADD) and Students Against Drunk Drivers (SADD) are examples of
organizations that have promoted trauma prevention through education successfully. It is essential that physicians network with these and other sympathetic organizations in their efforts to promote trauma prevention in their communities. An
example of such involvement by physicians is the THINK Foundation, founded initially as the National Head and Spinal Cord Injury Prevention Program of the
American Association of Neurosurgeons and the Congress of Neurological Surgeons.

Despite the limitations of educational approaches to trauma prevention, their value
may far exceed the narrow focus measured in outcome studies concentrating on
behavioral changes in high-risk groups. Certain high-risk groups may not change
their behavior, but the general public is considerably more educable. As the public becomes more aware of the medical and economic consequences of risk-taking

behavior, the more likely they are to accept legislative changes that reduce such risks. Educating the public about and increasing their awareness of unsafe products can lead to improvements in product design. Although years of education may be required before changes in attitudes translate into changes in behavior, physicians should take a leadership role in supporting educational programs designed to reduce risk-taking behaviors and promote trauma prevention.

VIII. ACS Committee on Trauma Prevention Programs

The Ad Hoc Committee on Trauma Prevention to the ACS Committee on Trauma has developed a series of trauma prevention programs that are revised on a regular basis. Physicians and other health care providers are encouraged to utilize these programs, thereby enabling them to promote and develop trauma prevention strategies in their communities.

Each program consists of a 30- to 40-minute lecture/slide presentation, and includes written texts, bibliographies, handout materials, and evaluation forms. The lecture series and slides are available on a rental/return basis. The programs are coordinated by the ACS Trauma Department and are distributed through the ACS Committee on Trauma State/Provincial Chairmen. Additional information concerning these programs and how to contact your State/Provincial Committee on Trauma Chairman can be obtained by communicating with the ACS Trauma Department at 55 East Erie Street, Chicago, Illinois 60611-2797, (312) 664-4050, extension 380.

These topics are available for presentation.

A. Alcohol and Trauma

This program describes the basic pathophysiologic effects of alcohol on the central nervous system and focuses on the relationship between alcohol and trauma. Various legislative approaches to reducing the toll of alcohol-related trauma and suggestions for innovative legislation are outlined.

B. Bicycle Helmet Safety

This program stresses the benefits of bicycle helmet usage among children and adults. It describes the successful Seattle program and provides a step-by-step approach for developing similar programs at the community level.

C. Motorcycle Helmet Legislation

This program describes the role of motorcycle helmets in reducing the morbidity and mortality of motorcycle injuries. It emphasizes the value of mandatory helmet laws, especially in those states that lack such legislation.

D. Trauma Prevention

This program outlines general issues related to trauma prevention, focuses on costs associated with preventable trauma, and encourages trauma prevention at the local level.

IX. Summary

Despite aggressive efforts by health care professionals, trauma continues to be the number one killer of young people, constituting one of the major health care challenges in the 1990s. Research breakthroughs, improvements in hands-on care, and improvements in regional trauma systems provide only a partial solution to this staggering health care problem. Supporting aggressive trauma prevention programs is the key to reducing the tragic loss of life and the emotional and economic toll of trauma. The missing ingredient in trauma prevention programs has been strong leadership from health care professionals. The opportunity to influence the broader fabric of society exists now. Health care professionals must provide the necessary direction and inspiration to assure the success of innovative and well-designed prevention campaigns. In so doing, the ultimate goal of significantly reducing trauma morbidity and mortality can be achieved.

Bibliography

1. ACS Pre and Postoperative Care Committee: **Care of the Surgical Patient** 1988-1991; Vol I: Section IV, Chapter 6, pp 3-4.

2. Comparative evaluation of three childhood injury prevention demonstration projects. Silver Springs, Maryland, Birch and Davis Associates, 1983.

3. Eyster EF, Watts C: The National Head and Spinal Cord Injury Prevention Program. **Journal of the Medical Association of Georgia** 1989;78:333-338.

4. Gorman RL, Charney E, Holtzman NA, et al: A successful city-wide smoke detector giveaway program. **Pediatrics** 1985;75:14-18.

5. Haddon W Jr: On the escape of titers: an ecological note. **American Journal of Public Health** 1970; 60:2229-2234.

6. Haddon W Jr: The pre-crash, crash, and post-crash parts of the highway safety problem, in Proceedings of the 11th Annual Meeting of the AAAM. Springfield, Illinois, Charles C. Thomas, 1970.

7. McLaughlin E: Injury Prevention Network Newsletter 1987-1988; 4:1-13.

8. McSwain NE Jr, Petrucelli E: Medical consequences of motorcycle non-usage. **Journal of Trauma** 1984; 24(3):233-236.

9. Miller RE, Reesinger KS, Blaller MM, et al: Pediatric counseling and its subsequent care of smoke detectors. **American Journal of Public Health** 1982;72:392-395.

10. Neuwelt E: Oregon Head and Spinal Injury Prevention Program. **Neurosurgery** 1989;24:453-458.

11. Rice DP, MacKenzie EJ, et al: Cost of injury in the United States: a report to Congress. San Francisco, California, Institute for Health and Aging, University of California and Injury Prevention Center, The Johns Hopkins University, 1989; Chapter 5.

12. Sanders RS, Dan BB: Bless the seats and the children: the physician and the legislative process, editorial. **Journal of the American Medical Association** 1984;252:2613-2614.

13. Thomas KA, Hassanein RS, Christophersen ER: Evaluation of group well-children care for improving burn prevention practices in the home. **Pediatrics** 1984;74:879-882.

14. Thompson RS, Frederick PR, Diane C, et al: A case controlled study of the effectiveness of bicycle safety helmets. **New England Journal of Medicine** 1989;320:1361-1367.

15. Trunkey DD: Trauma. **Scientific American** 1983; 249(2):28-35.

16. US Department of Transportation, National Highway Traffic Safety Administration: The effects of helmet law repeal on motorcycle fatalities. **DOT HS** 1986;807:065.

17. Wintemute GJ: Prevention. In: Cales RH, Heilig RW Jr (eds): **Trauma Care Systems.** Rockville, Maryland, Aspen Systems Corporation, 1986.

18. Wood T, Milne P: Head injuries to pedal cyclist and the promotion of helmet use in Victoria, Australia. **Accident Analysis and Prevention** 1988; 20:177.

Resource Document 2: Prehospital Triage Criteria

Optimally, patients should be triaged or sorted in the field to facilitate the rapid transport of patients with life-threatening injuries to verified trauma centers. Perfect triage criteria do not exist. The Triage Decision Scheme, published by the American College of Surgeons (ACS) Committee on Trauma, necessarily over-triages trauma patients by approximately 30%. In essence, 30% of patients sent to trauma centers as a result of these criteria eventually prove to have no life-threatening traumatic injuries. Until better criteria exist, on-the-line specificity is needed to assure reasonable sensitivity, ie, patients needing trauma centers are transported to them in almost every case. (See Flow Chart 1, Triage Decision Scheme.)

Flow Chart 1
Triage Decision Scheme

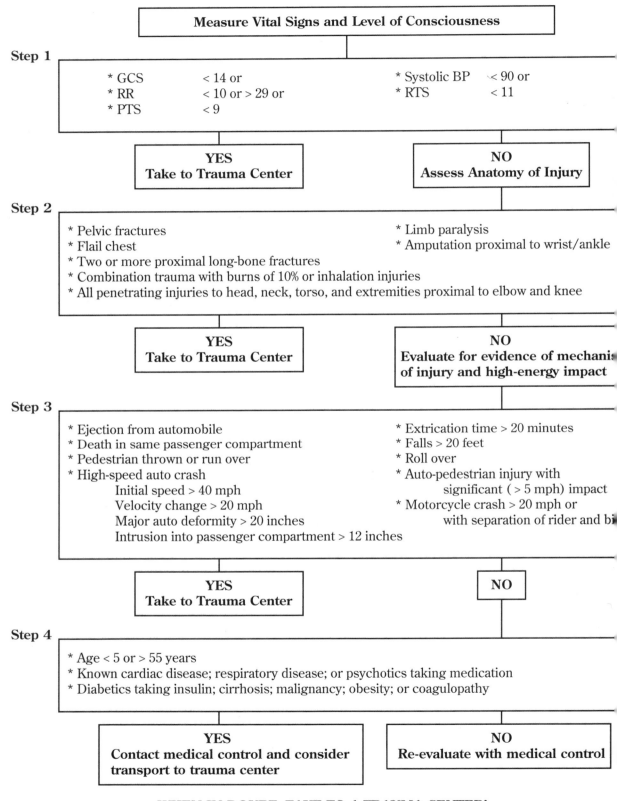

Measure Vital Signs and Level of Consciousness

Step 1

* GCS   < 14 or
* RR   < 10 or > 29 or
* PTS   < 9

* Systolic BP   < 90 or
* RTS   < 11

YES
Take to Trauma Center

NO
Assess Anatomy of Injury

Step 2

* Pelvic fractures
* Flail chest
* Two or more proximal long-bone fractures
* Combination trauma with burns of 10% or inhalation injuries
* All penetrating injuries to head, neck, torso, and extremities proximal to elbow and knee

* Limb paralysis
* Amputation proximal to wrist/ankle

YES
Take to Trauma Center

NO
Evaluate for evidence of mechanism
of injury and high-energy impact

Step 3

* Ejection from automobile
* Death in same passenger compartment
* Pedestrian thrown or run over
* High-speed auto crash
    Initial speed > 40 mph
    Velocity change > 20 mph
    Major auto deformity > 20 inches
    Intrusion into passenger compartment > 12 inches

* Extrication time > 20 minutes
* Falls > 20 feet
* Roll over
* Auto-pedestrian injury with
    significant (> 5 mph) impact
* Motorcycle crash > 20 mph or
    with separation of rider and bike

YES
Take to Trauma Center

NO

Step 4

* Age < 5 or > 55 years
* Known cardiac disease; respiratory disease; or psychotics taking medication
* Diabetics taking insulin; cirrhosis; malignancy; obesity; or coagulopathy

YES
Contact medical control and consider
transport to trauma center

NO
Re-evaluate with medical control

WHEN IN DOUBT, TAKE TO A TRAUMA CENTER!

Adapted with permission ACS Committee on Trauma: *Resources for Optimal Care of the Injured Patient,* Chapter 4, 1993.

Resource Document 3: Kinematics of Trauma

I. Introduction

In trauma, as other diseases, an accurate and complete history, correctly interpreted, can lead to an indication or suspicion of 90% of a patient's injuries. The history begins with information that occurred in the precrash phase, eg, alcohol and/or other drugs ingested. History related to the crash phase should include:

1. The type of traumatic event, eg, automobile or motorcycle collision, fall, penetrating injury

2. An estimation of the amount of energy exchange that occurred, eg, speed of vehicle at time of impact, distance of fall, and caliber and size of weapon

3. The collision or impact of the patient with the object, eg, car, tree, knife, baseball bat, bullet

Generally, the causes of injury are divided into blunt, penetrating, and blast injuries. Several energy laws need to be considered when obtaining the crash-phase history.

1. Energy is neither created nor destroyed; however, it can be changed in form.

2. A body in motion or a body at rests tends to remain in that state until acted on by an outside source.

3. Kinetic energy is equal to mass multiplied by velocity squared divided by two.

4. Force is equal to mass times deceleration (acceleration).

For a moving object to lose speed, its energy of motion must be transmitted to another object. This energy transfer occurs when the human body tissue cells are placed in motion directly away from the site of impact by the energy exchange—cavitation. Rapid movement of tissue particles away from the point of impact creates damage by tissue compression, and at a distance as the cavity expands by stretch. (See Figure 1, Cavitation.)

These same factors are involved whether the skin is penetrated. Assessing the extent of injury is more difficult when no skin penetration is apparent than when an open wound is present. For example, swing a baseball bat with equal force into a steel barrel and into a similar sized and shaped piece of foam rubber. After impact, the barrel shows the site and depth of the impact, but no indentation is visible in the foam rubber.

Figure 1
Cavitation

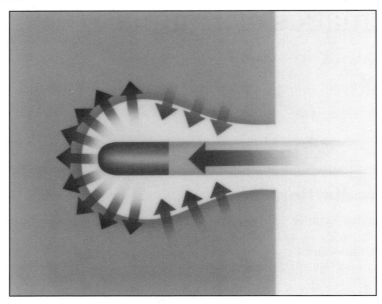

This same concept holds true with the trauma patient. For example, a fist driven into the abdominal area may sink in deeply but leaves no visible depression after the fist is removed. If bones are fractured, the significance of the impact may be visible, but if no fractures occur or if the bones rapidly resume a normal position, the extent of injury cannot be determined by physical examination alone. A history of the injury-producing event also must be obtained. A visible cavity after impact is referred to as a permanent cavity, and an invisible cavity is referred to as a temporary cavity. The amount of elastic tissue determines the size of each cavitation, since the energy exchange is the same.

The size of cavitation is determined by the amount of energy exchange. Energy exchange is determined by the number of tissue particles impacted by the moving object. The number of tissue particles impacted is determined by the density of the tissue in the path of the impacting object. The larger the surface area and the denser the tissue, the greater number of particles affected. The reverse also is true. A narrow object, with a small surface area, passing through tissue that is not very dense, eg, small bowel or lung, does not create much of a cavity because only a few tissue particles are affected. Bone is very dense, and when impacted by an object with a large cross-section area, it breaks, shatters, and frequently travels some distance from the initial impact and surrounding structures. These two scenarios represent the extremes. Most energy exchange lies somewhere between the two.

II. History

Information obtained from prehospital personnel related to the vehicle's interior and exterior damage frequently are clues to injuries sustained by its occupants. Prehospital care personnel are trained to make such observations. Knowledge of these facts facilitates the identification of occult or difficult-to-diagnose injuries.

For example, a bent steering wheel indicates chest impact; a bull's eye fracture of the windscreen indicates head impact and possible cervical spine injury; an indentation on the lower dashboard indicates a knee impact and possible dislocation of the knee, femur fracture, or posterior hip dislocation; and door intrusion into the passenger compartment indicates a lateral injury to the patient's chest, abdomen, pelvis, and/or neck.

III. Blunt Trauma

The common injury patterns and types of injuries identified with blunt trauma include:

1. Vehicular impact in which the patient is inside the vehicle

2. Pedestrian impact

3. Motorcycle crashes

4. Assaults

5. Falls

6. Blasts

A. Vehicular Impact

Vehicular collisions can be subdivided further into (1) collision between the patient and the vehicle, and (2) the collision between the patient's organ(s) and the external framework of the body (organ compression).

The interactions between the patient and the vehicle depends on the type of crash. Five crashes depict the possible scenarios—frontal, lateral, rear, angular (front quarter or rear quarter), and rollover.

1. Occupant collision
a. Frontal impact

A frontal impact is defined as a collision with an object in front of the vehicle that suddenly reduces its speed. The unrestrained occupant in the vehicle continues to travel forward (Newton's First Law of Motion) until some portion of the passenger compartment slows the occupant or the occupant is ejected.

On impact, the patient may follow a down-and-under pathway with the lower extremities being the initial point of impact and the knees or feet receiving the initial energy exchange. The forward motion of the torso onto the extremity may cause these injuries:

1) Fracture-dislocation of the ankle

2) Knee dislocation as the femur overrides the tibia and fibula

3) Femur fracture

4) Posterior dislocation of the acetabulum as the pelvis overrides the head of the femur

The second component of this down-and-under motion is a forward rotation of the torso into the steering column or dashboard.

If the structure of the seat and the patient's position are such that the head becomes the lead point of the "human missile," the skull impacts with the windscreen or the framework around the windscreen. The cervical spine absorbs some of the initial energy while the chest and abdomen impact the steering column or the dash board. (See Figure 2, Frontal Impact, Unrestrained Driver.)

Figure 2
Frontal Impact, Unrestrained Driver

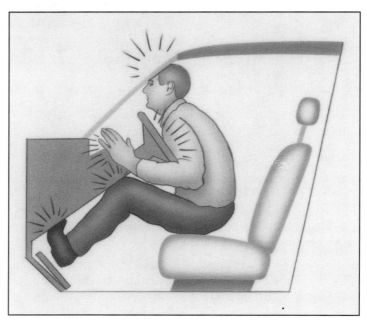

b. Lateral impact

Lateral impact is defined as a collision against the side of a vehicle that accelerates the occupant away from the point of impact (acceleration as opposed to deceleration). Many of the same type of injuries occur as with a frontal impact. In addition, compression injuries to the torso and pelvis may occur. Internal injuries are related to the side struck, the position of the occupant (driver or passenger), and force of impact (intrusion). The driver who is struck on the driver's side is at greater risk for left-sided injuries, eg, left rib fractures, splenic injury, and left skeletal fractures, including the pelvis. A passenger struck on the passenger side will have similar right-sided involvement, with liver injuries being a particular risk.

In lateral impacts, the head acts as a large mass that rotates and laterally bends the neck as the torso is rapidly pushed away from the side of collision. Basic biomechanics are the same with both frontal and lateral collisions. However, the examining physician also must consider acceleration versus deceleration forces and lateral anatomic considerations when examining the patient.

c. Rear impact

A rear impact represents a different type of biomechanics. More commonly, this type of impact occurs when a vehicle is at a complete stop and is hit from behind by another vehicle. The vehicle, including its occupant, is moved forward as it picks up energy from the impacting vehicle behind it. Because of the placement of the seats, the torso usually is accelerated forward along with the car. The occupant's head often is not accelerated with the rest of the body, because the headrest has not been elevated. The body accelerates, the head does not, and the neck is hyperextended back across the unused headrest. Such hyperextension stretches the supporting structures of the neck, producing a "whiplash" injury. (See Figure 3, Rear Impact, Improper and Proper Headrest Use.) A frontal impact also may occur as there often is a second car in front of the vehicle originally hit.

d. Quarter panel impact

A quarter panel impact, either front or rear, produces a variation of lateral and frontal impact collision injury patterns or lateral and rear impact collision injury patterns.

e. Rollover

During a rollover, the unrestrained occupant can impact any part of the interior of the passenger compartment. Injuries may be predicted from the impact points on the patient's skin. The general rule is that this type of collision produces more severe injuries because of the violent and multiple motions that occur during the rollover.

f. Ejection

The injuries sustained as the occupant is ejected from the vehicle may be greater than when the ground is impacted. Nevertheless, the likelihood of injury from this type of mechanism is increased by more than 300%. The examining physician must be attentive to the possibility of occult injuries.

Figure 3
Rear Impact,
Improper and Proper Headrest Use

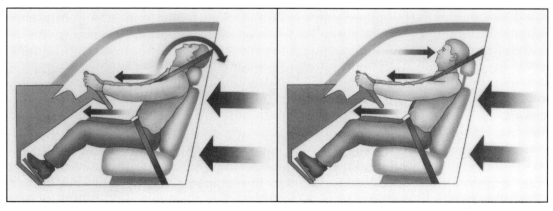

Improper Headrest Use   Proper Headrest Use

B. Organ Collision

1. Compression injury

Compression injuries occur when the anterior portion of the torso (chest and abdomen) ceases to move forward and the posterior portion continues to travel onward. The organs are trapped from behind by the continued motion of the posterior thoracoabdominal wall and the vertebral column, and in front by the impacted anterior structures. Myocardial contusion is a typical example of this type of injury mechanism. (See Figure 2, Frontal Impact, Unrestrained Driver.)

A similar injury can occur with the lungs or abdominal organs. The lungs and abdominal cavity represent a particular variation of this type of injury—the paper bag effect. Blowing up a paper bag, holding it tight at the neck, and crushing it with the opposite hand causes the bag to rupture. In a collision situation, it is instinctive for the patient to take a deep breath and hold it, thereby closing the glottis. Compression of the thoracic cage then produces a rupture of the alveoli and a pneumothorax and/or tension pneumothorax. (See Figure 2, Frontal Impact, Unrestrained Driver.) In the abdominal cavity, the same overpressure problem produces a rupture of the diaphragm resulting in translocation of the abdominal contents into the thoracic cavity.

Compression injuries inside the skull result from the brain being damaged by fractured bone intruding into the intracranial vault or the posterior portion of the brain compressing the anterior part against the skull.

2. Deceleration injury

Deceleration injuries occur as the stabilizing portion of an organ, eg, renal pedicle, ligamentum teres, or descending thoracic aorta ceases forward motion with the torso while the movable body part, eg, spleen, kidney, or heart and arch of the aorta, continues forward. For example, the heart and aortic arch continue to rotate forward while the descending aorta, attached to the thoracic spine, slows rapidly with the torso. The shearing forces are greatest where the movable aortic arch and the stable descending aorta join near the ligamentum arteriosum. This same type of injury may occur with the spleen and kidneys at their pedicle junctions, with the liver as the right and left lobes decelerate around the ligamentum teres splitting the liver down the middle, and in the skull when the posterior part of the brain separates from the skull tearing vessels and producing space-occupying lesions.

3. Restraint injury

The increasing availability of the air bag may reduce some frontal injuries significantly. However, air bags work only in about 70% of collisions. These devices must not be thought of as a replacement for the safety belt, but as supplemental protective devices. Occupants in head-on collisions may benefit from the air bag, but only on the first impact. At the time of the second impact into another object, the air bag already is deployed and deflated. The air bag provides no benefit in rollovers, second crashes, or lateral and rear impacts. The lap and shoulder restraints must be worn for more complete protection.

In side impact collisions, the lap belt is an effective device, providing it is worn effectively. As the vehicle is moved laterally, the occupant is placed into lateral motion by the belt and not the door or the impact. When the occupant has begun to move away from the point of impact, intrusion into the passenger compartment through the door is less likely to produce injury.

When worn correctly, the safety belt can reduce injuries. Worn incorrectly and the device can produce some injuries, although it reduces the overall damage. To function properly, the belt must be below the anterior/superior iliac spines and above the femur. It must be tight enough to remain in place during the motion of the crash. If worn incorrectly, eg, above the anterior/superior iliac spines, the forward motion of the posterior abdominal wall and vertebral column traps the pancreas, liver, spleen, and duodenum against the belt in front. Burst fractures of the kidney, spleen, and liver can occur as well as pancreatic lacerations. Hyperflexion over an incorrectly applied belt can produce anterior compression fractures of the lumbar spine. (See Figure 4, Proper versus Improper Lap Belt Application.)

There may be so much energy exchange occurring in the chest that even a properly worn diagonal strap can cause clavicular fractures or myocardial contusion. In these instances, the patient would not have survived without the belt.

Figure 4
Proper versus Improper Lap Belt Application

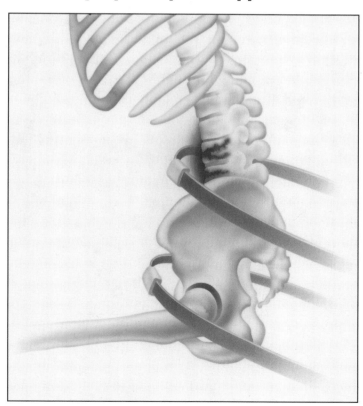

C. Pedestrian Injury

There are three impact phases to the injuries sustained by a pedestrian. (See Figure 5, Adult Pedestrian Injury Triad.)

1. Front vehicular bumper impact

Bumper height versus patient height is a critical factor in the specific injury produced. In the upright adult, the initial impact with the front bumper is usually against the legs and pelvis. Knee injuries are common as are injuries to the pelvis. Children are more likely to receive chest and abdominal injuries.

2. Vehicular hood and windscreen impact

Torso and head injuries occur as the patient impacts with the hood and windscreen.

3. Ground impact

Head and spine injuries result as the patient falls off the vehicle to the ground.

Organ compression injuries also occur—deceleration/acceleration—as described previously.

Figure 5
Adult Pedestrian Injury Triad

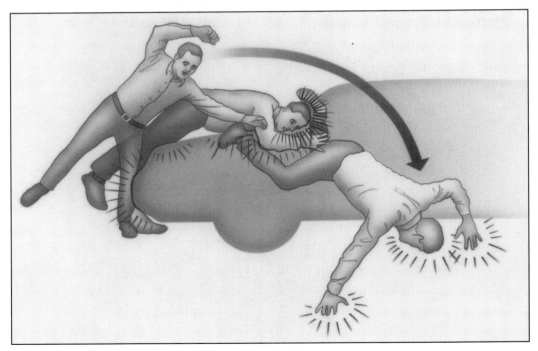

D. Motorcycle Collisions

Motorcyclists and/or their passengers also may sustain compression, acceleration/deceleration, and shearing-type injuries. However, the way they receive such injuries is different. Motorcyclists are not protected by the vehicle's structure or restraining devices as an occupant in a car would be protected. Motorcyclists are protected only by clothing and safety devices worn on their body—helmets, boots, or protective clothing. Obviously, the lesser protection that is worn, the greater the risk for injury. Therefore, the amount of and type of protective clothing worn by injured motorcyclists is important precrash information to obtain from prehospital personnel.

Mechanisms of injury that may occur with motorcycle collisions include frontal impact, lateral impact, ejection, and "laying the bike down."

1. Frontal impact/ejection

The motorcycle and cyclist travel at the same speed. The pivot point of the cycle is the front axle and the center of gravity is above this point, near the seat. If the front wheel of the motorcycle impacts with an object and stops, the motorcycle tends to tip forward and Newton's First Law of Motion is applied—the cyclist and the rest of the motorcycle continue their forward motion until they impact with an object or the ground. During this forward projection, the cyclist's head, chest or abdomen may impact with the handle bars. If the cyclist is projected over the handlebars and ejected off the bike, the upper legs may impact with the handlebars resulting in bilateral femur fractures. A variety of other injuries are sustained when the cyclist is ejected off the motorcycle and strikes an object or the ground.

2. Lateral impact/ejection

If a motorcyclist sustains a lateral impact, open and/or closed fractures or a crush injury to the lower extremity can occur. If the lateral impact is with a car or truck, the cyclist is vulnerable to the same type of injuries sustained by an occupant in an automobile involved in a lateral collision. Additionally, the cyclist can be ejected from the cycle and sustain a multitude of injuries on impact with an object or the ground.

3. "Laying the bike down"

To avoid entrapment between the motorcycle and a stationary object, the cyclist may turn the motorcycle sideways, dropping the bike and his inside leg down onto the ground. This strategy tends to slow the speed of the cyclist, separating him from the motorcycle. The motorcycle continues its forward motion and absorbs most of the energy of the collision with the stationary object. However, the cyclist can sustain rather significant tissue avulsion injuries and abrasions.

E. Falls

Falls are the leading cause of nonfatal injury in the United States and the second leading cause of both spinal and brain injury. The kinematics of motor vehicle crashes and falls are not dissimilar—both are deceleration-type injuries. Whenever an external force is applied to the human body, the severity of injury is the result of the interaction between the physical factors of the force and the body. If the body is in motion, eg, falling, and impacts a fixed surface, the extent of the injury is related to the ability of the stationary object to arrest the forward motion of the body. At impact, differential motion of tissues within the organism causes tissue disruption. Decreasing the rate of the deceleration and enlarging the surface area to which the energy is dissipated increase the tolerance to deceleration by promoting a more uniform motion of the tissues. The fall arresting contact surface also is important since concrete, asphalt, or hard firm surfaces increase the rate of deceleration, and are associated with more severe injuries.

Certain features of living tissue also must be considered, especially the combined cohesive properties of elasticity and viscosity of tissues. The tendency for a tissue following impact to presume its prestressed condition is related to its elasticity. Viscosity implies resistance to change of shape with changes in motion. The tolerance of the organism to deceleration forces is a function of these combined cohesive properties and the point beyond which additional force overcomes this tissue cohesion determines the magnitude of injury. Therefore, the severity of injury is closely related to the kinematics of vertical deceleration, the combined cohesiveness of the body's properties, and the consistency of the impact surface. The severity of the injury increases by increasing the rate of deceleration and decreasing the distance through which the body is decelerated. More severe injury occurs when deceleration forces are applied to the body in the vertical axis compared with the transverse, provided that mass, velocity, and stopping distance remain the same.

F. Blast Injury

Explosions result from extremely rapid chemical transformation of relatively small volumes of solid, semisolid, liquid, or gaseous materials into gaseous products that rapidly seek to occupy greater volumes than the undetonated explosive occupied. If unimpeded, these rapidly expanding gaseous products assume the shape of a sphere inside which the pressure is greatly increased compared with atmospheric pressure. The periphery of this sphere is a thin, sharply defined shell of compressed air that acts as a pressure wave. The pressure decreases rapidly as this pressure travels away from the site of detonation in proportion to the third power of the distance. As the pressure wave advances, the media through which it moves oscillates. The positive pressure phase may reach several atmospheres in magnitude, but it is of extremely short duration, whereas the negative phase that follows is longer in duration. This latter phenomenon accounts for the phenomenon of buildings falling inward.

Blast injuries may be classified into primary, secondary, or tertiary. **Primary blast injuries** result from the direct effects of the pressure wave and are most injurious to gas-containing organs. The eardrum is the most vulnerable to the effects of primary blast and may rupture if pressures exceed two atmospheres. The lungs also are vulnerable with changes of contusion, edema, and pneumothorax commonly seen. Rupture of alveoli and pulmonary veins creates the potential for air embolism, which may result in sudden death. Intraocular hemorrhage, retinal detachments, and rupture of intestines also may occur but are more common in underwater blasts. **Secondary blast injuries** result from flying objects striking the individual. Shrapnel wounds represent a typical secondary blast injury. **Tertiary blast injury** occurs when the individual becomes the missile and is thrown against a solid object or to the ground. Both secondary and tertiary blast injury may cause trauma typical of penetrating and blunt mechanisms, respectively.

IV. Penetrating Trauma

Cavitation, described previously, is the result of energy exchange between the moving object and body tissues. The amount of cavitation or energy exchange is proportional to the surface area of the point of impact, the density of the tissue, and the velocity of the projectile at the time of impact. (See Figure 6, Cavitation Results.) The wound at the point of impact is determined by:

1. The shape of the missile ("mushroom")

2. Its relation and position to the impact site, (tumble, yaw) (see Figure 7, Ballistics Tumble and Yaw)

3. Fragmentation (shotgun, bullet fragments, special bullets)

Figure 6
Cavitation Results

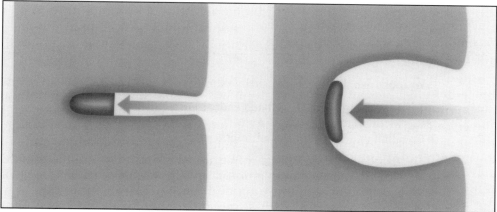

Sharp missiles with small, cross-sectional fronts slow with tissue impact, resulting in little injury or cavitation.

Missiles with large, cross-sectional fronts (eg, hollow-point bullets that expand or mushroom on impact) cause more injury or cavitation.

Figure 7
Ballistics Tumble and Yaw

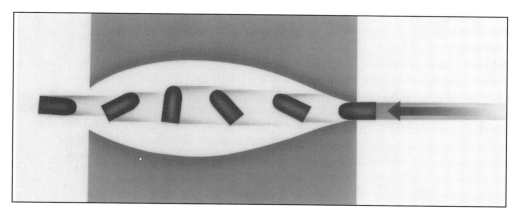

A. Bullets

Lead bullets cannot be propelled above the velocity of 2000 feet per second, because the lead melts. Semijacketed bullets with lead noses or hollow points are designed to mushroom when they strike the target. This effect increases the cross-sectional area of the missile, resulting in more rapid deceleration of the bullet and release of kinetic energy more rapidly. Higher-velocity missiles, eg, military ammunition, are fully jacketed, using copper-nickel or steel. Teflon bullets, which penetrate flexible body armor, are available as are Glasser Safety Slugs, a lightweight, hollow bullet filled with bird shot pellets. On impact, this bullet ruptures, releases its pellets, and produces severe wounds. Magnum rounds refer to cartridges with a greater amount of gunpowder than the normal round, which increases the muzzle velocity of the missile.

B. Velocity

The velocity of a missile is a significant determinant of its wounding potential. The importance of velocity is demonstrated by the formula relating mass and velocity to kinetic energy. Examples of this relationship are listed in Table 1, Missile Kinetic Energy.

$$\text{Kinetic Energy} = \frac{(\text{Mass})\ (\text{Velocity}^2)}{2}$$

Weapons usually can be divided into three types based on their initial energy.

1. Low energy—Knife or hand energized missiles
2. Medium energy—Hand guns
3. High energy—Hunting or military rifles

The final determinant is distance from the missile pathway, ie, as the distance increases the kinetic energy is dissipated. The wounding capability of a bullet increases markedly above a critical velocity. This velocity may be as low as 2000 feet per second. At these speeds the bullet creates a temporary cavity due to tissue being compressed radially, outward from the bullet tract. This temporary cavity can have a diameter of up to 30 times that of the diameter of the missile. The maximum diameter occurs at the area of the greatest resistance to the bullet (greatest decrease in velocity and greatest transfer of kinetic energy). The handgun (medium energy) may produce a temporary cavity only five to six times the diameter of the bullet. Knife injuries (low energy) result in little or no cavitation. Therefore, the damage from a high-velocity bullet can occur at a fairly great distance from the bullet tract itself. The difference in the size of the temporary and the permanent cavity is the amount of elastic tissue that can return the organ to its original shape, size, and position.

Other effects of missiles are important in determining the amount of energy dissipated and the injuries produced. **Yaw** (the deviation of a bullet from its longitudinal axis) and **tumble** increase the area it presents to the tissue and subsequently, the kinetic energy release. (See Figure 7, Ballistics Tumble and Yaw.) The later after tissue penetration the bullet tends to yaw, the deeper the maximum injury. Bullet deformation and fragmentation (semijacketed) increase area also, thereby increasing the primary tract and the release of kinetic energy.

Table 1
Missile Kinetic Energy

Caliber and Manufacturer	Bullet Weight (Grains)	Velocity (Feet/ Second)	Energy (Feet/ Pound)
Rifle Ammunition			
.22 Remington Rim Fire	40	1180	124
6 mm, 243 Winchester	75	3500	2037
.300 H and L Magnum	180	3670	3670
.375 H and H Magnum	270	2720	4440
Handgun Ammunition			
.25 Remington Automatic	50	810	73
.32 Short Remington	80	745	100
.32 Automatic Remington	71	960	140
.357 Magnum Remington	158	1410	540
.38 Special Remington	158	855	255
9 mm Automatic	140	935	270
10 mm Automatic	170	1340	680
.44 Magnum Remington	240	1470	1150
.45 Automatic Remington	230	850	370

Shotgun wounds present a different wounding potential. The muzzle velocity of this weapon is generally 1800 feet per second. However, due to air resistance acting on the spherical pellets, their velocity decreases rapidly. Deceleration also occurs rapidly after impact for the same reason, causing the maximum injury relatively superficially. The shot radiates in a conical distribution from the muzzle. With a choked or narrowed muzzle, 70% of the pellets are deposited in a 30-inch diameter circle at 40 yards. This weapon is lethal at a close range, but it is relatively ineffective at greater distances. Shotgun blasts carry clothing and wadding (paper or plastic separating the powder and pellets in the shell) deep into the wound, which is a source of infection if not removed.

C. Entrance versus Exit Wounds

Caution must be exercised when commenting on whether a bullet wound represents an entrance or exit wound. The type of projectile, jacketed or unjacketed, hollow-point or ball ammunition, velocity, yaw (angle) of the projectile at the time of the strike, and the type of underlying tissue, eg, bone, all influence the appearance of a bullet wound. A bullet wound can be identified as an entrance wound with certainty in only two instances. The first instance is when there is only one wound. The second is when there is histologic documentation of powder burns around the bullet wound. Because of the multiplicity of factors that influence the appearance of a bullet wound, statements that a wound is an entrance wound may be difficult to ascertain assuredly for legal purposes.

However, it may be very important for clinical reasons to make such a determination. Two holes may indicate two separate gunshot wounds or the entrance and exit of one bullet, pointing out the pathway the missile followed through the body. In either instance, the identification of the anatomic structures that may have been damaged and even the type of surgical procedure that needs to be done may be influenced by such information.

Weapons most commonly used in the civilian sector cause a round or oval entrance wound with a surrounding 1- to 2-mm blackened area of burn or abrasion from the spinning bullet passing through the skin. If the weapon muzzle was close to the skin, gases may have been forced into the subcutaneous tissue. A blast within a few inches of the skin leaves a visible burn on the skin. Stippling or tattooing from the burning particles of the gunpowder may be visible with a blast from four to six inches. The exit wound usually is stellate in appearance and does not have any of the other features. Like the physical examination and clinical tests, a finding that is present provides information. An absent finding is inclusive and yields no information, either positive or negative.

Bibliography

1. Fackler ML: Physics of missile injuries. In: McSwain NE Jr, Kerstein MD (eds): **Evaluation and Management of Trauma**. East Norwalk, Connecticut, Appleton-Century-Crofts, 1987, pp 25-53.

2. Feliciano DV, Wall MJ Jr: Patterns of injury. In: Moore EE, Mattox KL, Feliciano DV: **Trauma, Second Edition**. East Norwalk, Connecticut, Appleton & Lange, 1991, pp 81-96.

3. Mackay M: Kinematics of vehicle crashes. In: Maull KI, Cleveland HC, Strauch GO, et al (eds): **Advances in Trauma, Volume 2**. Chicago, Illinois, Year Book Medical Publishers Inc, 1987, pp 21-41.

4. Maull KI, Whitley RE, Cardea JA: Vertical deceleration injuries. **Surgery, Gynecology and Obstetrics** 1981;153:233.

5. McSwain NE Jr: Abdominal trauma. In: McSwain NE Jr, Kerstein MD (eds): **Evaluation and Management of Trauma**. East Norwalk, Connecticut, Appleton-Century-Crofts, 1987, pp 129-166.

6. McSwain NE Jr: Mechanisms of injury in blunt trauma. In: McSwain NE Jr, Kerstein MD (eds): **Evaluation and Management of Trauma**. East Norwalk, Connecticut, Appleton-Century-Crofts, 1987, pp 1-24.

7. Rozycki GS, Maull KI: Injuries sustained by falls. **Archives of Emergency Medicine** (in press).

8. Weigelt JA, McCormack A: Mechanism of injury. In: Cardona VD, Hurn PD, Mason PJB, et al: **Trauma Nursing From Resuscitation Through Rehabilitation**. Philadelphia, Pennsylvania, WB Saunders Company, 1988, pp 105-126.

Resource Document 4: Protection of Personnel From Communicable Diseases

Although there is great concern about the spread of Acquired Immune Deficiency Syndrome (AIDS) among health care personnel, there are also serious problems of death and disability in health care personnel each year from hepatitis. Recommendations from agencies such as the Centers for Disease Control (CDC) call for strict precautions in all cases when dealing with human body fluids and items contaminated with human body fluids.

Contact with human fluids is particularly a problem in the trauma patient, especially during initial resuscitation. AIDS can be transmitted by body fluids, wounds, needle sticks, and in some cases by contact with individuals with severe dermatitis. Protection against these fluids is absolutely necessary. The use of the following protective devices is recommended:

1. Goggles

2. Gloves

3. Fluid-impervious gowns or aprons

4. Shoe covers and fluid-impervious leggings

5. Mask

6. Head covering

Every patient entering the emergency department or trauma center should be considered a potential carrier of communicable disease. The use of such protective materials should be made a mandatory part of the trauma center activities. Careful management of hypodermic needles, knife blades, surgical needles, body fluids and tissues, etc, should be strictly enforced. Biohazard containers in the emergency department or trauma center should be provided for such materials.

The US Department of Labor Occupational Safety and Health Administration (OSHA) published a new standard (Part 1910.1030 of Title 29 of the *Code of Federal Regulations*) on bloodborne pathogens in the *Federal Register* on December 6, 1991 (29 CFR 1910.1030) for implementation during 1992. All health care personnel should be knowledgeable of and must comply with this mandate, and any future modifications.

A copy of **Occupational Exposure to Bloodborne Pathogens**, *Federal Register* 56(235): 64004-64182, December 6, 1991, Order No. 069-001-00040-8, may be obtained from the US Government Printing Office (GPO), Washington, DC 20402, (202) 783-3238. The following related materials may be obtained from the OSHA Publications Office, 200 Constitution Avenue, NW, Room N3101, Washington, DC 20210, (202) 523-9667.

**Resource
Document 4:
Protection of
Personnel
From
Communicable
Diseases**

OSHA 2056—All About OSHA

OSHA 3021—Employee Workplace Rights

OSHA 3047—Consultation Services for the Employer

OSHA 3077—Personal Protective Equipment

OSHA 3084—Chemical Hazard Communication

OSHA 3088—How to Prepare for Workplace Emergencies

OSHA 3110—Access to Medical and Exposure Records

OSHA 3127—Occupational Exposure to Bloodborne Pathogens

OSHA 3128—Bloodborne Pathogens and Acute Health Care Workers

OSHA 3129—Bloodborne Pathogens and Dental Workers

OSHA 3130—Bloodborne Pathogens and Emergency Responders

OSHA 3131—Bloodborne Pathogens and Long-Term Health Care Workers

Bibliography

1. Centers for Disease Control: Recommendations for preventing transmission of human immunodeficiency virus and hepatitis B virus to patients during exposure-prone invasive procedures. **ACS Bulletin** 1991;76:9,29-37.

2. Hill CJ: College joins ADA in OSHA petition. **ACS Bulletin** 1992;77:4,33.

3. Hill CJ: What surgeons should know about...OSHA regulation of bloodborne pathogens. **ACS Bulletin** 1992;77:6,6-9.

Resource Document 5: Roentgenographic Studies

The law of inverse proportionality: The number of x-ray films allowed in the emergency room must be inversely proportional to the severity of the injury.

Yoram Ben-Menachem, MD

I. Introduction

Roentgenograms should be obtained judiciously and must not delay patient resuscitation or transfer. Three roentgenograms should be obtained during the secondary survey—cervical spine (c-spine), anterior/posterior (AP) chest, and AP pelvis. These films can be taken in the resuscitation area, usually with a portable x-ray unit, during hiatuses in the resuscitation process. Equipment in the resuscitation room should be restricted to the basic portable or overhead x-ray unit.

Radiology on the triage table must be limited to survey films. It may be necessary to transport the patient to the radiology department for repeated plain films, contrast studies, or computed tomography (CT) or ultrasound. Transport of the patient to the radiology department should be viewed as an intrahospital patient transfer. (See Chapter 12, Stabilization and Transport.) Care must be taken to ensure airway management, continuous fluid resuscitation, spinal immobilization, and stabilization of potential and recognized fractures. The patient must be accompanied at all times by trained medical personnel and the appropriate equipment to manage changes in the clinical condition of the patient.

All radiographs must be labeled with the date and time they are obtained and the patient's name. If the patient is transferred to another institution, all radiographs must accompany the patient.

This document includes an outline of roentgenograms obtained during the initial assessment and resuscitation of the multiple-trauma patient—spine, chest, pelvis, abdomen, head, and extremities. It does not include radiographic interpretation of CT of the abdomen and head, other contrast studies (including arteriography), sonography, nuclear scans, and magnetic resonance imaging (MRI).

II. Spine

A. Indication

A lateral c-spine roentgenogram should be obtained on every patient sustaining multiple trauma. In addition, a lateral c-spine film should be obtained on every patient sustaining an injury above the clavicle, and especially a head injury. Films of the thoracic and lumbar spine should be obtained on any patient suspected of sustaining multiple trauma, especially to the trunk. (See Chapter 7, Spine and Spinal Cord Trauma for specific spine injuries.)

B. When to Obtain

A lateral c-spine roentgenogram should be obtained as soon as life-threatening problems are identified and controlled. Thoracic and lumbar films should be obtained during or after the secondary survey.

C. How to Obtain

1. Cervical spine

The first and most important film to obtain of the c-spine is a well-positioned, adequately penetrating, crosstable, brow up, lateral projection of the c-spine in a neutral position. The base of the skull, all seven cervical vertebrae, and the first thoracic vertebrae **must** be visualized. The patient's shoulders are routinely pulled down when obtaining the lateral c-spine film, preventing missed fractures or fracture-dislocations in the lower c-spine. If all seven cervical vertebrae are not visualized on the lateral roentgenogram, a lateral swimmer's view of the lower cervical and upper thoracic area may be obtained.

After adequate demonstration of all seven cervical and the first thoracic vertebrae, the physician can obtain chest and open-mouth odontoid films. Other roentgenograms that can be obtained after the first hour to further evaluate the c-spine include AP and oblique cervical views. These or more sophisticated studies should be done for any patient with a normal crosstable lateral roentgenogram who is suspected (by signs and symptoms or mechanism of injury) of having a cervical injury. Even the best portable films miss 5% to 15% of the injuries.

A CT scan may be needed to determine the presence of bone fragments in the spinal canal. Alternatively, tomograms may be obtained to confirm a c-spine injury and determine its stability. Lateral flexion and extension roentgenograms of the c-spine may be dangerous and should be done under the direct supervision and control of a knowledgeable physician.

2. Thoracic and lumbar spine

AP films of the thoracic and lumbar areas of the spine are standard. Because the crosstable lateral diameter of the body is usually greater than the AP diameter, most portable x-ray equipment used in the emergency department provides better bony definition in the AP view. Subsequent films may be obtained in the more elective environment of the radiology department. Oblique thoracic films seldom add further information. Lateral and oblique films of the lumbar spine are obtained if indicated.

D. Interpretation

(See Table 1, Spine Roentgenographic Suggestions.)

1. Cervical Spine

a. Roentgenograms of the c-spine should be examined for the following:

1) AP diameter of the spinal cord
2) Contour and alignment of the vertebral bodies
3) Displacement of bone fragments into the spinal canal

    4) Linear or comminuted fractures of the laminae, pedicles, or neural arches

    5) Soft-tissue swelling

b. Anatomic assessment

    1) Alignment — Identify and assess the four lordotic curves

       a) Anterior vertebral bodies

       b) Anterior spinal canal

       c) Posterior spinal canal

       d) Spinous process tips

    2) Bone—Assess these areas:

       a) Vertebral body—contour and axial height

       b) Lateral bony mass

          (1) Pedicles

          (2) Facets

          (3) Laminae

          (4) Transverse processes

       c) Spinous process

    3) Cartilage—Assess these areas:

       a) Intervertebral discs

       b) Posterolateral facet joints

    4) Soft-tissue spaces—Assess for the following:

       a) Prevertebral space

       b) Prevertebral fat stripe

       c) Space between spinous processes

c. Assessment guidelines for detecting abnormalities

    1) Alignment

       a) Vertebral malalignment > 3.0 mm—dislocation

       b) AP spinal canal space < 13 mm—spinal cord compression

       c) Angulation of intervertebral space > 11 degrees

    2) Bones

       a) Vertebral body

          (1) Anterior height < 3 mm posterior height—compression fractures

          (2) Lucency through the odontoid process of C-2—fracture

       b) Lack of parallel facets of the lateral mass—possible lateral compression fracture

       c) Lucency through the tip of the spinous process—avulsion fracture

       d) Atlas and axis (C-1 and C-2)

          (1) Distance between posterior aspect of C-1 to anterior odontoid process > 3 mm—dislocation

          (2) Lucency through the odontoid process of C-2 fracture

3) Soft-tissue space

   a) Widening of the prevertebral space > 5 mm—hemorrhage accompanying spinal injury

   b) Obliteration of prevertebral fat strip—fracture at same level

   c) Widening of space between spinous processes—torn interspinous ligaments and likely spinal canal fracture anteriorly

2. Thoracic and lumbar spine

During the early evaluation of the patient with suspected thoracic and/or lumbar vertebral injuries, it usually is sufficient to view only the AP film of the vertebral column. This film should be examined for the following:

a. Bilateral symmetry of the pedicles

b. Height of the intervertebral disc spaces

c. Central alignment of the spinous processes

d. Shape and contour of the vertebral bodies

e. Alignment of the vertebral bodies, if a lateral film is available

Table 1
Spine Roentgenographic Suggestions

Abnormal Findings	Diagnoses to Consider
Any c-spine bony abnormality	Cord compromise
C-spine injury	Airway compromise
Facial fracture	C-spine injury
Upper rib fracture	C-spine injury Upper thoracic spine injury Great vessel injury
Clavicular fracture	C-spine injury Upper thoracic spine injury Great vessel injury
Head injury	C-spine injury Upper thoracic spine injury
Lower thoracic spine fracture	Pancreatic injury

E. Roentgenographic Considerations in Children

A normal radiographic finding, in approximately 40% of children younger than seven years of age, is an anterior displacement of C-2 on C-3 (pseudosubluxation). Although this radiographic finding is seen less commonly at C-3 to C-4, more than 3 mm of movement can be seen when these joints are studied by flexion and extension maneuvers.

Increased distance between the dens and the anterior arch of C-1 occurs in about 20% of young children. Gaps exceeding the upper limit of normal for the adult population are frequently seen.

Skeletal growth centers can resemble fractures. Basilar odontoid synchrondrosis appears as a radiolucent area at the base of the dens, especially in children younger than five years of age. Apical odontoid epiphyses appear as separations on the odontoid roentgenogram and are usually seen between the ages of five and 11 years. The growth center of the spinous process may resemble fractures of the tip of the spinous process.

Children may sustain spinal cord injury without radiographic abnormality more commonly than adults. A normal spine series can be found in up to two-thirds of children sustaining spinal cord injury. Therefore, if spinal cord injury is suspected, based on history or the results of neurologic examination, normal spine roentgenograms do not exclude significant spinal cord injury. When in doubt about the integrity of the c-spine, assume that an unstable injury exists, maintain immobilization of the child's head and neck, and obtain appropriate consultation.

III. Chest Roentgenogram

A. Indications

A chest roentgenogram should be obtained on all patients who have sustained torso trauma—blunt or penetrating, and who are unconscious, going to the operating room, and/or are in respiratory distress.

B. When to Obtain

A chest roentgenogram should be obtained during the primary survey/resuscitation phase or the secondary survey.

C. How to Obtain

An AP film should be obtained with the patient in a supine position. An AP film may be obtained with the patient in an upright position; however, adequate immobilization of the patient's spine, particularly the c-spine, must be maintained.

D. Interpretation

(See Table 2, Chest Roentgenographic Suggestions.)

1. Soft tissues—chest wall

The soft tissues may be contused, lacerated, perforated, or avulsed. The physician should examine the film for displacement or disruption of the tissue planes and for evidence of subcutaneous emphysema.

2. Bony thorax

a. Ribs

Rib fractures are the most common injury seen on a chest film. However, 50% are missed due to the position or lack of the fracture displacement.

Fractures of the upper three ribs indicate severe trauma and require careful evaluation of the patient and the chest film for evidence of bronchial or aortic injury. Ribs four through nine are fractured most commonly. Two rib fractures in two or more places result in an unstable chest wall (flail chest). Fractures of the lower two ribs should cause the examiner to suspect an intra-abdominal injury, eg, spleen, liver, and/or kidney.

b. Scapula

Scapular fractures are associated with significant mortality due to associated injuries. Most scapular fractures are difficult to detect on a chest film. A high index of suspicion and knowledge of the mechanism of injury are required when examining chest films for scapular fractures. Special views are often required to identify such an injury.

c. Sternum

Most sternal fractures involve the sternomandibular junction or sternal body, and are often confused on the AP film as a mediastinal hematoma. A coned-down view, overpenetrated film, lateral film, or CT scan clarify this. The forces required to fracture the sternum also may produce myocardial contusion.

3. Pleural space

Abnormal accumulation of fluid may represent a hemothorax or chylothorax. On an upright or frontal chest film, a pneumothorax is seen usually as an apical lucent area absent of bronchial or vascular markings. This area separates the superior and lateral margins of the lung from the chest wall. Films obtained on full expiration may assist in identifying a small pneumothorax. Abnormal accumulations there constitute a pneumothorax.

The pneumothorax may progress to a tension pneumothorax, which can collapse more lung tissue. The increase in pleural pressure can restrict the inflow and outflow hemodynamics of the heart resulting in hypotension. Tension pneumothorax is **not** a radiographic diagnosis.

Pulmonary contusion appears as air space consolidation that can be irregular and patchy or homogeneous, diffuse, or extensive. Lacerations appear as a hematoma, vary according to the magnitude of the injury, and appear as areas of consolidation. Roentgenographic findings of inhalation injury appear late.

4. Trachea, bronchi

Tracheal lacerations present as pneumomediastinum, pneumothorax, and subcutaneous and interstitial emphysema of the neck or pneumoperitoneum. Bronchial fractures with free pleural communication produce a massive pneumothorax with a persistent air leak that is not responsive to thoracostomy.

5. Diaphragm

The diagnosis of a diaphragmatic rupture requires a high index of suspicion. An elevated, irregular, or obscure hemidiaphragm in a patient with multiple trauma requires close observation and further studies to evaluate the diaphragmatic integrity. The roentgenographic changes listed herein suggest diaphragmatic injury:

a. Elevation, irregularity, or obliteration of the diaphragm—segmental or total

b. Mass-like density above the diaphragm due to a fluid-filled bowel, omentum, liver, kidney, spleen, or pancreas—may appear as a "loculated pneumothorax"

c. Air- or contrast-containing stomach or bowel above the diaphragm

d. Contralateral mediastinal shift

e. Widening of the cardiac silhouette if the peritoneal contents herniate into the pericardial sac

f. Pleural effusion

g. The inferior border of the liver may appear higher than expected. Lower rib fractures, pulmonary contusions, and the appearance of foreign bodies in the chest cavity may be associated with diaphragmatic injury. Splenic, pancreatic, renal, and liver injuries also may be associated with diaphragmatic injury.

h. A nasogastric tube coiled in the chest may represent a stomach herniated into the chest or a hole in the esophagus

Initial chest roentgenograms may not suggest clearly a diaphragmatic injury, and sequential films may be needed to assist in this determination. Additional studies include oral barium, barium enema, or CT. Magnetic resonance imaging can show the diaphragm; however, the study is usually time consuming and is not indicated for a patient in respiratory distress. Ultrasonography also may be used to confirm the diagnosis of diaphragmatic injury.

6. **Mediastinum**

Mediastinal structures may be displaced by air or blood and may dissect out along the bronchial structures, either displacing those structures or blurring the demarcation between tissue planes or outlining them with radiolucency. Air or blood in the pericardium appears to enlarge the cardiac silhouette. Progressive changes in the cardiac size may represent an expanding pneumopericardium or hemopericardium. Radiologic signs that suggest aortic rupture include:

a. Widened mediastinum—most reliable finding
b. Fractures of the first and second ribs
c. Obliteration of the aortic knob
d. Deviation of the trachea to the right
e. Presence of a pleural cap
f. Elevation and rightward shift of the right mainstem bronchus
g. Depression of the left mainstem bronchus
h. Obliteration of the space between the pulmonary artery and the aorta
i. Deviation of the esophagus (nasogastric tube to the right)

Arteriography is the appropriate modality to make the definitive diagnosis.

Table 2
Chest Roentgenographic Suggestions

Abnormal Findings	Diagnoses to Consider
Any rib fracture	Pneumothorax
Fracture, first 3 ribs	Airway or great vessel injury
Lower ribs, 9 to 12	Abdominal injury
Two or more rib fractures in two or more places	Flail chest, pulmonary contusion
GI gas pattern in the chest (Loculated air)	Diaphragmatic rupture
NG tube in the chest	Diaphragmatic rupture or ruptured esophagus
Air fluid level in the chest	Hemothorax or diaphragmatic rupture
Loss of diaphragmatic contour	Diaphragmatic rupture
Sternal fracture	Myocardial contusion, head injury, c-spine injury
Mediastinal hematoma	Great vessel injury, sternal fracture
Disrupted diaphragm	Prompt celiotomy
Respiratory distress without roentgenographic findings	CNS injury, aspiration
Persistent large pneumothorax after chest tube insertion	Bronchial tear, esophageal disruption
Mediastinal air	Esophageal disruption, pneumoperitoneum, tracheal injury
Scapular fracture	Airway or great vessel injury, or pulmonary contusion
Free air under the diaphragm	Ruptured hollow abdominal viscus

IV. Pelvis

A. Indications

Indications for pelvic roentgenogram include patients with significant blunt trauma to the torso, pelvic instability, gross blood and/or disrupted prostate on rectal examination, gross blood on vaginal examination, gross hematuria, and unexplained hypotension.

B. When to Obtain

Pelvic films are obtained during the secondary survey.

C. How to Obtain

An AP pelvic film is obtained with the patient in a supine position. All bones of the pelvis must be visualized. A lateral view rarely is used and is difficult to obtain in the trauma patient. Oblique or angulated views are used to evaluate the sacroiliac joints and to further define fractures, particularly of the rami. Other imaging techniques used to delineate the pelvic anatomy include retrograde urethrogram and cystograms, intravenous pyelogram (IVP), ultrasonography, and CT.

D. Interpretation

(See Table 3, Pelvic Roentgenographic Suggestions.)

The anatomy of the pelvis is arranged primarily as a ring. If a fracture in any one portion is identified, there is generally a second disruption of the ring. The examining physician should be alerted to any disruption in the symmetry of the pelvic ring and the possibility of a fracture or significant soft-tissue injury. Avulsed fragments and comminuted wing fractures may be difficult to identify as well as fractures of the coccyx and sacroiliac joints.

Table 3
Pelvic Roentgenographic Suggestions

Abnormal Findings	Diagnoses to Consider
Any fracture of the pelvis	Hemorrhage, urethral trauma, bladder trauma, rectal injury
Pelvic fracture in a pregnant woman	Abruption placenta, uterine hematoma, or fetal distress
Widening of the sacroiliac joint	Urethral injury
Pubic diastasis	Urethral injury
Posterior hip dislocation	Sciatic nerve injury
Anterior hip dislocation	Vascular compromise
Pelvic fracture	Intra-abdominal visceral injuries, life-threatening thoracic injuries, diaphragmatic rupture, retroperitoneal vascular injury
Pelvic fracture	Femoral shaft fracture

V. Abdomen

A. Indications

Plain films of the abdomen are of limited use when evaluating the trauma patient. **Remember**, the information obtained on a roentgenogram is, for the most part, limited to the bony structures. Given the wide impact of blunt or penetrating trauma and the range of possible soft-tissue injuries in the abdomen, the limitations of the plain abdominal film must be recognized.

Plain films are useful in looking for foreign bodies, free air, and bony abnormalities. The interluminal gas pattern for the abdominal structures and the outline of solid soft-tissue organs are unreliable in the patient with multiple trauma. The air and soft-tissue patterns may be of indirect help in the assessment of structures contained in the peritoneum, retroperitoneum, and pelvis.

Abdominal films should be obtained on patients with (1) penetrating or blunt abdominal trauma who have suspected intra-abdominal injuries, (2) an altered sensorium and who are unable to provide a reliable history or responses to a physical examination, or (3) findings referable to the abdomen.

B. When to Obtain

Abdominal roentgenograms should be obtained during the secondary survey.

C. How to Obtain

1. Abdominal roentgenograms

AP plain or crosstable lateral decubitus films may be appropriate. Projection must include the top of the diaphragm and the entire pelvis. A chest film is an essential companion to the abdominal film. Repeated roentgenograms may be useful to detect shifts in fluid or air in the abdomen.

2. Contrast studies

a. Urethrography

Urethrography should be performed before inserting an indwelling urinary catheter when a urethral tear is suspected. The urethrogram can be performed with a #12-French urinary catheter secured in the meatal fossa by balloon inflation to 3 mL. Undiluted contrast material is instilled with gentle pressure.

b. Cystography

Bladder rupture is established with a gravity flow cystogram. A bulb syringe attached to the indwelling bladder catheter is held 15 cm above the patient, and 250 to 300 mL of water-soluble contrast is allowed to flow into the bladder. Anteroposterior, oblique, and postdrainage views are essential to definitively exclude injury. The order of an IVP versus cystography is governed by the index of suspicion for upper versus lower tract injury.

c. Excretory urogram

An IVP may be valuable for initial renal evaluation. High-dose intravenous bolus injection should provide evidence of relative kidney function at 5 to 10 minutes. In the stable patient, CT is preferable to the IVP if there is the suspicion of other intra-abdominal and/or retroperitoneal injuries. Intravenous contrast studies should not be performed in the hypotensive, unstable patient.

d. Computed tomography

Diagnostic peritoneal lavage can be performed rapidly and without delay in the emergency department. By comparison, CT requires transport of the patient to the scan area and time to perform the examination. A complete CT examination, usually using both intravenous and oral contrast material, must include the upper abdomen and pelvis. Therefore, the CT scan should be performed only on stable patients in whom there is no apparent indication for immediate operation. The CT scan, which provides information relative to specific organ injury and its extent, also can diagnose retroperitoneal and pelvic organ injuries that are difficult to assess by a physical examination or peritoneal lavage.

D. Interpretation

(See Table 4, Abdominal Roentgenographic Suggestions.)

1. Spleen

Intrasplenic hemorrhage, subcapsular hematoma, visceral fragments, and blood accumulation in the splenic fossa may appear as a radio-opaque mass in the left upper quadrant. Displacement or obliteration of the left kidney medially or the left transverse colon interiorly may be further signs. An upright roentgenogram with the patient in the right posterior oblique position may assist in the demonstration of the splenic mass and visceral displacement. Atelectasis, pleural effusion, irregularity, or prominence of gastric mucosal folds are additional signs. CT scan may provide more direct information. Radionucleotide scans and abdominal ultrasound also have been employed.

2. Hemoperitoneum

As blood fills the peritoneal cavity, the blood collects in the pelvis which constitutes approximately one third of the volume of the peritoneal cavity. Initially, perirectal and, later, perivesicle and perirectal pouches fill with blood, displacing the small intestine cephalad. This may appear as a homogenous density superior and lateral to the bladder. Free-flowing blood or other fluid in the lateral gutter displaces the colon medially and replaces the sacculations formed by the colonic haustra. Blood in the posterior subhepatic space (Morison's pouch) may obscure the outlines of the undersurface of the liver. CT demonstrates some of the anatomic subtleties of hemoperitoneum accurately.

3. Gastrointestinal tract

Bowel lacerations allow air, fluid, and food residue to escape into the bowel wall, peritoneum, and extraperitoneal spaces revealing itself as extraluminal air and alterations in the normal crisp outlines of the bowel air patterns. An upright chest film provides the best means of demonstrating free intraperitoneal air. A lateral decubitus of the abdomen is a second best plain film. Oral or rectally-administered water-soluble contrast material may assist in demonstrating perforation at either ends of the gastrointestinal tract. Barium is not used as its presence in the free peritoneal cavity increases the morbidity of perforation. Additional signs of free air under the diaphragm include the following:

a. Double wall sign, ie, intraluminal and extraluminal air outside the mucosal and serosal surfaces

b. A cap of air forming a lucency over fluid areas in the abdomen

c. Visualization of the falciform ligament as it is outlined by air

d. Subhepatic air

e. An accumulation of air in the central tendon of the diaphragm providing a curved, sharp interface with the inferior mediastinum

f. Subpulmonic pneumothorax with air apparently loculated between the base of the lung and the diaphragm

g. Mediastinal air that has dissected from the abdomen

h. An apparent large diverticulum arising from a subdiaphragmatic esophagus, the stomach, or the duodenum

4. Duodenum and pancreas

Duodenal and pancreatic injuries are difficult to diagnose. Intramural hematoma and air outlining retroperitoneal structures are suspicious of these problems. Extraluminal retroperitoneal gas may tend to the anatomic spaces outlined by facial planes. Air surrounding the right kidney may be an additional sign. Pancreatic injury is even less specific with elevation of the left hemidiaphragm, and basal atelectasis, pleural fluid, scoliosis, adynamic ileus, and loss of roentgenographic visualization of the normal retroperitoneal structures and facial planes are suggestive of this problem. Intramural duodenal hematomas are more common in children as their abdominal walls are less protective of the abdominal viscera.

5. Liver

There are few reliable signs of hepatic trauma. On a plain film, rib fractures in the area are of some assistance; however, CT scan is a more definitive imaging technique. Subcapsular hematomas may distort the liver outline and change the hepatic angle and displace the hepatic flexure of the colon interiorly. Additional measures include nuclear scanning and ultrasonography.

6. Kidney

Intravenous pyelogram is the most frequently performed contrast study in the patient with acute trauma. Renal injuries are divided as indicated herein:

a. Minor injury—compression of a collecting system; displacement by retroperitoneal hematoma; some delay in excretion

b. Major injury—contrast leakage from the collecting system; tear in the renal capsule; perinephric hematoma; obliteration of the renal outline or psoas muscle

c. Catastrophic injury—appears as the shattered kidney with extensive hemorrhage and displacement and disruption of the renal parenchyma

Roentgenographic signs include:

1) Loss of the psoas margin on the side of the injury

2) Concomitant fracture of the ribs, pelvis, or spine—suggestive of severe abdominal trauma

3) Concavity of the spine on the side of the trauma

4) Unilateral hypoconcentration

5) Absence or delayed function

6) Filling defects in the renal pelvis, parenchyma ureter, or bladder suggesting blood clots

7) A flank mass with displacement of the bowel loops

8) Fluid collection above the renal calyces representing a subcapsular collection

9) Hemorrhage into the perirenal fat

10) A striated nephrogram

11) Extravasation of contrast

Table 4
Abdominal Roentgenographic Suggestions

Abnormal Findings	Diagnoses to Consider
Lower rib fractures	Hepatic or splenic trauma
Pelvic fracture	Rectal laceration, diaphragmatic rupture, hemorrhage
Lumbar spine fracture	Renal injury
Free air	Ruptured hollow viscus
Apparent displacement of bowel gas patterns, eg, stomach or small bowel	Hemoperitoneum
Effacement of mucosal folds of the duodenum	Intramural hematoma of the duodenum
Loss of psoas shadow	Retroperitoneal hematoma
Retroperitoneal air	Duodenal rupture
Lower thoracic spine injuries	Pancreatic injury
Extraluminal air	Prompt celiotomy
Intraperitoneal perforation of urinary bladder	Prompt celiotomy

VI. Head Trauma

A. Skull Roentgenograms

Skull roentgenograms are of little value in the early management of patients with obvious head injuries, except in cases of penetrating injuries. The unconscious patient should have skull roentgenograms only if precise care of the cardiorespiratory system and continuing reassessment can be assured.

Physical examination is usually more valuable than skull roentgenograms. Clinical signs of basal fractures are more useful than radiographs of the skull base in diagnosing fracture. Increasingly, skull films are not being obtained on patients with minor head injuries because the information obtained is rarely helpful. When in doubt about the patient's condition, the physicians should obtain neurosurgical consultation.

B. Computed Tomography

The CT scan has revolutionized diagnosis in patients with head injuries and is the diagnostic procedure of choice for patients who have or are suspected of having a serious head injury. Although not perfect, the CT scan is capable of showing the exact location and size of most lesions. Specific diagnosis allows more precise planning of definitive care, including operation. The CT scan has supplanted less specific and more invasive tests such as cerebral angiography.

Except for patients with trivial head injuries, all head-injured patients require CT scanning at some time. The more serious the injury, the earlier and more emergent is the need for the scan. Consequently, injured patients seen first at facilities without CT capability may require transfer to a trauma center.

Once initial resuscitation has been undertaken and the need for a CT scan determined, care must be taken to (1) maintain adequate resuscitation during the scan, and (2) assure the best possible quality of the scan. The patient must be attended constantly in the CT suite to monitor his vital signs closely, and immediate treatment must be initiated should the patient's status deteriorate.

Patient movement results in artifacts and a poor-quality scan. This artifact may mask significant intracranial lesions requiring urgent surgical intervention. Movement artifact can be eliminated by sedating restless or unco-operative patients. However, extreme caution must be exercised to avoid sedating patients whose restlessness or lack of cooperation is a clinical manifestation of hypoxia. Often endotracheal intubation with controlled ventilation becomes necessary if the scan is considered mandatory and the patient can be rendered motionless only with paralyzing drugs. Ideally, the neurosurgeon should examine the patient before the patient is iatrogenically paralyzed or has a CT scan. However, efficient and correct management of the patient in certain situations may dictate otherwise.

C. Isotope Scan

Isotope scanning has no role in the early management of head trauma.

VII. Extremities

A. Indications

Indications for obtaining extremity roentgenograms on the trauma patient include blunt or penetrating trauma to the extremity, extremity deformity, or evidence of vascular or neurologic compromise of the extremity.

B. When to Obtain

Roentgenograms of the extremities are obtained during the secondary survey.

C. How to Obtain

Anterior, posterior, and lateral extremity films may be obtained. Comparison views visualizing the contralateral extremity are helpful, particularly in children. Patterns of bone injury may be helpful in predicting associated extremity injuries other than the one that is first seen, eg, a suspected fracture of the tibia with a less obvious fracture of the fibula or dislocation of a joint proximal or distal to an obvious long bone fracture. Because of the three-dimensional nature of the extremity, views in at least two projections, preferably at right angles, are desirable. These may be supplemented by oblique views. Specific anatomic areas include the shoulder, scapula, clavicle, elbow, forearm, wrist, hand, knee, leg, ankle, and foot. Special imaging may be necessary for smaller bones such as the wrist, patella, foot, and hand. Stress fractures or small fracture lines may be best visualized in days or weeks after the injury incident.

When obtaining and viewing extremity roentgenograms, these items should be reviewed.

1. Is this the correct patient and the correct side to be filmed?

2. Do the roentgenograms cover the entire area of injury, including one joint above and one joint below the injury?

3. Have proper projections been obtained?

4. Are the roentgenograms properly exposed?

5. Is the detail adequate?

6. Are the contours of the bones in the cortical surfaces?

7. Inspect the cortical margins of each bone completely as the bones may be superimposed. Look for secondary soft-tissue signs.

8. If there is an obvious lesion, disregard it until you have looked at the remainder of the film.

9. Document findings and opinions.

D. Roentgenographic Considerations in Children

1. General

Roentgenographic diagnoses of fractures and dislocations in the younger child are difficult because of the lack of mineralization around the epiphysis and the presence of a physis (growth plate). Information about the magnitude, mechanism, and time of injury facilitates better correlation of the physical findings and roentgenograms. Radiographic evidence of fractures of different ages should alert the physician to possible child abuse.

2. Physeal (growth plate) fractures

Bones lengthen as new bone is laid down by the physis near the articular surfaces. Injuries to or adjacent to this area before the physis has closed can potentially retard the normal growth or alter the development of the bone in an abnormal way. Crush injuries, which are often difficult to recognize roentgenographically, have the worst prognosis.

3. Unique fractures

The immature, pliable nature of bones in children may lead to a so-called "greenstick" fracture. Such fractures are incomplete, with angulation maintained by cortical splinters on the concave surface. The torus or "buckle" fracture, seen in small children, involves angulation due to cortical impaction with a radiolucent fracture line. Supracondylar fractures at the elbow or knee have a high propensity for vascular injury as well as injury to the growth plate.

Table 5
Extremity Roentgenographic Suggestions

Abnormal Findings	Diagnoses to Consider
Extremity fracture	Arterial injury Nerve injury Hemorrhage with or without shock Compartment syndrome Fat embolization Some anaerobic soft-tissue infections Fracture fragments within the joint Thromboembolism Continued soft-tissue injury Joint dislocation about and below fracture site Growth plate injury
Femoral fracture	Acetabular fracture, hip dislocation, pelvic ring fracture
Calcaneal fracture	Vertebral column injuries
Shoulder girdle fracture	Thoracic injuries
Soft-tissue signs without fracture	Ligamentous injury
Multiple long-bone fractures in a child	Child abuse
Multiple fractures of different ages	Child abuse

Bibliography

1. Ben-Menachem Y: Radiology. In: Moore EE (ed): **Early Care of the Injured Patient.** Philadelphia, Pennsylvania, BD Decker Inc, 1990, pp 84-90.

2. Berquist TH: Spinal Trauma. In: McCort J (ed): **Trauma Radiology.** New York, 1990, pp 131-154.

3. Guyott DR, Manoli II: Upper extremity trauma. In: McCort J (ed): **Trauma Radiology.** New York, 1990, pp 381-340.

4. Gehweiler JA, Osbornee RL, Becker RF: **The Radiology of Vertebral Trauma.** Philadelphia, Pennsylvania, WB Saunders Company, 1980.

5. Keats TE: **Emergency Radiology**. Chicago, Illinois, Year Book Medical Publishers Inc, 1984.

6. McCort J: Gastrointestinal tract trauma. In: McCort J (ed): **Trauma Radiology**. New York, 1990, pp 159-166, 194-198, 249-257, 303-313, 343-357.

7. Mitchell MJ, Ho C, Howard BA, et al: Lower extremity trauma. In: McCort J (ed): **Trauma Radiology**. New York, 1990, pp 435.

8. Swischuk LE: **Emergency Radiology of the Acutely Ill or Injured Child**. Baltimore, Maryland, Williams & Wilkins, 1986.

**Resource
Document 5:
Roentgeno-
graphic
Studies**

Resource Document 6: Tetanus Immunization

I. Introduction

Attention must be directed to adequate tetanus prophylaxis in the multiply injured patient, particularly if open-extremity trauma is present. The average incubation period for tetanus is 10 days; most often it is four to 21 days. In severe trauma cases, tetanus can appear as early as one to two days. All of the medical profession must be cognizant of this important fact when providing care to the injured patient.

Tetanus immunization depends on the patient's previous immunization status and the tetanus-prone nature of the wound. The following guidelines have been adapted from *A Guide to Prophylaxis Against Tetanus in Wound Management*, prepared by the ACS Committee on Trauma, and information available from the Centers for Disease Control (CDC). Because this information is reviewed and updated as new data become available, the Committee on Trauma recommends contacting the CDC for the latest information and detailed guidelines related to tetanus prophylaxis and immunization for the injured patient.

II. General Principles

A. Individual Assessment

The attending physician must determine the requirements for adequate prophylaxis against tetanus for each injured patient individually.

B. Surgical Wound Care

Regardless of the active immunization status of the patient, meticulous surgical care—including removal of all devitalized tissue and foreign bodies—should be provided immediately for all wounds. If doubt exists about the adequacy of the debridement of the wound or a puncture injury is present, the wound should be left open and not closed by sutures. Such care is essential as part of the prophylaxis against tetanus.

C. Human Tetanus Immune Globulin (TIG)

Passive immunization with 250 units of tetanus immune globulin (TIG), administered intramuscularly, must be considered individually for each patient. TIG provides longer protection than antitoxin of animal origin and causes few adverse reactions. The characteristics of the wound, conditions under which it occurred, its age, TIG treatment, and the previous active immunization status of the patient must be considered (Table 2). When tetanus toxoid and TIG are given concurrently, separate syringes and separate sites should be used.

If the patient has ever received two or more injections of toxoid, TIG is not indicated, unless the wound is judged to be tetanus prone and is more than 24 hours old. Do not administer equine tetanus antitoxin, except when the human toxin is not available, and only if the possibility of tetanus outweighs the potential reactions of horse serum.

D. Documentation

For every injured patient, information about the mechanism of injury, the characteristics of the wound, age, previous active immunization status, history of a neurologic or severe hypersensitivity reaction following a previous immunization treatment, and plans for follow-up should be documented. Each patient must be given a written record describing treatment rendered and follow-up instructions that outline wound care, drug therapy, immunization status, and potential complications. The patient should be referred to a designated physician who will provide comprehensive follow-up care, including completion of active immunizations.

A wallet-sized card documenting the immunization administered and date of immunization should be given to every injured patient. The patient should be instructed to carry the written record at all times and complete active immunization, if indicated. For precise tetanus prophylaxis, an accurate and immediately available history regarding previous active immunization against tetanus is required. Otherwise, rapid laboratory titration is necessary to determine the patient's serum antitoxin level.

E. Antibiotics

The effectiveness of antibiotics for prophylaxis of tetanus is uncertain. In patients who need TIG as part of the treatment to prevent tetanus, and it is not available for any reason, antibiotics like penicillin delay the onset of tetanus. This allows a period of two days in which to obtain the TIG and institute proper passive immunization.

F. Contraindications

The only contraindication to tetanus and diphtheria toxoids in the wounded patient is a history of neurologic or severe hypersensitivity reaction following a previous dose. Local side effects alone do not preclude continued use. If a systemic reaction is suspected to represent allergic hypersensitivity, immunization should be postponed until appropriate skin testing is undertaken at a later time. If a tetanus toxoid-containing preparation is contraindicated, passive immunization against tetanus should be considered for a tetanus-prone wound.

Contraindications to pertussis vaccination in infants and children younger than seven years old include either a previous adverse reaction after DTP or single-antigen pertussis vaccination and/or the presence of a neurologic finding. If such a contraindication to using pertussis vaccine adsorbed (P) exists, diphtheria and tetanus toxoid adsorbed (for pediatric use) (DT) is recommended. A static neurologic condition, such as cerebral palsy or a family history of convulsions or other central nervous system disorders, is not a contraindication to giving vaccines containing the pertussis antigen.

G. Active Immunization for Normal Infants and Children

For children younger than seven years of age, immunization requires four injections of diphtheria and tetanus toxoids and pertussis vaccine adsorbed (DTP). A booster (fifth dose) injection is administered at four to six years of age. Thereafter, a routine booster of tetanus and diphtheria toxoids adsorbed (Td) is indicated at 10-year intervals.

H. Active Immunization for Adults

Immunization for adults requires at least three injections of Td. An injection of Td should be repeated every 10 years throughout the individual's life, providing no significant reactions to Td have occurred.

I. Active Immunization for Pregnant Women

Neonatal tetanus is preventable by active immunization of the pregnant mother during the first six months of pregnancy, with two injections of Td given two months apart. After delivery and six months after the second dose, the mother should be given the third dose of Td to complete the active immunization.

An injection of Td should be repeated every 10 years throughout life, providing no significant reactions to Td have occurred. In the event that a neonate is born to a nonimmunized mother without obstetric care, the infant should receive 250 units of TIG. Active and passive immunization of the mother also should be initiated.

J. Previously Immunized Individuals

1. Fully immunized

When the attending physician has determined that the patient has been previously and fully immunized, and the last dose of toxoid was given **within 10 years**:

a. Administer 0.5 mL of adsorbed toxoid for tetanus-prone wounds, if more than five years has elapsed since the last dose.

b. This booster may be omitted if excessive toxoid injections have been given before.

2. Partially immunized

When the patient has received two or more injections of toxoid, and the last dose was received more than ten years ago, 0.5 mL adsorbed toxoid is administered for both tetanus-prone and nontetanus-prone wounds. Passive immunization is not necessary.

K. Individuals Not Adequately Immunized

When the patient has received only **one or no** prior injections of toxoid or the immunization history is unknown:

1. Nontetanus-prone wounds: Administer 0.5 mL of adsorbed toxoid for nontetanus-prone wounds.

2. **Tetanus-Prone wounds**

   a. Administer 0.5 mL adsorbed toxoid.

   b. Administer 250 units TIG.

   c. Consider administering antibiotics, although their effectiveness for prophylaxis of tetanus remains unproved.

   d. Administer medication using different syringes and sites for injection.

L. Immunization Schedule

1. **Adult**
   a. Three injections of toxoid
   b. Booster every 10 years

2. **Children**
   a. Four injections of DTP
   b. Fifth dose at four to six years of age
   c. Booster every 10 years

III. Specific Measures for Patients With Wounds

Recommendations for tetanus prophylaxis are based on (1) condition of the wound, and (2) the patient's immunization history. Table 1 outlines some of the clinical features of wounds that are prone to develop tetanus. A wound with any one of these features is a tetanus-prone wound.

Table 1
Nontetanus- and Tetanus-Prone Wounds

Clinical Features	Nontetanus-Prone Wounds	Tetanus-Prone Wounds
Age of wound	≤ 6 hours	> 6 hours
Configuration	Linear wound	Stellate wound, avulsion, abrasion
Depth	≤ 1 cm	> 1 cm
Mechanism of injury	Sharp surface (eg, knife, glass)	Missile, crush, burn, frostbite
Signs of infection	Absent	Present
Devitalized tissue	Absent	Present
Contaminants (dirt, feces, soil, saliva, etc)	Absent	Present
Denervated, and/or ischemic tissue	Absent	Present

Table 2
Summary of Tetanus Prophylaxis for the Injured Patient

History of Adsorbed Tetanus Toxoid (Doses)	Nontetanus-Prone Wounds		Tetanus-Prone Wounds	
	Td[1]	TIG	Td[1]	TIG
Unknown or ≤ three	Yes	No	Yes	Yes
≥ Three[2]	No[3]	No	No[4]	No

Key to Table 2

1   For children younger than seven years old: DTP (DT, if pertussis vaccine is contraindicated) is preferred to tetanus toxoid alone. For persons seven years old and older, Td is preferred to tetanus toxoid alone.

2   If only three doses of fluid toxoid have been received, a fourth dose of toxoid, preferably an adsorbed toxoid, should be given.

3   Yes, if more than 10 years since last dose.

4   Yes, if more than five years since last dose. (More frequent boosters are not needed and can accentuate side effects.)

Td   Tetanus and diphtheria toxoids adsorbed—for adult use.

TIG   Tetanus immune globulin—human.

**Resource
Document 6:
Tetanus
Immunization**

Resource Document 7: Pediatric Trauma Score

Correct triage is essential to effective function of regional trauma systems. Overtriage inundates trauma centers with minimally injured patients who then impede care for severely injured patients. Undertriage can produce inadequate initial care and may cause preventable morbidity and mortality.

Unfortunately, the perfect triage tool does not exist. Experience with adult trauma scoring systems illustrates this problem by the multiplicity of scoring systems that have been proposed over the last decade. None of these scoring protocols is universally accepted as a completely effective triage tool. At present, most of adult trauma surgeons utilize the Revised Trauma Score (RTS) as a triage tool and the weighted variation of this score as a predictor of potential mortality. This score is based totally on physiologic derangement on initial evaluation and entails a categorization of blood pressure, respiratory rate, and the Glasgow Coma Scale.

Application of these three components to the pediatric population is difficult and inconsistent. Respiratory rate is often inaccurately measured in the field and does not necessarily reflect respiratory insufficiency in the injured child. The Glasgow Coma Scale is an extremely effective neurologic assessment tool; however, it requires some revision for application to the preverbal child. These problems, in association with the lack of any identification of anatomic injury or quantification of patient size, undermine the applicability of the Revised Trauma Score to effective triage of the injured child. For these reasons, the Pediatric Trauma Score (PTS) was developed. The PTS is the sum of the severity grade of each category and has been demonstrated to predict potential for death and severe disability reliably. (See Table 1, Pediatric Trauma Score.)

Size is a major consideration for the infant-toddler group, in which mortality from injury is the highest. **Airway** is assessed not just as a function, but as a descriptor of what care is required to provide adequate management. **Systolic blood pressure** assessment primarily identifies those children in whom evolving preventable shock may occur (50 mm Hg to 90 mm Hg systolic blood pressure [+1]). Regardless of size, a child whose systolic blood pressure is below 50 mm Hg (-1) is in obvious jeopardy. On the other hand, a child whose systolic pressure exceeds 90 mm Hg (+2) probably falls into a better outcome category than a child with even a slight degree of hypotension.

Level of consciousness is the most important factor in initially assessing the central nervous system. Because children frequently lose consciousness transiently during injury, the "obtunded" (+1) grade is given to any child who loses consciousness, no matter how fleeting the loss. This grade identifies a patient who may have sustained a head injury with potentially fatal—but often treatable—intracranial sequelae.

Skeletal injury is a component of the PTS because of its high incidence in the pediatric population and its potential contribution to mortality. Finally, **cutaneous injury**, both as an adjunct to common pediatric injury patterns and as an injury category that includes penetrating wounds, is considered in the computed PTS.

The PTS serves as a simple checklist, ensuring that all components critical to initial assessment of the injured child have been considered. It is useful for paramedics in the field, as well as for physicians in facilities other than pediatric trauma units. As a predictor of injury, the PTS has a statistically significant inverse relationship with the Injury Severity Score (ISS) and mortality. Analysis of this relationship has identified a threshold PTS of eight, below which all injured children should be triaged to an appropriate pediatric trauma center. Children with a PTS of > 8 have the highest potential for preventable mortality, morbidity, and disability. According to the National Pediatric Trauma Registry statistics, they represent approximately 25% of all pediatric trauma victims, clearly requiring the most aggressive monitoring and observation.

Recent studies comparing the PTS with the Revised Trauma Score (RTS) have identified similar performances of both scores in predicting potential for mortality. Unfortunately, the RTS produces unacceptable levels of undertriage which is an inadequate trade-off for its greater simplicity. Perhaps more importantly, however, the PTS's function as an initial assessment checklist requires that each of the factors that may contribute to death or disability is considered during initial evaluation and becomes a source of concern for those individuals responsible for the initial assessment and management of the injured child.

Table 1
Pediatric Trauma Score

ASSESSMENT	SCORE		
	+ 2	**+ 1**	**− 1**
Weight	> 44 lbs (> 20 kg)	22-44 lbs (10-20 kg)	< 22 lbs (< 10 kg)
Airway	Normal	Oral or nasal airway	Intubated, tracheostomy invasive
Blood pressure	> 90 mm Hg	50-90 mm Hg	< 50 mm Hg
Level of consciousness	Completely awake	Obtunded or any LOC*	Comatose
Open wound	None	Minor	Major or penetrating
Fractures	None	Minor	Open or multiple fractures
Totals:			

*Loss of consciousness.

Resource Document 8:
Sample Trauma Flow Sheet*

NAME:

DATE: ARRIVAL
                        TIME:

CHIEF COMPLAINT:

PREHOSPITAL INFORMATION

TRANSPORT

☐ Scene   ☐ Police
☐ Auto   ☐ Ambulatory
☐ Ambulance _____   ☐ Wheelchair
☐ Helicopter _____   ☐ Ref. Hospital _____
☐ Ref. Physician _____

MECHANISM OF INJURY

☐ MVA: ☐ Driver or ☐ Passenger: ☐ Front ☐ Back
    ☐ Seat belt on ☐ Air bag inflated
☐ MCA: ☐ Driver or ☐ Passenger
    ☐ Helmet worn ☐ Protective clothing worn
☐ Speed _____ mph
☐ BCA: ☐ Front ☐ Back ☐ Helmet worn
☐ Pedestrian vs. auto
☐ Fall _____ feet
☐ GSW   ☐ Stab
☐ Crush   ☐ Burn
☐ Assault ☐ Other _____

PROCEDURES BEFORE ARRIVAL

☐ Oral airway   ☐ Nasal airway
☐ ET Tube # _____   ☐ NT Tube # _____
☐ Crico # _____   ☐ EOA ☐ PTL
☐ O₂ @ _____ L/min via _____
Breath Sounds: Left: Right:
☐ IVs # ____ : ☐ Peripheral ☐ Central ☐ Intraosseous
☐ IV fluids 1 2 3 4 5 6   ☐ Blood 1 2 3 4 5
☐ CPR   ☐ PASG ☐ Legs ☐ Abd
☐ Urinary Cath   ☐ NG Tube
☐ Chest tubes ☐ R ☐ L ☐ Both
☐ Medication _____
☐ C-collar
☐ Spine Immobilization Device: Time on: _____
☐ Other _____
☐ Splints; Type _____
☐ Other procedures: _____
_____

PERSONNEL RESPONSE

Service	Name	Time Called	Time Arrived
ED Physician			
Trauma Surgeon			
Neurosurgery			
Orthopedics			
Anesthesia			
Pediatrics			
ENT/OMFS			
Plastics, Burns			
OB/GYN			
Urology			
Med/ICU			
RN			
RN			
RN			

AMPLE HISTORY

Allergies:

Medications:

Past Illnesses:

Last Meal: Last Tetanus:

Events:

Pregnant? ☐ Yes ☐ No LMP: _____

Backboard: Time off: _____

INITIAL ASSESSMENT

AIRWAY/BREATHING

☐ Patent   ☐ Obstructed
☐ Symmetrical   ☐ Asymmetrical
☐ Unlabored   ☐ Labored
Trachea midline?   ☐ Yes ☐ No
Breath Sounds: R   L
   Present   ☐   ☐
   Clear   ☐   ☐
   Decreased   ☐   ☐
   Absent   ☐   ☐
   Rales/rhonchi   ☐   ☐
Crepitus: ☐ Yes   ☐ No

INITIAL ASSESSMENT

CIRCULATION

Skin/mucous
membrane color:
□ Pink ☐ Pale
☐ Flushed ☐ Jaundiced
☐ Ashen ☐ Cyanotic

Pulses:
☐ Normal: Site _____
☐ Bounding: Site _____
☐ Weak: Site _____
☐ Absent: Site _____
Rate: _____ Rhythm: _____

Skin temp: ☐ Warm ☐ Hot ☐ Cool/Cold

Skin moisture: ☐ WNL ☐ Dry ☐ Moist

DISABILITY

GCS	Score	RTS	Score
1. Eye Opening		1. Respiratory Rate	
Spontaneous	4	10 - 24	4
To voice	3	25 - 35	3
To pain	2	≥ 36	2
None	1	1 - 9	1
		0	0
2. Verbal			
Oriented	5	2. Systolic BP	
Confused	4	> 89 mm Hg	4
Inappropriate words	3	70 - 89	3
Incomprehensive	2	50 - 69	2
None	1	1 - 49	1
		0	0
3. Motor			
Obeys command	6	3. GCS Score	
Purposeful move	5	13 - 15	4
Withdrawn	4	9 - 12	3
Flexion	3	6 - 8	2
Extension	2	4 - 5	1
None	1	3	0
Total GCS	_____	Total RTS	_____

PUPIL REACTION

	OS	Size	OD	Size
Brisk	☐	___mm	☐	___mm
Constricted	☐	___mm	☐	___mm
Sluggish	☐	___mm	☐	___mm
Dilated	☐	___mm	☐	___mm
Nonreactive	☐	___mm	☐	___mm

1 ● 2 ● 3 ● 4 ● 5 ● 6 ● 7 ● 8 ●

IDENTIFY INJURY SITE BY NUMBER

1. Laceration	2. Abrasion	3. Hematoma
4. Contusion	5. Deformity	6. Open fx
7. GSW	8. Stab	9. Burn
10. Cold	11. Edema	12. Amputation
13. Avulsion	14. Pain	

Head:

Maxillofacial:

C-spine/neck:

Chest:

Abdomen:

Perineum:

Musculoskeletal:

TRAUMA RESUSCITATION ORDERS

Resource Document 8: Sample Trauma Flow Sheet

TIME	LABORATORY	TIME	X-RAYS	TIME	PROCEDURES
	Type/cross # units		Lateral c-spine		O$_2$ @ L/min via
	Type/hold		Swimmers		ET # By:
	CBC Screen		Chest: Erect / Supine		NT # By:
	ETOH		Pelvis		Crico # By:
	Drug screen		Thoracic spine		Needle thoracostomy by:
	PT/PTT		Lumbar spine		Chest tube # R L
	ABGs		Odontoid		Right return:
	Urinalysis		Skull		Left return:
	DPL fluid		Facial series		ED Thoracotomy by:
	Pregnancy test + -		Mandible		Autotransfuser
	HIV + -		Abdomen		RIV: Site: Size:
			Extremity: LUE / RUE		RIV: Site: Size:
			Extremity: LLE / LRE		LIV: Site: Size:
	Other:		IVP		LIV: Site: Size:
			Cystogram		CVP: Site: Size:
			Urethrogram		Pericardiocentesis by:
			Arteriogram / Aortogram		ECG
			CT Head		NG # Return Color
			CT Chest		Rectal tone: Guaiac
			CT ABD / pelvis		Foley # Return Color
					Urine dip + -
					Spont. void: Dip + -
					DPL: + - ? By:
					Gardner Wells by:
					Suturing by:
					Restraints: UE LE Type:

FLUID INTAKE/OUTPUT

INTAKE
Ringer's Lactate
Total prehospital _____ mL
ED: 1 2 3 4 5
6 7 8 9 10 12 _____ mL

Blood Products
Total prehospital _____ mL

ED: PRBCs 1 2 3 4 5 6
7 8 9 10 12 13 _____ mL

FFP 1 2 3 4 5 6
7 8 9 10 11 _____ mL

Platelets _____ mL
Total _____ mL

OUTPUT
Urine _____ mL
NG _____ mL
Blood _____ mL
Total _____ mL

ABGs

Time	pH	PCO$_2$	PO$_2$	O$_2$ LPM

MEDICATIONS

Time	Med	Dose	Route/Site	By
	Tetanus			

Time										
Cuff BP										
Pulse										
Rhythm										
Respirations										
Temperature										
A-line										
Oximetry (O_2 Sat)										
Carboximetry										
CVP										
Urinary output										
Glasgow Coma Scale										
1. Eyes										
2. Verbal response										
3. Motor response										
Total (1 + 2 + 3)										
R Pupil size + react										
L Pupil size + react										

Time	NOTES

DISPOSITION: ☐ Alive: Time out:_____ To:_____ Service:_____

☐ Dead: Time out:_____ To:_____

Operative permit signed: ☐ Yes ☐ No Family Notified: ☐ Yes ☐ No

Pastoral service notified: ☐ Yes ☐ No ☐ NA Social service notified: ☐ Yes ☐ No ☐ NA

Valuables/Clothing:_____ Forensic evidence:_____

Physician's Signature:_____

*NOTE: This flow sheet is only an example of information that may be required. All institutions that receive trauma patients should develop their own forms that meet the needs of the institution.

Resource Document 9: Transfer Agreement

This document is a sample transfer agreement. It is presented for educational purposes only and is not intended to provide legal advice or to serve as the basis for a specific transfer arrangement. The ACS Committee on Trauma recommends that institutions entering into a specific agreement seek the assistance of legal counsel in the preparation of such a document.

This agreement is made as of the _____ day of _____, 19 ____by and between (referring hospital) generally at (city, state), a nonprofit corporation, and (receiving hospital) at (city, state), a nonprofit corporation.

Whereas, both the (referring hospital) and the (receiving hospital) desire, by means of this Agreement, to assist physicians and the parties hereto in the treatment of trauma patients; and whereas the parties specifically wish to facilitate: (a) the timely transfer of such patients and medical and other information necessary or useful in the care and treatment of trauma patients transferred, (b) the determination as to whether such patients can be adequately cared for other than by either of the parties hereto, and (c) the continuity of the care and treatment appropriate to the needs of trauma patients, and (d) the utilization of knowledge and other resources of both facilities in a coordinated and cooperative manner to improve the professional health care of trauma patients.

Now, therefore, this agreement witnesseth: That in consideration of the potential advantages accruing to the patients of each of the parties and their physicians, the parties hereby covenant and agree with each other as follows:

1. In accordance with the policies and procedures of the (referring hospital) and upon the recommendation of the attending physician, who is a member of the medical staff of the (referring hospital) that such transfer is medically appropriate, a trauma patient at the (referring hospital) shall be admitted to (receiving hospital) of (city, state) as promptly as possible under the circumstances, provided that beds are available. In such cases, the (referring hospital) and (receiving hospital) agree to exercise their best efforts to provide for prompt admission of the patients.

2. The (referring hospital) agrees that it shall:

   a. Notify the (receiving hospital) as far in advance as possible of impending transfer of a trauma patient.

   b. Transfer to (receiving hospital) the personal effects, including money and valuables, and information relating to same.

c. Effect the transfer to (receiving hospital) through qualified personnel and appropriate transportation equipment, including the use of necessary and medically appropriate life support measures. (Referring hospital) agrees to bear the responsibility for billing the patient for such services, except to the extent that the patient is billed directly for the services by a third party.

3. The (referring hospital) agrees to transmit with each patient at the time of transfer, or in the case of emergency, as promptly as possible thereafter, an abstract of pertinent medical and other records necessary in order to continue the patient's treatment without interruption and to provide identifying and other information.

4. Bills incurred with respect to services performed by either the (referring hospital) or the (receiving hospital) shall be collected by the party rendering such services directly from the patient, third party, and neither the (referring hospital) nor the (receiving hospital) shall have any liability to the other for such charges.

5. This Agreement shall be effective from the date of execution and shall continue in effect indefinitely, except that either party may withdraw by giving thirty (30) days notice in writing to the other party of its intention to withdraw from this Agreement. Withdrawal shall be effective at the expiration of the thirty (30) day notice period. However, if either party shall have its license to operate revoked by the State, this Agreement shall terminate on the date such revocation becomes effective.

6. The Board of Directors of the (referring hospital) and the Governing Body of the (receiving hospital) shall have exclusive control of the policies, management, assets, and affairs of their respective facilities. Neither party assumes any liability, by virtue of this Agreement, for any debts or other obligations incurred by the other party to this Agreement.

7. Nothing in this Agreement shall be construed as limiting the right of either to affiliate or contract with any hospital or nursing home on either a limited or general basis while this Agreement is in effect.

8. Neither party shall use the name of the other in any promotional or advertising material unless review and approval of the intended use shall first be obtained from the party whose name is to be used.

9. The parties hereby agree to comply with all applicable laws and regulations concerning the treatment and care of patients designated for transfer from one health care institution to another, including but not limited to the Emergency Medical Treatment and Active Labor Act, 42 U.S.C. 1395dd.

10. This Agreement may be modified or amended from time to time by mutual agreement of the parties, and any such modification or amendment shall be attached to and become part of this Agreement.

In witness whereof, the parties hereto have executed this Agreement the day and year first above written.

By:_____   By:_____

Resource Document 10: Sample Transfer Record Information

A. Patient's Name

Address:
Address:
Age: Sex: Weight:

Next of Kin:
Address:
Address:
Phone Number:

B. Time

Of Injury:
Admitted to ED:
Admitted to OR:
Transfer:

C. History of Current Injury:

Mechanism of Injury:

AMPLE History:

D. Condition on Admission:

Pulse: Respiratory Rate:
Blood Pressure: Rhythm:
Temperature:

E. Initial Diagnostic Impressions:

F. Diagnostic Studies:

1. Laboratory Data—Attach all results to form

2. Basic Radiographic Studies— Send all films with patient

3. Electrocardiogram

4. Send appropriate specimens, eg, peritoneal lavage fluid

G. Treatment Rendered:

1. Medications: Amount and Time

2. IV Fluids: Type and Amount

3. Other:

H. Status of Patient When Transferred:

I. Management During Transport:

J. Referring Physician:
Referring Hospital:
Phone Number:

K. Receiving Physician:
Receiving Hospital:

**Resource
Document 10:
Sample
Transfer Record
Information**

American College of Surgeons

Resource Document 11: Organ and Tissue Donation

Of the fewer than 4% of all deaths that result in potentially suitable donors, less than 15% of these suitable donors actually donate organs. The major factor in this discrepancy and the resultant shortage of organs is the lack of donor referrals by responsible physicians, nurses, or hospital administrators. Seventy percent to 80% of families will consent to organ donation if approached. Most states now require that organ donation be offered to the families of dying or brain-dead patients. The referral of an organ or tissue donor begins with the recognition by a physician that a patient may be a suitable organ or tissue donor. A computer registry of potential recipients of renal and extrarenal organs is maintained by the United Network for Organ Sharing (1-800-446-2726).

All patients should be considered initially as organ and/or tissue donors until they are excluded for medical reasons. Cadaveric organ donors are previously healthy patients who have suffered irreversible, catastrophic brain injury of a known etiology; most commonly head trauma, a subarachnoid hemorrhage, primary brain tumors, or cerebral anoxia. Organs and tissues that may be donated are:

1. Bone
2. Bone marrow
3. Corneas (eyes)
4. Skin
5. Soft tissues
6. Heart
7. Heart/lungs
8. Kidneys
9. Liver
10. Pancreas
11. Intestines
12. Endocrine tissue

If a patient may ultimately become a donor, it is critically important to follow several principles that will optimize the patient as a donor. These principles include:

1. Resuscitation
2. Adequate organ perfusion
3. Vigorous hydration
4. Diuresis
5. Avoidance of infection
6. Avoidance of hypothermia

Cadaveric organ donors can be any age. All solid organ donors should have intact cardiac function, and brain death should be confirmed by the number of physicians required by state law. Many organs may be donated from patients without cardiac function: skin, corneas, bone and bone marrow, fascia, dura, and thyroid and and pituitary glands.

Contraindications to organ donation include:

1. Insulin-dependent diabetes mellitus
2. Systemic sepsis
3. Autoimmune diseases
4. Intravenous drug abuse
5. Transmissible infections
6. Malignancies other than brain or skin
7. Severe, chronic hypertension
8. History of trauma or disease involving the organs considered for donation

Brain death is defined as irreversible cessation of brain function, including the cerebellum and brain stem. Brain death prevails in patients in whom other organ functions are maintained by artificial ventilation and pharmacologic support. Brain death can be confirmed through clinical examination, apnea tests, electroencephalogram, and cerebral blood flow studies.

Organ donation is covered in all 50 states of the United States by the Uniform Anatomical Gift Act (UAGA). The UAGA states that persons older than 18 years of age can donate via a donor card, minors can donate with the consent of their parents, or the family of the deceased can allow donations of the organs.

Consent from the donor's relatives is obtained primarily through the use of a specifically drafted consent form. The UAGA also provides a method for securing relatives' consent through a recorded telephone conversation that must be witnessed by two or more people. However, discussion of the opportunity for organ donation is enhanced by direct contact with the family.

Donor referrals are usually accepted 24 hours a day, and potential donors can be discussed by contacting the regional organ procurement agency. Early referral is recommended in order to assess donor suitability, coordinate medicolegal requirements, initiate necessary laboratory tests, and assure the collection of complete data. Referrals can be expedited if the following patient data are available:

1. Patient history
2. Diagnosis and date of admission
3. Patient height and weight
4. ABO group
5. Hemodynamic data
6. Urinalysis
7. Laboratory data (including serum creatinine and serum urea nitrogen levels)
8. Current medications
9. Culture results

Transplant coordinators usually are available to assist with donor evaluation and donor maintenance, to discuss organ donation with next of kin, to arrange donor surgery, to provide educational materials, and to coordinate the referral process.

Resource Document 12: Preparations for Disaster

I. Introduction

These guidelines for disaster preparation were adapted directly from *Early Care of the Injured Patient*, by the Committee on Trauma of the American College of Surgeons, Alexander J. Walt, MD (Editor), 1982, "Disaster Planning for Mass Casualties," Chapter 24, page 377.

II. Planning and Preparation

Disaster planning, whether at the state, regional, or local level, involves a wide range of individuals and resources. **All plans:**

A. Should involve high-level officials of the local police, fire, and civil defense agencies.

B. Must be written and tested (at least twice a year) in advance.

C. Must provide for communication arrangements, taking into account the likely overtaxing of existing telephone systems. Designated telephone lines inside and outside the hospital, and portable radio receivers obviate the need for routing messages through switchboards, which by nature of the situation are almost certain to become overtaxed.

D. Must provide for storage of special equipment and supplies.

E. Must provide for routine first aid.

F. Must provide for definitive care.

G. Must prepare for transfer of casualties to other facilities by prior agreement, should the location in question be overtaxed or unusable.

H. Must consider the urgent needs of patients already hospitalized for conditions unrelated to the disaster.

III. Hospital Planning

Although a regional approach to planning is ideal for the management of mass casualties, circumstances may require that each hospital function with little or no outside support. Earthquakes, floods, riots, or nuclear contamination may force the individual hospital to function in isolation. The crisis may be instantaneous, as with an explosion, or may develop slowly, as do most civil disturbances, malfunctions of nuclear reactors, and floods. Developments that cannot be predicted may have great influence on preventing access to designated disaster facilities. Once a state of disaster has been declared by civil authorities or internally by the hospital director, specific hospital procedures should be performed automatically. These include:

A. Notification of personnel

B. Preparation of treatment areas

C. Classification to differentiate emergency department and hospital patients

D. Checking of supplies of blood, fluids, medications, food, potable water, and other materials essential to hospital operation

E. Provision for decontamination procedures, which take high priority in nuclear accidents

F. Institution of security precautions

G. Control of visitors and press

Resource Document 13: Ocular Trauma

(Optional Lecture)

Objectives:

Upon completion of this topic, the physician will be able to:

A. Obtain patient and event histories.

B. Perform a systematic examination of the orbit and its contents.

C. Identify and discuss those eyelid injuries that can be treated by the primary care physician, and those that must be referred to an ophthalmologist for treatment.

D. Discuss how to examine the eye for a foreign body, and how to remove superficial foreign bodies to prevent further injury.

E. Identify a corneal abrasion, and discuss its management.

F. Identify a hyphema, and discuss the initial management and necessity for referral to an ophthalmologist.

G. Identify those eye injuries requiring referral to an ophthalmologist.

H. Identify a ruptured globe injury, and discuss the initial management required prior to referral to an ophthalmologist.

I. Evaluate and treat eye injuries resulting from chemicals.

J. Evaluate a patient with an orbital fracture, and discuss the initial management and necessity for referral.

K. Identify a retrobulbar hematoma, and discuss the necessity for immediate referral.

**Resource
Document 13:
Ocular Trauma**

**(Optional
Lecture)**

I. Introduction

The initial assessment of a patient with ocular injury requires a systematic approach. The physical examination should proceed in an organized, step-by-step manner, and does not require extensive, complicated instrumentation in the multiple-trauma setting. Simple therapeutic measures often can save the patient's vision and prevent severe sequelae before an ophthalmologist is available. This optional lecture provides that pertinent information about early identification and treatment of ocular injuries that enhances the physician's basic knowledge and may save the patient's sight.

II. Assessment

A. History

Obtain a history of any pre-existing ocular disease.

1. Does the patient wear corrective lenses?
2. Is there a history of glaucoma?
3. What medications does the patient use, ie, pilocarpine?

B. Injury Incident

Obtain a detailed description of the circumstances surrounding the injury. This information often raises the index of suspicion for certain potential injuries and their sequelae, ie, the higher risk of infection from certain foreign bodies—wood versus metallic.

1. Was there blunt trauma?
2. Was there penetrating injury? In motor vehicular crashes there is potential for glass or metallic foreign bodies.
3. Was there a missile injury?
4. Was there a possible thermal, chemical, or flash burn?

C. Initial Symptoms/Complaint

1. What were the patient's initial symptoms?
2. Did the patient complain of pain or photophobia?
3. Was there an immediate decrease in vision that has remained stable or is it progressive?

The physical examination must be systematic so that function as well as anatomic structures are evaluated. As with injuries to other organ systems, the pathology also may evolve with time, and the patient must be periodically re-evaluated. A directed approach to the ocular examination, beginning with the most external structures in an "outside-to-inside" manner, ensures that injuries will not be missed.

D. Visual Acuity

Visual acuity is evaluated first by any means possible and recorded, eg, patient counting fingers at three feet.

E. Eyelids

The most external structures to be examined are the eyelids. The eyelids should be assessed for the following: (1) edema; (2) ecchymosis; (3) evidence of burns or chemical injury; (4) laceration(s)—medial, lateral, lid margin, canaliculi; (5) ptosis; (6) foreign bodies that contact the globe; and (7) avulsion of the canthal tendon.

F. Orbital Rim

Gently palpate the orbital rim for a step-off deformity and crepitus. Subcutaneous emphysema may result from a fracture of the medial orbit into the ethmoids or a fracture of the orbital floor into the maxillary antrum.

G. Globe

The eyelids should be retracted to examine the globe without applying pressure to the globe. The globe is then assessed anteriorly for displacement resulting from a retrobulbar hematoma and for posterior or inferior displacement due to a fracture of the orbit. The globes also are assessed for normal ocular movement, diplopia at the extremes of the patient's gaze, and evidence of entrapment.

H. Pupil

The pupils are assessed for roundness with regular shape, equality, and reaction to light stimulus.

I. Cornea

The cornea is assessed for opacity, ulceration, and foreign bodies. Fluorescein and a blue light facilitate this assessment.

J. Conjunctiva

The conjunctivae are assessed for chemosis, subconjunctival emphysema (indicating probable fracture of the orbit into the ethmoid or maxillary sinus), subconjunctival hemorrhage, and nonimpaled foreign bodies.

K. Anterior Chamber

Examine the anterior chamber for a hyphema (blood in the anterior chamber). The depth of the anterior chamber can be assessed by shining a light into the eye from the lateral aspect of the eye. If the light does not illuminate the entire surface of the iris, a shallow anterior chamber should be suspected. A shallow anterior chamber may result from an anterior penetrating wound. A deep anterior chamber may result from a posterior penetrating wound of the globe.

L. Iris

The iris should be regular in shape and reactive. Assess the iris for iridodialysis, a tear of the iris or iridodensis, and a floppy or tremulous iris.

M. Lens

The lens should be transparent. Assess the lens for possible anterior displacement into the anterior chamber, partial dislocation with displacement into the posterior chamber, and dislocation into the vitreous.

N. Vitreous

The vitreous also should be transparent, allowing for easy visualization of the fundus and retina. Visualization may be difficult if vitreous hemorrhage has occurred. In this situation, a black rather than red reflex is seen by ophthalmoscopy. A vitreous bleed usually indicates a significant underlying ocular injury. The vitreous also should be assessed for an intraocular foreign body.

O. Retina

The retina is examined for hemorrhage, possible tears, or detachment. A detached retina is opalescent, and the blood columns are darker.

III. Specific Injuries

A. Lid

Lid injuries often result in marked ecchymosis, making examination of the globe difficult. However, a more serious injury to the underlying structures must be ruled out. Look beneath the lid as well to rule out damage to the globe. Lid retractors should be used if necessary to forcibly open the eye to inspect the globe. Ptosis may be secondary to edema, damage to the levator palpebrae, or oculomotor nerve injury.

Lacerations of the upper lid that are horizontal, superficial, and do not involve the levator may be closed by the examining physician using five (6-0 to 8-0 silk) sutures. The physician also should examine the eye beneath the lid to rule out damage to the globe.

Lid injuries to be treated by an ophthalmologist include: (1) wounds involving the medial canthus that may have damaged the medial canaliculus; (2) injury to the lacrimal sac or nasal lacrimal duct, which can lead to obstruction if not properly repaired; (3) deep horizontal lacerations of the upper lid that may involve the levator and result in ptosis if not repaired correctly; and (4) lacerations of the lid margin that are difficult to close and may lead to notching, entropion, or ectropion.

Foreign bodies of the lid result in profuse tearing, pain, and a foreign-body sensation that increases with lid movement. The conjunctiva should be injected, and the upper and lower lids should be everted to examine the inner surface. Topical anesthetic drops may be used, but only for initial examination and removal of the foreign body.

Impaled, penetrating foreign bodies are not disturbed and are removed only in the operating room by an ophthalmologist or appropriate specialist. If the patient requires transport to another facility for treatment of this injury or others, apply a dressing about the foreign body to stabilize it.

B. Cornea

Corneal **abrasions** result in pain, foreign body sensation, photophobia, decreasing visual acuity, and chemosis. The injured epithelium stains with fluorescein.

Corneal **foreign bodies** sometimes can be removed with irrigation. However, if the foreign body is embedded, the patient should be referred. Corneal foreign bodies are treated with antibiotic drops or ointment (eg, sulfacetamide or neomycin combination, bacitracin, or polymyxin). The eye should then be patched to prevent movement, minimize pain, and promote faster healing in the case of an abrasion or prevent further injury if there is an embedded foreign body. Patients with embedded foreign bodies should be referred to an ophthalmologist.

C. Anterior Chamber

Hyphema is blood in the anterior chamber that may be difficult to see if there is only a small amount of blood. In extreme cases, the entire anterior chamber is filled. The hyphema can often be seen with a pen light. Hyphema usually indicates severe intraocular trauma.

Glaucoma develops in 7% of patients with hyphema. Corneal staining also may occur. **Remember**, hyphema may be the result of serious underlying ocular injury. Even in the case of a small bleed, spontaneous rebleeding often occurs within the first five days, which may lead to total hyphema. Therefore, the patient must be referred. Both eyes are patched, the patient is usually hospitalized, placed at bed rest, and re-evaluated frequently. Pain after hyphema usually indicates rebleeding and/or acute glaucoma.

D. Iris

Contusion injuries of the iris may cause traumatic mydriasis or miosis. There may be a disruption of the iris from the ciliary body, causing an irregular pupil and hyphema.

E. Lens

Contusion of the lens may lead to later opacification. Blunt trauma can cause a break of the zonular fibers that encircle the lens and anchor it to the ciliary body. This results in subluxation of the lens, possibly into the anterior chamber, causing a shallow chamber and acute, closed-angle glaucoma. In cases of posterior subluxation, the anterior chamber deepens. Patients with this injury should be referred to an ophthalmologist.

F. Vitreous

Blunt trauma also can lead to vitreous hemorrhage. This is usually secondary to retinal vessel damage and bleeding into the vitreous, resulting in a sudden, profound visual loss. Funduscopic examination may be impossible, and the red reflex, seen with an ophthalmoscope light, is lost. A patient with this injury should be placed at bed rest with binocular patches and referred to an ophthalmologist.

G. Retina

Blunt trauma also causes retinal hemorrhage. The patient may or may not have decreased visual acuity, depending on involvement of the macula. Superficial retinal hemorrhages appear cherry red in color; the deeper lesions appear gray.

Retinal edema and detachment can occur with head trauma. A white, cloudy discoloration is observed. Retinal detachments appear "curtain-like." If the macula is involved, visual acuity is affected. An acute retinal tear usually occurs in conjunction with blunt trauma to an eye with a pre-existing vitreoretinal pathology. Retinal detachment most often occurs as a late sequelae of blunt trauma. The patient describes light flashes and a curtain-like defect in peripheral vision.

A rupture of the choroid (blood supply of the retina) initially appears as a beige area at the posterior pole. Later it becomes a yellow-white scar. If it transects the macula, vision is seriously and permanently impaired.

Resource
Document 13:
Ocular Trauma

(Optional
Lecture)

H. Globe

A patient with a ruptured globe has marked visual impairment. The eye is soft due to a decreased intraocular pressure, and the anterior chamber is flattened or shallow. If the rupture is anterior, ocular contents may be seen extruding from the eye.

The goal of initial management of the ruptured globe is to protect the eye from any additional damage. A sterile dressing and eye shield should be applied carefully to prevent any pressure to the eye that may cause further extrusion of the ocular contents. The patient should be instructed not to squeeze his eye shut. If not contraindicated by other injuries, the patient may be sedated while awaiting transport or treatment. Do not remove foreign objects, tissue, or clots before dressing placement. No topical analgesics are used—only oral or parenteral, if not contraindicated by any other injuries.

An intraocular foreign body should be suspected if the patient complains of sudden sharp pain with a decrease in visual acuity. Inspect the surface of the globe carefully for any small lacerations and possible sites of entry. These may be difficult to find. In the anterior chamber, tiny foreign bodies may be hidden by blood or in the crypts of the iris. A tiny iris perforation may be impossible to see directly, but with a pen light the red reflex may be detected through the defect (if the lens and vitreous are not opaque).

I. Chemical Injuries

Chemical injuries require immediate intervention if sight is to be preserved. Acid precipitates proteins in the tissue and sets up somewhat of a natural barrier against extensive tissue penetration. However, alkali combines with lipids in the cell membrane, leading to disruption of the cell membranes, rapid penetration of the caustic agent, and extensive tissue destruction. Chemical injury of the cornea causes disruption of stromal mucopolysaccharides, leading to opacification.

The treatment is **copious and continuous irrigation**. Attempts should not be made to neutralize the agent. Intravenous solutions (sterile saline or Ringer's lactate) and tubing can be used to improvise continuous irrigation. Blepharospasm is extensive, and the lids must be manually opened during irrigation. Analgesics and sedation should be used, if not contraindicated by coexisting injuries.

Thermal injuries usually occur to the lids only and rarely involve the cornea. However, burns of the globe occasionally occur. A sterile dressing should be applied and the patient referred to an ophthalmologist. Exposure of the cornea **must** be prevented or it can perforate, and the eye can be lost.

J. Fracture

Blunt trauma to the orbit causes rapid compression of the tissues and increased pressure within the orbit. The weakest point is the orbital floor, which fractures, allowing the periorbital fat and possibly the inferior rectus and/or inferior oblique muscles to herniate into the antrum—hence the term, "blow out" fracture.

Clinically the patient presents with pain, swelling, and ecchymosis of the lids and periorbital tissues. There may be subconjunctival hemorrhage. Facial asymmetry and possibly enophthalmos might be evident or masked by surrounding edema. Limitation of ocular motion and diplopia secondary to edema or entrapment of extraocular muscles may be noted. Palpation of the infraorbital rim often reveals a step-off. Subcutaneous and/or subconjunctival emphysema can occur when the fracture is into the ethmoid or maxillary sinuses. Hypoesthesia of the cheek occurs secondary to injury of the infraorbital nerve.

The Waters view and Caldwell view (straight on) are very helpful for evaluating orbital fractures. Examine the orbital floor, and look for soft tissue density in the maxillary sinus or an air fluid level (blood). Computed tomographic scans also are helpful and may be considered mandatory.

Exophthalmometry must be performed as soon as possible. Treatment of fractures may be delayed up to a week. If entrapment is suspected, a forced duction test should be performed. (The inferior rectus is grasped with a forceps to test for entrapment.) Watchful waiting has avoided unnecessary surgery by allowing the edema to decrease, allowing more accurate evaluation of the cosmetic or functional deficit.

K. Retrobulbar Hematoma

A retrobulbar hematoma requires immediate treatment by an ophthalmologist. The resulting increased pressure within the orbit compromises the blood supply to the retina and optic nerve, resulting in blindness if not treated.

L. Fat Emboli

Patients with long-bone fractures are at risk for fat emboli. Remember, this is a possible cause of a sudden change in vision for a patient who has sustained multiple injuries.

IV. Summary

Thorough, systematic evaluation of the injured eye results in few significant injuries being missed. Once the injuries have been identified, treat the eye injury using simple measures, prevent further damage, and help preserve sight until the patient is in the ophthalmologist's care.

Resource
Document 14:
ATLS and the
Law

(Optional
Lecture)

Resource Document 14:
ATLS and the Law

(Optional Lecture)

Objectives:

Upon completion of this topic, the student will be able to:

A. Apply practical knowledge of basic medicolegal principles to delivery of trauma patient care.

B. Identify possible sources of liability exposure.

**Resource
Document 14:
ATLS and the
Law**

**(Optional
Lecture)**

American College of Surgeons

I. Introduction

Resource
Document 14:
ATLS and the
Law

(Optional
Lecture)

The Committee on Trauma of the American College of Surgeons emphasizes that trauma is a disease of all ages; swift in onset and slow in recovery. Each year accidents disable approximately nine million Americans and kill another 145,000. The ATLS Course is designed to prepare physicians to exercise a quantum of basic knowledge and skills such as rapid assessment, resuscitation, stabilization, appropriate use of consultation, and transfer where necessary.

The overriding principle of the ATLS Course is *primum non nocere*; that is, first do no harm. *Primum non nocere* also implies that a physician who fails to properly exercise advanced trauma life support principles may negligently cause avoidable, unnecessary injury. In the final analysis, the physician must develop "first-hour competence," which demands the proper exercise of ATLS principles in order to save lives, reduce morbidity, and avoid unnecessary harm.

The ideas behind ATLS enhance societal expectations that many lives will be saved and morbidity will be reduced if the proper techniques are exercised. When societal expectations are enhanced by the advancements and claims of the medical profession, there is a corresponding concern that where unexpected injury occurs, someone may have malpracticed.

Note: This optional lecture is not to be considered legal advice, nor is it a substitute for advice of counsel. This presentation is an overview of certain areas of the law and of particular interest to participants in the ATLS Program.

II. Objectives of ATLS and the Law

Liability exposure occurs when any physician attempting trauma care fails to exercise that degree of knowledge, skill, and due care expected of a reasonably competent practitioner in the same class, acting in the same or similar circumstances. This standard of care, particularly applicable to ATLS, will be discussed more completely later in this text.

The objective of "ATLS and the Law" is to provide an understandable, practical, applicable knowledge of basic medicolegal principles. Upon completion, each participant should be able to identify possible sources of liability exposure. **Remember, good medicine is good law**. Physicians need not fear the law when they exercise diligence (attentiveness) and due care (carefulness or caution) during the diagnostic and treatment processes.

III. Medicolegal Principles

The following medicolegal principles are reviewed in this text.

1. Physician/patient relationship
2. Consent
3. Right to refuse treatment
4. Artificial life support
5. Negligence

IV. Physician/Patient Relationship

A. Contract

Mutual consent is the principle applied to the traditional physician/patient relationship. The patient requests diagnosis and treatment; the physician agrees to provide professional services; the patient agrees to pay; the physician accepts a duty to provide appropriate medical care. Ordinarily, recovery for malpractice against a physician is allowed only where an express or implied contractual relationship exists between the physician and the patient. However, the duty of a physician to bring skill and care to the diagnosis and treatment of a patient does not arise out of contract, but out of policy considerations based on the nature of a physician's function.

B. Undertaking to Treat

Situations have arisen in which the traditional contract theory does not seem to apply, yet courts have found that a physician/patient relationship exists by applying the "undertaking to treat" theory. Advanced trauma life support is a specialty to which this theory is particularly appropriate. In many situations, physicians "undertake to treat" by immediately providing emergency medical care in the absence of any mutual assent. Nevertheless, a binding physician/patient relationship begins the moment the physician undertakes the treatment.

1. Telephone

In a well-known New Jersey case, *O'Neill v. Montefiore Hospital*, 202 NY S2d 436 1960, a patient presented to the emergency department of Montefiore Hospital complaining of chest pain. The emergency department physician examined the patient and requested the on-call physician cardiologist to review the case. The cardiologist elected to discuss the case over the telephone with the patient, and decided the patient could go home. One hour later, while disrobing at home, the patient "dropped dead." The patient's estate sued the hospital, the emergency department physician, and the cardiologist. The cardiologist contended that he was not liable because no contract was made with the patient.

The Supreme Court of New Jersey rejected the contention, outlining that the cardiologist had established a physician/patient relationship by discussing the case with the patient via the telephone, and advising the patient to go home.

The morals of this case are: Do not talk to patients on the telephone while on call to the emergency department, and do not engage in therapeutic endeavors with unknown patients via the telephone. The physician may be concerned that this admonition would apply to any patient, particularly patients who are well-known to the physician. Even when the patient is known, telephone advice may create liability exposure. The individual physician should consider this factor as part of his medical judgment.

2. Subordinate physician

In another case, *Smart v. Kansas City*, 105SW 709 (Mo 19907), the chief of orthopedics was searching the outpatient department for teaching materials. He observed one of the residents examining a patient, walked over, examined the patient, and advised the resident to amputate below

Resource
Document 14:
ATLS and the
Law

(Optional
Lecture)

the knee. The resident did and committed malpractice. The patient sued the hospital, the resident, and the chief of orthopedics. The chief of orthopedics contended that he was not liable because he did not enter into a physician/patient contract. The state supreme court disagreed, stating the chief of orthopedics was "in charge," ordered the resident to amputate, and subsequently was responsible for the resident's actions, and indeed had entered into a physician/patient relationship.

3. Medical staff conference

Is a presiding physician at a medical staff conference liable for advising a staff physician during a case presentation, if such advice allegedly leads to medical malpractice? A California court ruled that where a practicing physician seeks advice "from a professor" by presenting a case at a regularly scheduled medical staff conference, the physician, acting as professor, will not be liable. The court reasoned that the professor is not "in control" of the practicing physician's activities, because the physician is free to disregard the professor's advice. Therefore, the plaintiff cannot reach the professor by contending that his physician followed professorial advice. *Rainer v. Grossman*, 31 Cal. App. 3d 539, 107 Cal. Rptr. 469 (2nd Dist., 1973).

4. Gratuitous service

Gratuitous medical care is subject to liability. The mere fact that the physician does not collect a fee does not bar the patient from suing for medical malpractice. Treating a friend's child in the middle of the night creates liability exposure, and the courts will not accept a defense of, "I did it for nothing."

Once a physician gives his medical opinion regarding diagnosis or treatment, directly or indirectly, he places himself in a physician/patient relationship. This relationship also can arise if the actions of the patient and physician imply that such a relationship exists. In such instances, the courts have held that the physician's duty is not to abandon the case or abdicate his responsibility. He also has a duty to exercise the degree of skill, judgment, knowledge, and concern that would be expected of a reasonably competent medical practitioner acting under the same or similar circumstances.

C. Duty to Rescue

There is no legal duty to rescue another person. However, moral and ethical duties may exist and must be distinguished from legal duties.

1. Moral duty

A moral duty is self-imposed, originating from family and ethnic mores, religious exposure, and personal philosophical principles.

2. Ethical duty

An ethical duty arises from membership in unions, associations, or societies. Such organized groups have ethical standards by which they expect their members to act.

Resource
Document 14:
ATLS and the
Law

(Optional
Lecture)

3. Legal duty

A legal duty is imposed by law, which expects a person to behave in a certain manner under certain circumstances. The common law (law of the courts) does not impose a legal duty on a person to rescue another person. Therefore, if a physician encounters a stranger on the street who needs CPR, the law would not impose a duty on the physician to attempt a rescue. The physician may have difficulty dealing with his ethical and moral duties by refusing to do anything, but the law will not hold him responsible.

In some situations, the law does impose a duty to rescue. For example, if a physician encounters his own patient on the street, and that patient needs CPR, the physician is under legal duty to render emergency care. A parent is under legal duty to rescue his child. A public servant, such as a policeman or fireman, is under legal duty to rescue persons in distress. A lifeguard or physician in a hospital is under legal duty by virtue of his employment to rescue patients. It should be noted that once a person undertakes the rescue, he is under a legal duty to do all he can to complete the rescue without causing injury to himself. However, the law does not expect anyone to lose his own life, even when there is a legal duty to rescue.

D. Good Samaritan Statutes

Good Samaritan statutes exist in every state, not because of any evidence that rescuers have been successfully sued, but to encourage potential rescuers to render aid in an emergency. Several states have mandates for rescue. However, legislative exceptions to the mandate raise a question about the enforceability to such laws, because no one is expected to injure himself, or even stop, if he must attend to matters of greater import.

Physicians and health care providers should not refuse to rescue for fear of legal liability, because the potential for a successful suit is virtually nonexistent unless the physician performs in a grossly or shockingly negligent manner. The following scenario is an example of such gross negligence.

A physician encounters a patient lying in the street who has just been ejected through a car's windshield. He observes that the patient has no apparent breathing or circulatory difficulties or any signs of external hemorrhage. Yet the physician decides to examine the patient, inadvertently moves the head, and causes the patient to become quadriplegic.

Based on these facts, the physician committed gross negligence. Every physician knows or should know that patients sustaining head injuries may have a concomitant cervical-spine injury. Conversely, if the same patient had an obstructed airway or hemorrhage requiring immediate treatment to prevent death, and the physician followed the basic principles of ATLS, the physician would not be liable for gross negligence or even ordinary negligence, because the risk of death was greater than the risk of quadriplegia.

Resource
Document 14:
ATLS and the
Law

(Optional
Lecture)

V. Consent

A. Battery

Traditionally, the concept of consent is governed by the law of battery. A person is liable for the tort of battery whenever there is an intentional and unpermitted touching of another person. A person does not have to engage in fisticuffs to commit a battery. The mere intentional touching of a person without consent is a battery. A patient who has specifically consented to a panhysterectomy has not consented to an appendectomy. Patients have successfully sued physicians for battery when an unrequested incidental appendectomy has been performed. Liability in such cases depends on whether the patient has implied consent in some way to the additional procedure.

B. Implied Consent in an Emergency

The law usually presumes consent. In an action for malpractice based on lack of consent, the plaintiff must prove that the physician did not obtain consent. If it is practicable to obtain actual consent for treatment from the patient or someone authorized to consent for him, this must be done. However, in an emergency situation in which immediate action is necessary for the protection of the patient's life, the law will imply consent if it cannot be obtained. The law presumes that most reasonable persons under the same or similar circumstances would want their lives saved, if at all possible. This presumption is generally true even when the patient is not competent to consent for himself, as in the case of a minor or someone under the care of a third party, such as a natural guardian, a legal guardian, or a person whom the law of the state allows to substitute consent for the patient. If the emergency immediately endangers the life or permanent health of the patient, a physician should do what the occasion demands.

C. Consent: Competence and Capacity

A physician must understand the difference between capacity and competence. A fully conscious minor is usually not considered to consent to surgery, even if he understands what is happening. Some states have created exceptions to this rule, but generally his parents must consent for him. However, a competent adult may lack the capacity to consent due to a comatose state. Whether someone lacks the capacity to consent depends on the facts in each case, for courts have even held that an intoxicated adult has the capacity to consent. The general standard given by the courts in cases involving questions of capacity to consent is whether the patient understands the risks involved in consenting to treatment and in refusing to consent to treatment.

D. Third-party Consent

1. Minors

The common-law doctrine is clear in stating that minors cannot consent to treatment unless their parents or natural or legal guardians consent. One parent is usually enough, but some states may require both parents to consent. A number of exceptions to this rule are statutory in nature, governed by state legislative law. Therefore, the state statutes should be reviewed to determine those situations in which a minor can consent without parental permission. Generally, minors may consent without parental permission if they are emancipated, pregnant, seeking contra-

Resource
Document 14:
ATLS and the
Law

(Optional
Lecture)

ception, seeking treatment for drug abuse, parents themselves, or married. However, tubal ligation or any type of major surgery usually requires parental consent.

2. Spouses

As a general rule, one spouse cannot exercise consent rights for another spouse. A number of cases emphatically underscore the principle that one spouse cannot interfere with the consent rights of another spouse to undergo treatment, including the right of a woman to have an abortion during the first trimester of pregnancy.

3. Next of kin

The patient's next of kin usually does not have a right to substitute consent for the patient. This is true even though the next of kin is the designee for permission to perform an autopsy on a relative in most states. On July 1, 1984, the state of Maryland passed a law providing that the next of kin may give substitute consent for an incompetent patient or the patient in the emergency situation. The Maryland law states that the available next of kin, in the following order of preference, may give the necessary consent: (1) the spouse; (2) an adult child; (3) a parent; (4) a sibling; (5) a grandparent; or (6) an adult grandchild. The Maryland law probably represents a trend. The purpose of such laws is to avoid legal entanglements in order to obtain consent to effectively treat an incompetent patient.

4. Family members

In the absence of a legally granted authority of "next-of-kin" substitute-consent statute, the common law does not permit family members to exercise the consent rights of another family member, even if the patient is incompetent.

E. Informed Consent

Most courts emphatically hold that consent to treatment, to be effective, must be informed. Informed consent is rarely an issue during life-saving processes. Acute trauma incapacitates many patients, rendering them incapable of communicating or understanding the emergency treatment. The more urgent the medical situation, the less likely that consent of any kind will be an issue. Therefore, informed consent will not be discussed in detail. Remember, where the patient or his third-party substitute can give consent, that consent must be based on knowledge and understanding of the treatment to be given and the risks involved in either undergoing or failing to undergo recommended treatment.

F. Physician Defenses to Lack of Consent

1. Consent implied

The patient's lack of capacity and its effect on consent has already been discussed and is self-evident. A second defense, closely related to the first, is that the consent was implied from the circumstances. The physician may contend that he reasonably inferred that the patient's voluntary submission to the treatment indicated consent. The inference may be drawn only if the patient, or a reasonable person in similar circumstances, should have been aware that this passive submission to an obvious procedure constitutes consent to treatment.

2. Disclosure unduly alarming

Another defense, usually used in cases regarding informed consent, is that the disclosure of information concerning the adverse effects of treatment would unduly alarm a patient. The courts have fashioned this defense for the physician by pointing out that situations arise in which the physician knows the patient would become unduly alarmed when informed of the treatment risks, and would probably reject essential treatment that would reduce morbidity or mortality. In those situations, the physician is generally not liable for failing to obtain fully informed consent.

VI. Right to Refuse Treatment

A. Source of Right

The right to refuse treatment is derived from the common law, the principles of democracy, and the United States (US) Constitution.

1. Common law

The common-law doctrine states that "every human being of adult years and sound mind has a right to determine what shall be done with his own body; and a (physician who administers treatment) without his patient's consent commits a battery for which he is liable in damages."

2. Democracy

Courts also have used the principles of democracy to enforce the right to refuse treatment. They point out that the American democratic system promises us the implied fundamental right to make choices about our personal existence.

3. Constitution

The right to refuse treatment also arises from the US Constitution as interpreted by the US Supreme Court. The Constitution's Bill of Rights promises us freedom of speech, freedom of religion, freedom to assemble, the right against unlawful searches and seizures, the right not to have soldiers housed in our homes during peacetime, and the right against self-incrimination. The US Supreme Court has noted that we have other, unwritten constitutional guarantees implied from that Bill of Rights. In a number of decisions, the Supreme Court has emphasized the right of privacy and the right against bodily invasion by protecting the right to use and receive contraceptives, the right to marry a person of another race, the right to possess pornographic literature at home, and the right to terminate pregnancy.

B. Right of Self-determination

Clearly, the competent patient has a right to refuse treatment if that patient understands the consequences of such refusal, and no substantial state interests exist to override this right. The courts balance the competent patient's right to self-determination against state interests, which override the patient's right to refuse under certain circumstances. How this occurs will be discussed later in this text.

**Resource
Document 14:
ATLS and the
Law**

**(Optional
Lecture)**

C. Policy Trend—Competent Patient

Abe Perlmutter was a 73-year-old man suffering from progressive, terminal amyotrophic lateral sclerosis. He was unable to move his extremities except for several fingers on one hand. At one time he had disconnected himself from his respiratory tubing; however, the alarms signaled the nurses to reconnect it. He asked that the machines be removed, and he be allowed to die. The physicians refused because they recognized that Florida law was not clear on the issue of disconnecting an artificial life-support system without being liable for homicide. The Florida Supreme Court reviewed the case in terms of compelling state interests. They found Mr. Perlmutter a competent individual. He had no minor dependents and his family members supported his desire to discontinue his life-prolonging treatment. The court finally held that Mr. Perlmutter's right to refuse treatment outweighed the state's interests, and ordered that his wishes be obeyed. The court cautioned, however, that his adoption of this principle was limited to the specific facts of this case. *Satz v. Perlmutter*, 379 So2d 359 (Fl 1980).

D. Compelling State Interests

1. Duty to preserve human life

The state has a paramount duty to preserve human life, particularly where that life has value to the person and society.

2. Duty to protect innocent third party

The state has a duty to protect innocent third parties, such as children who are unable to make their own choices, and therefore may prevent a parent or guardian from exercising the right to refuse treatment on behalf of the minor.

3. Duty to prevent suicide

The state has a duty to prevent suicide. Preventing suicide must be distinguished from allowing patients to die from the natural course of a disease. Abe Perlmutter was not committing suicide when he requested that his advanced life-support systems be discontinued. He had no possible chance of recovery, and he simply requested that nature take its course. Suicide is an act of specific intent in which the patient exercises his right to refuse treatment for a clearly reversible illness, solely to end his life.

4. Duty to help maintain the integrity of the medical profession

American courts are duly concerned that the right-to-refuse-treatment doctrine shall not be a "club" to coerce a physician either to abandon established medical therapy or to become an "executioner." Where judges sense a compromise of medical integrity, they will either override the patient's right to refuse or declare that the physician shall not be criminally liable.

E. State Interest Applied

1. Preschool vaccination

Preschool vaccination requirements have been validated by the Supreme Court, because no individual citizen has the right to jeopardize the health of the populace.

Resource
Document 14:
ATLS and the
Law

(Optional
Lecture)

2. Court order to treat minors

The courts have ordered the treatment of minor children when parents have refused to permit them life-saving treatment.

3. Court order to an adult's guardian

The courts also have ordered blood transfusions for a retarded adult patient who was not terminally ill and whose guardian had refused consent.

4. Court order to undergo treatment

Cases are on record in which the courts have ordered a competent adult to undergo treatment so that his or her minor children would not be denied the benefits of a supporting parent.

5. Court order to prevent deliberate suicide

A California court recently rejected the plea of a quadriplegic to be allowed to reject all nourishment and not be force-fed by hospital personnel. The court ruled that the state's interest in the preservation of life and the prevention of suicide outweighed the woman's desire to "die with dignity," because she would probably live another 15 to 20 years.

6. Court order to protect a fetus

An unusual case is on record in which a woman, pregnant with a viable fetus, was ordered to undergo a transfusion in order to protect the fetus.

VII. Artificial Life Support

A. Incompetent Patient/Substituted Judgment

The incompetent patient has the same substantive rights as the competent patient. The question is how does the law protect the rights and fulfill the wishes of those who cannot act in their own behalf? The following cases demonstrate how the courts have either appointed a guardian to decide whether to terminate the artificial life-support system of an incompetent person or have made that decision themselves. Many factors weigh in the court's decision in such cases. One factor is a clear and convincing statement by the patient, while competent, that he never wished to prolong his life by artificial means.

Another factor is the physical condition of the patient coupled with the physician's medical judgment regarding possibility of recovery. Finally, the wishes of the patient's family must be considered.

B. Legal Precedents

1. Quinlan case

The doctrine of substituted judgment is applied when a third party is allowed to step into the shoes of an incompetent patient. That third party may be the court, a natural guardian, or a court-appointed guardian. The famous Karen Quinlan case is an example of a situation in which the court appointed Karen's father as guardian, and allowed him to decide that her artificial life-support system should be discontinued. This case is also an example of the common-law doctrine that prevents one adult from exercising rights over another adult's body, whether competent or incompetent. Mr. Quinlan

**Resource
Document 14:
ATLS and the
Law**

**(Optional
Lecture)**

did not have the legal right to have the artificial life-support system discontinued until he was appointed the legal guardian of his adult, incompetent daughter. *In Re Quinlan*, 355 A2d 647 (1976).

2. Saikewicz case

The Saikewicz case is one example in which the court directly substituted its own judgment for that of the patient. A court will always presume that the patient wants his life extended, but the particular circumstances of Mr. Saikewicz's case overcame that presumption. In this case, the superintendent of Belchertown petitioned the court to appoint him the guardian of Mr. Saikewicz in order to prevent the patient from undergoing treatment for acute myelogenous leukemia. The court decided it was the best judge, and would have the greatest concern for Mr. Saikewicz, who was severely mentally retarded since birth.

The court, as guardian, then decided that Mr. Saikewicz should not be forced to undergo treatment, because he was mentally incompetent and could not cooperate during the painful treatment process. Moreover, he would probably not live beyond six months, even with treatment.

This case caused a great deal of consternation in the medical profession, because the language of the decision implied that a physician would have to go to court in every case in which it was medically imprudent to treat a patient. *Supt. of Belchertown v. Saikewicz*, 370 NE2d 417 (1977). The Massachusetts court, however modified the Saikewicz decision in *Dinnerstein*.

3. Dinnerstein case

The Saikewicz case brought about the hospital's decision to petition the court concerning Shirley Dinnerstein, because the physician did not want to write a "do not resuscitate" (DNR) order for her. The court determined that Shirley Dinnerstein, a noncognitive, vegetative patient who was suffering from Alzheimer's disease, was in the terminal phase of a terminal illness. The court reasoned that a physician did not have to petition the court to write a DNR order if the patient suffered from an irreversible, noncognitive illness, and was in the terminal phase of that illness, provided the physician wrote the DNR order on the chart and wrote a progress note explaining his decision. The physician was also required to seek consultation from colleagues to substantiate his medical judgment. *Dinnerstein*, 380 NE2d 134 (1978).

C. Clear and Convincing Evidence

1. Legally brain-dead

A growing number of courts have adopted a clear-and-convincing-evidence doctrine to permit physicians to go beyond writing a DNR order, and to withdraw artificial life support altogether. When a patient is legally brain-dead, life has ended and there is no question that the law will permit physicians to withdraw artificial life support without fear of either criminal or civil prosecution. However, if the patient is brain-alive, a legal dilemma arises.

Resource
Document 14:
ATLS and the
Law

(Optional
Lecture)

2. Eichner case

In the *Eichner* case, the treating physicians determined that clear and convincing evidence existed that while competent, the patient—now 83-years old and permanently vegetative—expressed a desire not to be coded or put on artificial life support. The New York court held that physicians can discontinue artificial life-support systems in such circumstances without fear of criminal or civil liability. The court went on to say that guardians of incompetent patients like Eichner were not required to petition the court to decide whether to discontinue life-support treatments. But should a disagreement arise among the treating physician, his colleagues, the family members of the patient, or other interested persons, the physician should always seek legal counsel in deciding whether to terminate life support. *In the Matter of Eichner and In the Matter of Storar*, 438 NYS2d 266 (1981).

3. Right to die

Many states have responded to the dilemma of the brain-alive, incompetent patient by enacting statutes recognizing the right of individuals to privacy and dignity in establishing for themselves an appropriate level of medical care in specified medical situations. These "right-to-die" statutes provide a formal method by which a person can express his desire not to be put on artificial life support. However, euthanasia is never authorized by such laws.

D. Can Physicians Terminate Artificial Life Support?

In spite of cases like *Eichner* and "right-to-die" statutes, the law is still not completely clear with regard to the possible liability of a physician who discontinues the artificial life support for a patient in the terminal phase of a terminal illness, when the patient is brain-alive. In the *Eichner* case, the patient was in a permanent vegetative state, and clear and convincing evidence was present that the patient would not have wanted artificial life support continued. If no such clear and convincing evidence exists, the physician has no clear mandate from the law to be allowed to terminate artificial life support in a situation in which medical judgment is clear, the family agrees, and a hospital ethics committee concurs. Some states have adopted this standard, but if a question exists concerning the solution to this dilemma, one should always seek legal guidance or even petition the court.

E. Policy Trend—Family Involvement

More and more courts, dealing with the problems of terminating artificial life support for an incompetent patient, recommend that the family be involved in such a decision. The courts are not clear as to whether they are changing the common-law doctrine regarding the ability of the next of kin to consent for the patient. Some speculate that the courts are suggesting family involvement in order to avoid civil and criminal lawsuits. In any event, the family of the patient, the hospital ethics committee, the treating physician, and his colleagues should all be in agreement that termination of artificial life support is the best solution for the patient before any action is even considered.

**Resource
Document 14:
ATLS and the
Law**

**(Optional
Lecture)**

F. Can Physicians Stop a Code?

Physicians are involved daily in discontinuing CPR and advanced cardiac life support. Physicians should not rely solely on physical signs in deciding whether to discontinue CPR on a patient. The legal definition of death is now considered brain death, but brain death cannot be diagnosed during CPR because an EEG cannot be performed. The best measure of CPR failure in these situations is cardiac unresponsiveness. In the event that a physician is confronted in the emergency department with a sudden unexpected death, a reasonable medical determination should be made that the patient is in the state of cardiac unresponsiveness. Only then should cardiac life support be discontinued. Judging from the standards noted in the cases presented herein, the courts will accord great weight to the physician's medical judgment concerning when life has ceased.

G. Reasonable Medical Judgment

This discussion on ATLS and the Law is premised on the idea that in every circumstance, as much as possible, a physician will exercise reasonable medical judgment. Reasonable medical judgment means that the physician has considered the medical facts and has drawn a logical medical conclusion after exercising diligence and due care during the diagnostic and therapeutic processes. Where medical judgment is reasonable, it can and will be readily substantiated by a colleague. Reasonable medical judgment must precede all decisions not to treat or withdraw life support. The physician must not allow himself to become a philosopher, an ethicist, a moralist, or a sociologist prior to making a reasonable medical judgment that will withstand the scrutiny of his colleagues. The ethics committees and nonphysician decision-makers involved in such decisions must rely on the treating physician's reasonable medical judgment as the source for their decision to withdraw treatment or terminate life support.

VIII. Negligence

A. Elements

All negligence actions require that the plaintiff patient prove all four elements of negligence. The plaintiff must first establish the **standard of care** by expert medical testimony. Second, the plaintiff must establish a **breach** of that standard by the defendant physician. Third, the plaintiff must have a **demonstrable physical injury**. Fourth, the plaintiff must establish that the breach of duty was the logical and legal **cause** of the claimed injury.

B. Malpractice Claim

The plaintiff patient must show by a preponderance of the evidence (51% or a featherweight in the plaintiff's favor) that the defendant physician breached the standard of care applicable to the particular alleged malpractice claim, and that the breach of duty, legally and logically, caused the alleged injury.

Resource
Document 14:
ATLS and the
Law

(Optional
Lecture)

C. Standard of Care

A physician has a legal duty to exercise that degree of knowledge, care, and skill that is expected of a reasonably competent practitioner in the same class in which he belongs, acting in the same or similar circumstances.

The key phrase in the standard of care, as defined by the courts, is **"in the same class in which he belongs."** This phrase would be a national standard enunciation if it referred to any specialist acting under the same or similar circumstances anywhere in the United States. For example, a member of a national society of dermatologists, whose members have met certain standards to belong to that society, will be held to the society's standards, regardless of where they practice. However, a small-town general practitioner in rural Idaho will typically not be held to the same standard as a general practitioner in New York City. The resources available to the two physicians are not comparable. However, available knowledge is comparable, especially the knowledge leading to the conclusion whether to transfer or refer the patient.

The rule cited herein is only a general rule, for some courts have held that certain aspects of medicine are so general in nature that English doctors may testify as expert witnesses as to those practices.

Other courts construe a standard of care whereby the physician will be compared with another physician who practices in the same geographic locality. In some states, a similarity rule even holds that the physician will be compared with another physician who practices in a similar locality under the same or similar circumstances. However, in those states, the presumption is that the similar locality may exist anywhere in the United States. The modern legal trend is moving toward a national standard of care, rather than one based strictly on regional or local practice.

Further, where a physician undertakes to treat a condition that would be referred to a specialist, the treating physician will be held to that standard of care required of the specialist. For example, a family practitioner was held to an orthopedic standard because he treated a comminuted fracture of the wrist that should have been referred to an orthopedist or treated according to orthopedic standards. *Larsen v. Yelle*, 246 NW2d 841 (1976), Supreme Court of Minnesota.

D. ATLS Standard

A physician rendering advanced trauma life support has a legal duty to exercise that degree of knowledge, care, and skill expected of a reasonably competent physician trained in ATLS and acting in the same or similar circumstances.

The application of this standard is not based on right or wrong, but on what a reasonably competent ATLS physician would do under the circumstances of a particular case. For example, a patient appears in the emergency department after being flipped off a motorcycle and has evidence of possible head and cervical spine injuries and shock. The ATLS physician has a duty to act reasonably, preventing further injury by properly immobilizing the patient's head and neck, obtaining crosstable, lateral cervical spine films, and initiating two, large-caliber intravenous lines with Ringer's lactate. The physician is expected to make a reasonable assessment and act accordingly. He is not expected necessarily to make the absolute correct diagnosis at the time, but to support life until the correct diagnosis can be made and the patient can be transferred to a facility providing a higher level of care.

The standard of care does not require the physician to be correct in his initial diagnosis, but that he act reasonably under the circumstances of the case by providing the appropriate measures for advanced trauma life support.

IX. Summary

A. Physician/Patient Relationship

Physician/patient relationship has been discussed in terms of two legal theories, the mutual assent contract and undertaking to treat. The law will usually find a physician/patient relationship whenever a physician is involved in the treatment of a patient.

B. Consent

Consent arises from the law of battery. The importance of obtaining consent has been emphasized. However, the unlikelihood that informed consent will ever be an issue in advanced trauma life support also has been discussed.

C. Right to Refuse Treatment

The right to refuse treatment is a modern problem closely related to the principles of consent and generally involves life-sustaining procedures. The competent patient has a right to refuse treatment. This right is based on common-law doctrine of the right of privacy, the democratic principles of free choice, and the constitutional right against bodily invasion, as espoused by the Supreme Court. The state also has interests in this area that may outweigh the patient's right to refuse treatment.

D. Artificial Life Support

The issues surrounding the question of when to terminate the artificial life support of a terminally ill or vegetative, noncognitive patient have been reviewed.

E. Negligence

Legal negligence has been discussed. The four elements of negligence are: (1) duty—standard of care; (2) breach of duty—defendant physician acts negligently or negligently fails to act; (3) physical injury—the plaintiff must demonstrate a physical injury; and (4) causation—a plaintiff must demonstrate a logical and legal connection between the breach of duty and the alleged injury.

In summary, ATLS physicians must never operate under fear of the law. **Remember**, good medicine is good law. Whenever a physician acts reasonably under the circumstances of the case, exercising reasonable medical judgment, the likelihood is slim that a patient can bring a successful legal action against the physician.